Contents

Preface

We were prompted to write this simple introduction to disease for two reasons. The first is that the accumulated data about disease are now so complex that nearly all students find it difficult at first to know which are the important messages and which are unnecessary detail. Therefore, for the beginner, we have ruthlessly eradicated the detail and concentrated on the principles.

The second reason is that, these days, most research into disease, and most caring for the sick, is not done by medical doctors. Therefore a number of scientists and carers might, we feel, welcome an elementary analysis of how diseases happen.

Medical and veterinary students will need to learn a lot more about disease than is provided here. They will also need practical experience of some of the techniques used. But at least this is a start.

The authors share the wish to make your first contact with disease processes as friendly as possible. In trying to do that, we have had the encouragement, over the years, of many valued colleagues and thousands of students. We thank them all. We also hope you will enter into that spirit by pointing out to us the areas where we fail in our aim.

M.J.M., J.A., P.A.W.E., R.W.F.LeP., A.C.M.

Essentials of Pathology

M.J. Mitchinson MA MD FRCPath

With
J. Arno MA BM BCh MRCPath
P.A.W. Edwards MA PhD
R.W.F. LePage MA PhD BVMS
A.C. Minson MA BSc PhD

All of the Department of Pathology
University of Cambridge

b
**Blackwell
Science**

© 1996 by
Blackwell Science Ltd
Editorial Offices:
Osney Mead, Oxford OX2 0EL
25 John Street, London WC1N 2BL
23 Ainslie Place, Edinburgh EH3 6AJ
238 Main Street, Cambridge
  Massachusetts 02142, USA
54 University Street, Carlton
  Victoria 3053, Australia

Other Editorial Offices:
Arnette Blackwell SA
  1, rue de Lille, 75007 Paris
  France

Blackwell Wissenschafts-Verlag GmbH
  Kurfürstendamm 57
  10707 Berlin, Germany

  Feldgasse 13, A-1238 Wien
  Austria

First published 1996

Set by Excel Typesetters, Hong Kong
Printed and bound in Great Britain
by BPC Paulton Books Ltd., Bristol,
a member of the British Printing Company

DISTRIBUTORS

  Marston Book Services Ltd
  PO Box 87
  Oxford OX2 0DT
  (*Orders*: Tel: 01865 791155
          Fax: 01865 791927
          Telex: 837515)

North America
  Blackwell Science, Inc.
  238 Main Street
  Cambridge, MA 02142
  (*Orders*: Tel: 800 215-1000
                 617 876-7000
          Fax: 617 492-5263)

Australia
  Blackwell Science Pty Ltd
  54 University Street
  Carlton, Victoria 3053
  (*Orders*: Tel: 03 9347-0300
          Fax: 03 9349-3016)

A catalogue record for this title
is available from the British Library

ISBN 0-632-02944-7 (BSL)
     0-86542-630-9
     (International Edition)

Library of Congress
Cataloging-in-Publication Data

Essentials of pathology/M.J. Mitchinson
  . . . [et al.].
      p.   cm.
  Includes index.
  ISBN 0-632-02944-7
  1. Pathology.   I. Mitchinson, M. J.
  [DNLM: 1. Pathology.
  QZ 4 E788 1996]
  RB25.E78   1996
  616.07 – dc20
  DNLM/DLC
  for Library of Congress   95-14348
                                  CIP

Acknowledgements

Among the many colleagues who have contributed directly or indirectly during the writing of this book we must thank in particular Drs Margaret Stanley, Carlos Hormaeche, David Bowyer, Nabeel Affara and Sathia Thiru. That the book has appeared at all is due largely to the secretarial skill of Mrs Virginia Mullins and the extraordinary patience and skill of the publishers.

Figure 2.20 (also reproduced on cover) copyright Boehringer Ingelheim International GmbH, photo Lennart Nilsson. Figures 7.3 and 7.4 are modified from Selyers, A.A. & Whitt, D.D. (1994), *Bacterial Pathogenesis—a Molecular Approach*, American Society for Microbiology, Washington, D.C. Table 13.2 is adapted from Warren, K.S. (1989), Selective primary health care and parasitic diseases, Chapter 12 in *New Strategies in Parasitology* (ed. K.P.W.J. McAdam), pp. 217–231, Churchill Livingstone. Figure 13.7 is reproduced, by permission of WHO, from *Weekly Epidemiological Record*, **69**(43), 318 (1994).

1

Disease and its causes

Patterns of human disease are different in New York and Nairobi. The geographical variations can be due to different genes in the population and differences in the environment influenced by factors such as diet, climate, wealth, politics and even social customs. If we add to these variables the thousands of different causes of disease and the complexity of the mammalian body, it is not surprising that there is still a lot about the subject that we do not understand. Nevertheless, the essential facts about how diseases happen are quite simple, as we shall see.

Any departure from the normal structure and function of an organism is disease

Disease is a broad term, and includes all sorts of abnormalities, even some that we do not usually refer to as disease, such as cuts and bruises. When we speak of **a disease**, on the other hand, we mean a particular abnormality, or group of abnormalities, recognized in some plants or animals. In this book we shall be discussing the basic facts about how diseases of humans and other mammals happen.

The first description of a human disease usually comes from doctors, who notice a **repeating pattern of findings in a number of patients**. This is particularly likely to be noticed during periods when a large number of people suffer the same disease—**epidemics**. **Plague** and **smallpox** are examples of epidemic diseases recognized and described long ago, centuries before their causes were understood. Essentially, in defining a disease, the doctor notices recurrent patterns of **symptoms** (what the patient complains of, such as a rash, or a pain) and **signs** (what the doctor finds on examination, such as a raised temperature, or a heart murmur).

Such definitions of obvious disease are **clinical**. But sometimes a disease may be present before either patient or doctor is aware of it; this is **subclinical** disease. For instance, coronary artery disease takes many years to develop, but it only becomes obvious when a complication, such as a heart attack, occurs. Nevertheless, the silent, subclinical stage is certainly disease.

When a disease has been described and defined, there comes the opportunity to find out more about it: ideally, what causes it, how it develops and, if possible, how it can be prevented or cured. Once a disease has been described, it may happen, sometimes years later, that it turns out to be not a single disease but a group of similar diseases with different causes. Bright's disease of the kidney, described in the 19th century,[1] is now classified using modern tech-

1 By Dr Richard Bright (1789–1858) of Guy's Hospital, London.

1

niques, into about twenty different diseases. The opposite can happen too. Scrofula (of the neck glands), consumption (of the lungs) and Pott's disease of the spine were shown, in the late 19th century, to be simply different forms of the same bacterial disease—**tuberculosis**.

Any disease is never exactly the same in all patients. Some may die, some recover. Clearly there must be many factors that influence how a disease develops, and understanding them makes a fascinating challenge. The study of disease is called **pathology**.[2]

Most people think of a pathologist as someone who does post-mortem examination of human bodies. Although this is a vital contribution to understanding disease, and is usually the first essential to defining a disease properly, the study of disease only begins there, and requires many other scientific investigations in addition.

Medical terms are sometimes ill-defined

Because pathology sprang from medicine, many of the terms used are inherited from medicine. Some of these terms are old and time-honoured, but incapable of accurate definition. For example, 'benign' means 'tends not to be fatal'; 'malignant' means 'tends to be fatal'—no more than that. Other terms, however, have been introduced more recently and have strict scientific definitions, such as the names of chemical substances involved in disease processes.

A disease is essentially the effect of some sort of injury and the reactions of the body to the injury

Before you have finished this book, you will wonder how you have managed to survive so far. There are so many harmful things, and so many devious ways that parasites of various sorts can do damage that the question is how we cope with them. The answer is that the living body has evolved really sophisticated mechanisms of reaction to injury. This interaction of injury and the reactions to it is the essence of how diseases happen.

The injury may come about because of a **genetic abnormality** or an **adverse environment**, or both. It is important at the outset to consider what degrees of environmental changes we are discussing. The normal adaptations of the mammalian body to mild variations, such as changes in temperature, humidity or diet, are themselves wonderfully efficient. They are certainly not disease. These fine inbuilt adjustments to slight environmental changes are entirely natural, and are known as **homeostasis**. What distinguishes disease is that **the nature or degree of the environmental change is sufficiently severe to cause significant damage to the structure or function of the body**.[3]

The first way to consider how diseases start is to look at the different forms of injury that we know about and consider first **how they can damage cells**. The cells that form the mammalian body are, by their nature, vulnerable structures composed of delicate membranes surrounding viscous fluids.[4]

2 From the Greek *pathos* (suffering), *logos* (discourse).

3 This is the distinction, in fact, between **physiology** and **pathology**, but the distinction is rather blurred.

4 It was the brilliant German pathologist, **Rudolf Virchow** (1821–1902), who taught us the benefit of analysing disease by considering the effects of injuries on cells.

2

Table 1.1 Causes of injury.

Physical
Trauma
Heat
Cold
Irradiation
Chemical
Poisons
Cooperative
Quantitative
Living agents
Bacteria
Viruses
Parasites
Others
Genetic
Inherited or germline
Acquired or somatic

Cells can be injured in many ways

Table 1.1 shows a list of things that can damage the structure or function of cells. We can look at each of them in turn.

Physical injuries include trauma, temperature extremes and irradiation (Fig. 1.1)

Trauma, or **mechanical injury**, usually comes about by accident, and includes cuts, grazes, fractures of bones and bruises. Bruises are due to leakage of blood into the tissue from damaged small vessels. More severe bleeding (**haemorrhage**) results if larger blood vessels are damaged.

If trauma results in breakage of the skin, or the mucous membranes lining such sites as the mouth, this very commonly leads to **infection**, especially by bacteria. This familiar event reveals two important facts. First, the intact skin and mucous membranes must normally be **an efficient defence against infection**: second, it is an illustration of an important principle—that **tissue damage from one form of injury often allows access to another harmful agent.** Even a wound from a rose-thorn can lead to a fatal infection!

Injury from heat (burns) can occur even at only a few degrees higher than body temperature, but the duration of heat is important. The higher the temperature, the quicker it kills cells. Death of the epidermis occurs in 3–4 min at 51 °C. The injury is mainly due to damage to the essential large molecules of the cells, such as proteins and DNA, and to the cell membranes. This thermal injury to the skin carries two additional secondary hazards—**infection** (again) and, if the area of skin loss is large, **dehydration** due to rapid evaporation of tissue fluid from the exposed tissues.

3

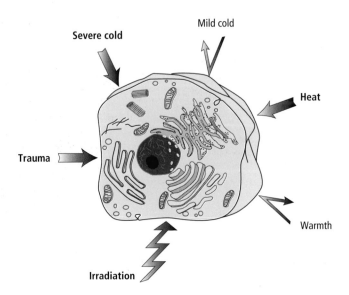

Figure 1.1 Physical injury to a cell.

Prolonged exposure of the body to less extreme heat (e.g. over 40 °C for some hours) can lead to **heat stroke** rather than burns. This is because certain neurons in the brain are damaged at these temperatures. As a result, their usual temperature-regulating function is impaired, and convulsions, coma and death can all follow.

Cold injures in two ways. Freezing directly damages cells by causing ice crystals to form inside and between the cells. However, in addition, low temperatures cause the blood vessels to constrict (become narrower). This leads to inadequate blood supply to the cold cells, worsening the outcome; this is the explanation of **frostbite**.

Irradiation may cause both immediate and delayed injuries. The cells most affected by radiation are those that divide regularly, such as those of the bone marrow or gut epithelium, because DNA is most vulnerable during cell division. The other immediate effect of radiation is that it causes the production of **free radicals**. These are chemical groups with unpaired electrons, signified with a dot. For instance, water (H_2O) may be split by irradiation into the hydrogen atom (H·) and the hydroxyl radical (OH·). Once formed, free radicals can cause considerable cell damage by setting up chain reactions that damage the essential large molecules of the cells, including DNA, proteins and membrane constituents.

The delayed effects of radiation appear to be due to more subtle changes in DNA. Survivors of atomic bombs and those exposed to irradiation in industry may develop cancer decades afterwards. Exposure to ultraviolet light is probably responsible for the high incidence of skin cancer, for example, in white Australians. It is thought that radiation induces genetic mutations, which predispose to the triggering of cancer by additional chance mutations later in life.

4

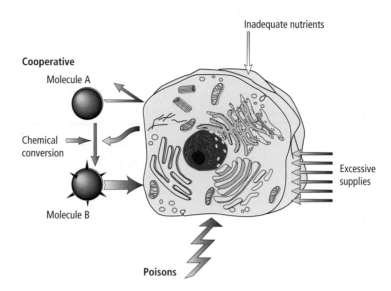

Figure 1.2 Chemical injury to a cell.

Chemical injury comes in various forms (Fig. 1.2)

Poisons are the most obvious source of chemical injury to cells, being chemicals that cause catastrophic damage even in low concentrations. **Cyanide**, for instance, destroys the activity of the vital enzyme, cytochrome oxidase, in all cells. Exposure to poisons is particularly common in industry. Some poisons, such as lead, are only dangerous when they accumulate due to repeated exposure.

Other chemicals are less toxic in themselves and injure cells only when they have been altered by chemical reactions in the body. This might be called **cooperative injury**, because it requires the body's cooperation. **Methanol**, for example, is only poisonous after enzymatic action within the cell converts it to **formaldehyde**. Similarly, some substances act indirectly by **triggering free radical formation**, for example, tobacco smoke and other chemicals, such as carbon tetrachloride, which causes liver cell injury in this way.

More common than either of these is cell damage caused by **quantitative variations** in supply of chemicals. Dietary deficiencies are a well-known example. But even substances that are vital for cell survival can be toxic in excess. For instance, even excessive oxygen exposure, in the course of medical treatment, can be harmful, particularly to the lungs and the eyes. **Fats** are essential in the diet, particularly for the maintenance of cell membranes, but excessive amounts can lead to obesity and its associated ailments, as well as arterial disease. **Glucose** is a vital nutrient, but excessive concentrations, as seen in **diabetes mellitus**, damage cells. Overdose of certain **vitamins**, as well as lack of them, can cause harm.

5

A variety of living organisms can cause disease

Most disease-causing organisms can only be seen under the microscope and are therefore often called **microorganisms** or **microbes**. Bacteria, for instance, have a diameter of only one-thousandth of a millimetre (a **micron**, or μm). Some organisms, however, are visible to the naked eye—the **macroparasites**. Some tapeworms can be a metre or more long! The organisms that can cause disease are referred to as **pathogenic organisms**, or pathogens, to distinguish them from the vast majority which do not cause disease.

Pathogenic organisms present an additional threat which is totally different to that of physical or chemical injury, because **they can multiply inside the body**. The damage that they cause therefore increases as they multiply, unless the body can defend itself.

Microorganisms can multiply very quickly. Most bacteria, for instance, have a generation time measured in minutes. As a result, mutations are common, and new characteristics evolve rapidly. Microorganisms are therefore a major threat to almost all forms of life. The defence mechanisms that we shall discuss later have evolved, it seems, mainly as a defence against microorganisms. Amongst the pathogenic microorganisms (Fig. 1.3), most are **bacteria**, **viruses** or **protozoa**. Fungi, yeasts and other varieties of microorganisms are also occasionally pathogenic.

Most bacteria are harmless. Uncountable types of bacteria are vital for degrading and recycling material in the environment, and many live harmlessly in and on the mammalian body. A few varieties, however, are pathogenic, including some that are normally found living harmlessly in close relationship with the host. A number of the important diseases of history, such as plague and tuberculosis, therefore had to await the invention of the microscope and bacterial culture techniques before their real cause became apparent. The varieties of ways in which bacteria can injure cells are fascinat-

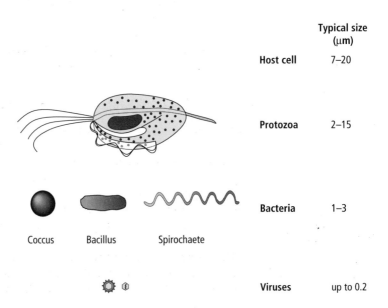

Figure 1.3 Some pathogenic microbes.

ing as well as worrying. Many bacteria cause disease by secreting toxic molecules called **exotoxins**, which are protein poisons, or by means of **endotoxins**, which are complex lipopolysaccharides of the cell wall. Some bacteria can even hide within cells and persist in the body for long periods. The discovery of antibiotics has by no means removed all the dangers that bacteria present.

Viruses are, of course, much smaller than bacteria (Fig. 1.3) and cannot be seen with the ordinary microscope. The other main difference is that they can only multiply inside living cells; and when they do so the effects can be devastating. From the common cold to acquired immunodeficiency syndrome (AIDS), the viruses present a complex series of problems, which are proving difficult to solve.

Parasites can be unicellular (**protozoa**, such as the malaria parasite) or multicellular (**metazoa**, such as tapeworms). The worst of the diseases they cause are seen in tropical climates, but no country is free from them.

Genetic factors influence virtually all diseases and are the sole cause of many of them

The contribution of genes to disease is all-important. In general terms, genetic makeup dictates the nature of the host. For instance, it was appreciated long ago that there seemed to be a natural resistance to certain diseases, on either an individual or racial basis. However, technological developments in the recent past have helped us to understand, in a more specific way, how genetic factors influence disease.

First, there are the inherited disorders caused by transmission of a **defective** or **absent gene** or genes. These abnormalities, present in the germ cells, often cause **congenital disease**, that is disease that is apparent from birth, such as cystic fibrosis. They can also bring about disorders that appear for the first time in adulthood, such as Huntington's disease. Second, cells may acquire changes in the arrangement or quantity of their genetic information, later in life (**somatic mutations**), sometimes interacting with inherited abnormalities already present. The study of somatic, or acquired mutations is helping our understanding of a number of diseases, in particular **cancer**.

Inherited genetic disorders vary considerably in their severity

Some inherited genetic abnormalities are severe. There may be whole extra chromosomes or pieces of one chromosome that are lost or duplicated or exchanged with a piece from another chromosome. Gross changes of this sort may be visible microscopically. Abnormalities in the number of chromosomes can result when chromosomes fail to separate normally during meiosis.[5] Such severe abnormalities usually result in death of the fetus; but when the sex chromosomes (X or Y) are the only ones affected, the individual is more likely to survive.

The presence of three rather than the usual pair of chromosomes is called **trisomy**. Trisomy 21 is compatible with life, causing what is known as Down's syndrome,[6] with varying degrees of mental and growth retardation. Many

5 The specific type of cell division which takes place in order to produce the haploid gamete.

6 John Down, London physician, 1828–1896.

of these patients have congenital heart disease, elevated risks of developing leukaemia and opacity of the lens of the eye (cataract) as well as characteristic facial features. They are also subject to premature ageing.

Other diseases have been linked with less severe abnormalities, for instance exchange of material between two different chromosomes—a **translocation**.

The majority of known inherited disorders result from changes in a single gene

Mutation at a single locus can alter the function of a single gene. Because this involves only a small change in the genetic information, many of these abnormalities are compatible with life and indeed more than 4000 such conditions have been described. The existence of these natural mishaps has helped to build up our knowledge of the function of individual genes. Single-gene disorders are classified as to whether or not they involve the X chromosome or a somatic chromosome and whether their effect is **dominant** or **recessive**.

Unfortunately, a number of the diseases caused by single-gene disorders of the autosomal[7] dominant type, although they may be very severe, such as Huntington's disease, polycystic kidney disease and familial polyps of the colon, sometimes do not become manifest until the third or fourth decade, when the affected individual has already had children. Thus the normal pressures which help to limit the handing-on of harmful mutations are side-stepped, sometimes with tragic consequences.

Worldwide, the most frequent diseases caused by mutations of genes are those which affect the structure of haemoglobin. These are referred to as **haemoglobinopathies**, all inherited disorders and, in more severe forms, associated with significant anaemia.

Other single mutations may affect the expression of receptors on the surface of cells, such as a defective low-density lipoprotein receptor, leading to the condition known as familial hypercholesterolaemia, which accelerates coronary artery disease. In others, the structure of connective tissue components in the body may be rendered abnormal and the sufferer has unusually brittle bones or the collagen is weak, leading to abnormally extensible skin, joints and blood vessels.

Some one in 25 people in Caucasian populations carry the gene responsible for the disease known as **cystic fibrosis**. It is inherited as an autosomal recessive and, as a result, about one in 2500 newborn babies are homozygous and suffer the disease, which is caused by the presence of two mutant genes in each cell. It is believed that their effect is to alter the transport of ions across cell membranes, and the result is a condition with profound effects in the digestive tract, lungs and other tissues.

Of course, the elucidation of the genetic basis of a disease is not only helpful in designing effective treatment; equally important is the detection of carriers and the possibility of advising individuals of the risks their children may run.

7 An autosome is a chromosome other than the X and Y chromosomes.

8

Variations in multiple genes contribute to a variety of diseases

These diseases are often much more difficult to understand. They may be referred to as **familial**, meaning that there is some degree of increased risk for blood relatives, but they have no definite pattern of inheritance. Examples include diabetes and coronary artery disease.

Cell injury affects tissues and organs

The analysis of how cells are injured is an important component of understanding disease, but not the only one. We must consider the broader effects upon the tissues of the body.

Some injuries are tissue-specific

Cells are, of course, mostly specialized, or differentiated, and organized into tissues; many forms of injury have to be considered at this level, rather than at the cellular level alone.

1 Some tissues are more vulnerable to particular injuries than others. For instance, the neurons in the central nervous system can survive lack of oxygen for only about 4 min, whereas liver cells may survive for over an hour.

2 Organotropism. Some harmful agents specifically target particular organs or tissues. Many chemical poisons, and the toxins of some bacteria, for instance, are specific for one cell type; some viruses too affect only one particular organ.

3 Opportunity. Clearly, the tissue damaged by a particular agent may well depend partly on chance. For microorganisms, the disease produced may be governed by the **portal of entry** — the way it gets in. Staphylococci are bacteria; they may cause a boil if they get into a hair follicle, but if they are inhaled into the lung they can cause pneumonia.

Some agents cause chain reactions (vicious circles) of injury

1 Damage to cells can cause secondary damage to nearby cells. For example, disruption of cells in the pancreas spills enzymes which damage nearby cells both in the pancreas itself, and in the adjacent tissue. The same sort of thing often happens when the phagocytes of the body are injured, and occurs to some extent after the death of any cell.

2 Secondary injuries. As we have seen, it is a general principle that anything that injures a tissue can predispose to damage by something else. The simplest example is that a cut in the skin often leads to bacterial infection. Virus infections, too, frequently damage tissues sufficiently to lead to bacterial invasion. Influenza epidemics, for example, cause many deaths not because of the infection by the influenza virus itself, but because of secondary bacterial infections of the lung.

3 Vital responses to injury, such as inflammation and immunity, can themselves sometimes cause cell damage.

Some agents injure the tissue matrix rather than the cells

One component of injury that must not be overlooked is damage to the **ground substance** between the cells, which is rich in **mucopolysaccharides**, and to the important fibres such as **collagen** and **elastin** that provide the framework that supports the cells. The tissues are dependent on this skeleton for their integrity, and some diseases, especially those affecting connective tissue, are caused at least partly by this type of damage. Some bacteria, such as streptococci, owe a good deal of their pathogenicity to their secretion of enzymes (such as hyaluronidase) that destroy this tissue skeleton and thereby enable the organisms to spread more widely.

Injuries affect the whole animal

Although a good deal of disease can now be analysed at the cellular or tissue level, it has to be considered also in the context of the whole animal. The specialization of tissues in higher animals means that **any one tissue is vitally dependent on many others**, and if one organ fails to do its job properly, others suffer. This is perhaps so obvious it hardly needs stating; adequate function of vital organs such as the heart, lungs or brain is necessary for all tissue function, but lesser degrees of inadequacy of distant organs can sometimes contribute subtly to disease processes—we shall see important examples when we consider cardiovascular disease. One such is **ischaemia** (inadequate blood supply) due to arterial narrowing, which is a common cause of tissue damage.

Last but not least, although this book does not address the problem, is the profound effect that disease can have upon the mind, and vice versa.

Disease in the population

The way that a disease affects human communities, rather than individuals, is an important component of the study of disease, for two reasons. The first is that it can provide information about patterns of incidence of disease, which is essential to the organization of health care, including the prevention and treatment of diseases. The second—more important for our purpose—is that it provides clues to the causes and modes of spread of a disease. The study of diseases in human populations is **epidemiology**.

Epidemiology began with the study of how infections occur. It was only too well known that diseases like plague were **epidemic**, spreading rapidly through a population in major outbreaks, with intervening periods in which the disease apparently disappeared. Some such infections spread rapidly across large parts of the world, and are called **pandemic**.[8] Influenza is one example. Diseases that occur constantly at a steady rate in the population are **endemic**. Those that only appear now and again, as isolated examples, are called **sporadic**.

Careful observations of how particular infections occur in populations have provided a great deal of knowledge as to the source of the infection **(the reservoir of infection)** and how the organisms spread through a community.

8 The adjectives pandemic and epidemic can also be nouns. Thus we can speak of an influenza pandemic, or an epidemic of measles.

But epidemiology is no longer concerned only with infections. The patterns of incidence of non-infective diseases have been the source of valuable clues about their causes. An example is the recognition of **risk factors** for cancer and coronary artery disease. Risk factors in a population are associated with a higher incidence of a disease, and may be contributing to it. Cigarette smoking is a strong risk factor for cancer; high-fat diets are a weak risk factor for coronary artery disease.

Summary

Disease is due, in the last analysis, to damage to cells or their supporting framework. Many different things can cause that damage, including new insults from outside the body and quantitative changes within. The damage may be local or, because of the interdependence of tissues, far-reaching.

The study of disease must take into account not only the molecular mechanisms of cell damage but also the effects on different tissues of the body and the pattern of its occurrence in the population.

Cell injury has recognizable results

Cell injury can sometimes only be detected by impaired function

Abnormal cell function, such as failure to synthesize a particular molecule normally, can sometimes be detected chemically. For instance, secretion of insulin by pancreatic islet cells is decreased in some patients with diabetes, and a decreased level of insulin can be detected in the plasma. Various forms of injury can affect the cell's integrity by impairing the function of its membranes. The result may be excessive cellular uptake of water and ions such as calcium, or excessive leakage of cell components such as enzymes.[9] Such chemical changes can sometimes be detected in the living patient, but can also be studied in more detail in cells cultured in the laboratory.

More severe injury leads to visible changes seen on histological examination

The opportunity to examine tissues microscopically arises either at post-mortem examination or when tissue is removed surgically. Thin sections of tissue can be cut, and stained in various ways to provide a permanent visual record of the appearance of the tissue. This **histological examination** is usually a vital step in the process of beginning to understand how a particular disease develops, and will constantly reappear in these pages as we consider various disease processes. The most useful staining procedure for sections of tissues is a combination of haematoxylin and eosin. In general, this stains nuclei purple and cytoplasm mauve-pink (Fig. 1.4). Many diseases produce visible changes in tissues that can be assessed in this way.

9 Different cell types often leak different enzymes, so this can sometimes be used clinically to indicate the site of damage, e.g. creatine kinase from muscle.

11

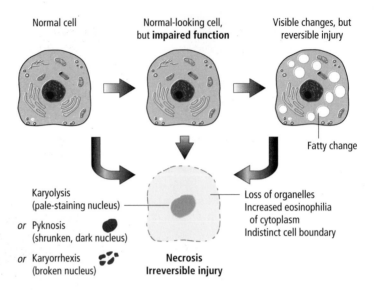

Normal cell

Normal-looking cell,
but **impaired function**

Visible changes, but
reversible injury

Fatty change

Karyolysis
(pale-staining nucleus)

or Pyknosis
(shrunken, dark nucleus)

or Karyorrhexis
(broken nucleus)

Loss of organelles
Increased eosinophilia
of cytoplasm
Indistinct cell boundary

**Necrosis
Irreversible injury**

Figure 1.4 Cell injury.

Severe injury to cells may result in visible swelling, organelle damage or fatty change. **Fatty change** is the appearance within a cell of cytoplasmic droplets of lipid, visible histologically (Fig. 1.4). This is most often seen in liver cells, because of their very active lipid metabolism; in the liver it may be due to excessive alcohol intake, anaemia and many other conditions, but it can also occur in other tissues. Essentially it is due to the fact that cells constantly take up lipids essential for their function and maintenance; many forms of mild injury do not affect the uptake, but slow down the usage of this lipid, which therefore accumulates as droplets in the cytoplasm.[10]

All these functional and visible changes indicate that the cell is injured, but not irreversibly so.

Irreversible injury causes cell death (necrosis)

Necrosis means death of cells, usually a large group of cells, during the lifetime of the animal. The word is therefore not used to describe the death and dissolution of cells which occurs after death. Necrotic cells not only lose all their functions; they also leak contents such as enzymes, as mentioned above. Finally they develop, over the course of 24 h or so, certain histological changes characteristic of necrosis (Fig. 1.4). These consist of a loss of cytoplasmic structure, so that the cytoplasm of a necrotic cell now stains bright pink rather than mauve; and nuclear changes become visible. Membrane damage often also leads to loss of definition of the edges of the cell; it may also cause loss of normal adhesive properties, e.g. a necrotic epithelial cell usually separates from its basement membrane. One particular cause of necrosis is dignified by a special name. Necrosis due to ischaemia (inadequate blood supply) is called **infarction**. The dead area is referred to as an **infarct**. A characteristic of necrosis that we shall discuss later is that it almost always causes an **inflammatory reaction**.

10 Another cause of fatty change in the liver is overloading with fat. In the Dordogne the Strasbourg goose is force-fed; its fatty liver is *pâté de foie gras*.

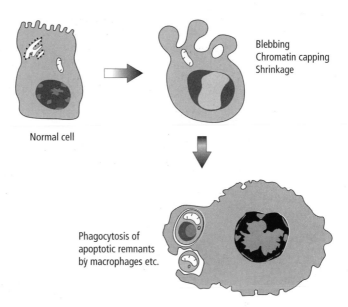

Blebbing
Chromatin capping
Shrinkage

Normal cell

Phagocytosis of
apoptotic remnants
by macrophages etc.

Figure 1.5 Apoptosis.

Strictly speaking, necrosis is used to mean only **unexpected** death of cells, usually in considerable numbers locally. In many tissues, such as epithelia, individual cells are normally constantly dying and being replaced by the multiplication of their neighbours. This natural process of **programmed cell death**, which also occurs extensively during fetal development, seems to be a sort of cell suicide, because it requires a controlled process of enzymatic activation leading to DNA fragmentation. This results in changes in histological appearance which are highly characteristic (Fig. 1.5) and referred to as **apoptosis**.[11] Apoptosis is quite different from necrosis and does **not** cause an inflammatory reaction. Curiously enough, it has now emerged that apoptosis occurs not only as a result of programmed cell death, but can also result from exposure to various toxic substances.

Summary

Various forms of injury affect cells. Some of these injuries are only quantitative changes in the environment. Depending on their severity these injuries may give rise to functional or visible reversible injury, or to cell death, by necrosis or apoptosis.

Simple defences against injury

Certain anatomical structures are a barrier to injury

The most obvious defences, as we have seen, are epithelial surfaces, mainly the skin and mucous membranes of the mouse, nose, vagina, etc. The best evidence

11 Apoptosis, from the Greek, means 'dropping off', like the leaves of a tree in autumn. (The second 'p' is silent.)

that a structure is useful in defence is what happens when it is defective. A break in those epithelial surfaces often leads to bacterial infection.

Also, a part of our bony so-called endoskeleton is, in fact, more like an exoskeleton – the skull and the ribcage can protect the vital organs within from severe trauma and occasionally other injuries.

Many physiological functions are defensive

Various parts of the body are protected by **movement**. For instance, movement of the mucus in the respiratory tract caused by the activity of cilia on the epithelial cells constantly tends to expel inhaled dusts and microbes. The coughing and sneezing reflexes have a similar effect, in response to a more powerful stimulus, such as after inhaling fluid or solid material.

This defence of the respiratory tract has analogies in other hollow organs draining to the exterior, such as the outward movements of the contents of the biliary, alimentary, genital and urinary tracts. This gives rise to the important principle – **if a hollow organ is blocked, infection develops behind the obstruction**.

Many simple reflexes such as blinking, the withdrawal reflex or vomiting noxious material are also clearly protective.

Normal resident microbes are protective

Microorganisms, mainly bacteria, are always found in large numbers in certain parts of the body, such as the gut, and are normally harmless. They also provide a protection against pathogenic organisms because, if these normal flora are depleted, pathogenic bacteria can sometimes multiply instead. For example, giving antibiotics by mouth can sometimes kill some of the normal flora, and thus lead to bacterial disease of the bowel.

Vital reactions to injury have evolved to provide further protection

Four vital reactions provide the last line of natural bodily defence against injury:

1 inflammation is a local response that tends to limit the injury, whatever the cause;

2 haemostasis (blood-clotting and vasoconstriction) minimizes the risk of haemorrhage;

3 regeneration is the capacity of most tissues to multiply to replace damaged cells;

4 the immune response is a means of boosting inflammation, mainly that caused by microbes.

All of these reactions tend to be protective, which explains how they evolved. They are central to the understanding of disease, and in due course we shall consider each of them in turn. We shall begin with inflammation.

2 Acute inflammation and healing

Inflammation is one of the four vital reactions of the body to injury. The others are **haemostasis** (blood clotting), **regeneration** and the **immune response**. These are all complex reactions, as we shall see, and therefore have to be distinguished from the basic inbuilt defences such as the skin. All these four reactions have evolved in animals because they tend usually to be protective in their effects, and are therefore sometimes called defence mechanisms. They are, however, blind reactions which unfortunately can also sometimes do harm.

Inflammation is the local reaction of living tissue to any severe cell injury

It is important to note that inflammation occurs no matter what causes the cell injury. So **inflammation is not the same thing as infection; it may result from infection, but may also follow when anything else disrupts cells.** The ancients understandably thought inflammation was a disease; it was left to John Hunter, the 18th century London surgeon, to point out that it was **not a disease, but a reaction** to a disease or injury.

As to the clinical nature of inflammation, the cardinal signs were described by the Roman patrician, Celsus,[1] as **rubor** (redness), **calor** (warmth), **tumor** (swelling) and **dolor** (pain). It is arguable that he could have included **fluor** (excessive secretion). All these signs are explicable by the microscopic dynamic events of inflammation, as we shall see.

Inflammation of a tissue is usually signified by the suffix -itis, thus appendicitis, peritonitis, gastritis, etc., but two old words are exceptions: pleurisy is inflammation of the pleura and pneumonia is inflammation of the lung. The word **acute** means of **relatively short duration**; it does **not** mean severe. In the context of acute inflammation it implies a few days' duration, whereas **chronic inflammation** lasts longer than a week or so, often for months or years. Here we shall discuss only acute inflammation.

Acute inflammation is a sequence of events that are similar, whatever the injury

The microscopic events of acute inflammation were described in the 19th century by Wharton-Jones and by Cohnheim, watching the reactions of transparent tissues (such as the web of a frog's foot) after experimental injury, under a microscope.

1 The head of a large Roman household, with relatives and slaves, was often called upon as a 'doctor'. Celsus's account of diseases is really impressive, although his remedies are not.

15

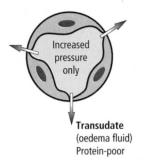

Transudate
(oedema fluid)
Protein-poor

Figure 2.1 Transudate.

First, when the tissue is damaged, there is **dilatation of all the nearby blood vessels**, resulting in increased capillary blood pressure and increased blood flow. This explains the local redness and increased temperature.

Second, these dilated vessels develop **increased permeability** to fluid, but the fluid which escapes is of a rather special kind. It should be contrasted with the effect of the increased hydrostatic pressure in a capillary which might result from blockage of a vein. When a vein is blocked, protein-rich fluid escapes from capillaries, but it does not include the largest plasma proteins, which the vascular endothelium retains, and the resulting fluid is referred to as **transudate**, or oedema fluid (Fig. 2.1). However, in acute inflammation, the **endothelial permeability** is actually **increased** so that **the largest molecules do escape**. This protein-rich fluid which collects outside the blood vessels is called **exudate** (Fig. 2.2) and contains the large plasma proteins, including **fibrinogen**. The large molecules in the exudate are broken down, by enzymes spilled from the damaged cells, into smaller molecules. This also tends to increase the flow of fluid from vessels to tissue spaces, because the osmotic pressure of the exudate increases.

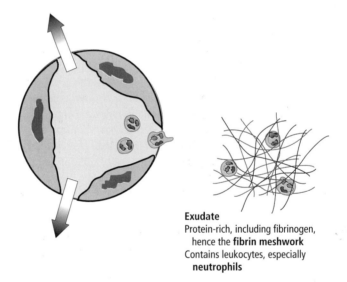

Exudate
Protein-rich, including fibrinogen,
hence the **fibrin meshwork**
Contains leukocytes, especially
neutrophils

Figure 2.2 Formation of exudate in acute inflammation.

When fibrinogen escapes from vessels, it encounters a substance in the tissues called **thromboplastin**,[2] which converts fibrinogen into solid strands of **fibrin**, forming a meshwork in the tissue. If a lot of fibrin is present in an exudate, it looks yellow to the naked eye, almost buttery, and is called a **fibrinous exudate**. The existence of the exudate explains the swelling and, at least partly, the pain of acute inflammation.

The third event in acute inflammation is emigration of leukocytes from the blood into the tissue. Figure 2.3 shows the types of leukocytes. The majority of the cells which emigrate in acute inflammation are neutrophils, although some monocytes and a few eosinophils may accompany them. First, the neutrophils adhere to the local endothelium (**margination** or **pavementing**) and then crawl out between endothelial cells to emerge into the injured tissue (Fig. 2.2).

2 Thromboplastin seems to be at least partly a tissue-derived, membrane-associated phospholipid–protein complex.

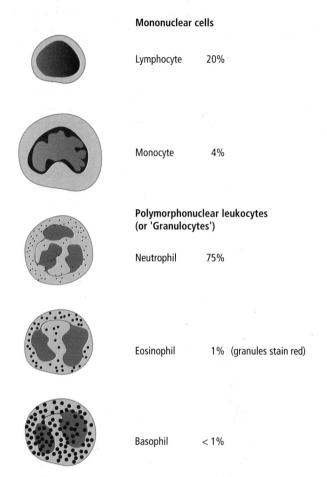

Mononuclear cells

Lymphocyte   20%

Monocyte   4%

Polymorphonuclear leukocytes
(or 'Granulocytes')

Neutrophil   75%

Eosinophil   1%   (granules stain red)

Basophil   < 1%

Figure 2.3 Types of leukocyte in blood. The sizes and percentages are variable and shown approximately. A lymphocyte might be typically 10–12 μm in diameter.

All three of these events of early inflammation are seen within an hour or so of the injury. It must be emphasized that they are all **local**, near the injured cells.

The components of acute inflammation are variable in amount

We have referred to the yellow buttery appearance of a fibrinous exudate. One variation seen occasionally is that the proportion of fibrin in the exudate is unusually low, and the exudate is more watery—**serous exudate**. This occurs in infection by certain bacteria such as **streptococci**, which produce **fibrinolysins**—enzymes that break down fibrin. Serous exudates are also a feature of **burns**.

Sometimes tissue injury, especially that caused by certain bacteria, leads to complete destruction of an area, with liquefaction of the tissue and a high content of living and dead neutrophils. The thick yellow fluid that results is called **pus**. This is referred to as **purulent inflammation**. Those bacteria, such as **staphylococci**, that commonly cause pus formation are called **pyogenic bacteria**.

Histologically, most inflammatory exudates contain both a good deal of fibrin and also many neutrophils. They are called **fibrinopurulent exudates**.

When the initial injury causes significant damage to the blood vessels themselves, the exudate also contains spilled blood—a **haemorrhagic exudate**.

One further component of inflammation is common but often overlooked—**fluor**, or **excessive secretion**. This refers to the increased activity of any exocrine glands near the acute inflammation. Examples include the excessive secretions of the nasal mucosa and glands in the common cold and in hayfever—hence the runny nose. It is beneficial to the host, however, because it flushes out pathogenic microorganisms. In turn, this is helpful to the microbes, because coughs and sneezes help them to find a new host.

The gross appearances of acute inflammation vary according to anatomical site

In a solid tissue, the amount of exudate that accumulates depends on the amount of dead tissue and is limited by how much the tissue can swell. Eventually the amount of exudate can increase no more, presumably when the pressure in the extravascular space equals that of the blood. If however the inflammation is next to a natural cavity such as the pleural or peritoneal cavity, more exudate may escape into the cavity (Fig. 2.4), where it forms yellowish buttery adhesions.

Within a solid tissue, if an abnormal cavity is formed, filled with pus, it is called an **abscess** (Fig. 2.5), usually due to bacterial infection. Damage to an

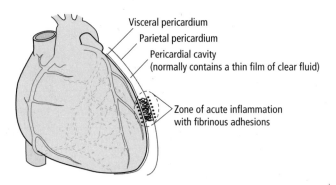

Visceral pericardium
Parietal pericardium
Pericardial cavity
(normally contains a thin film of clear fluid)

Zone of acute inflammation
with fibrinous adhesions

Figure 2.4 Acute exudate in a cavity, forming fibrinous adhesions.

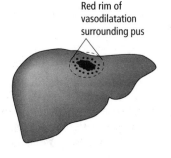

Red rim of
vasodilatation
surrounding pus

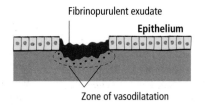

Fibrinopurulent exudate

Epithelium

Zone of vasodilatation

Figure 2.5 An acute abscess in a solid organ (left).

Figure 2.6 An acute ulcer (right).

(a)

(b)

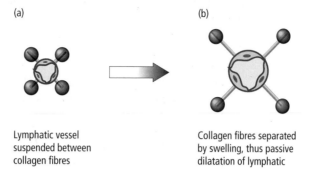

Lymphatic vessel
suspended between
collagen fibres

Collagen fibres separated
by swelling, thus passive
dilatation of lymphatic

Figure 2.7 Swelling of tissue
leads to lymphatic dilatation.

epithelial surface sufficient to cause a gap in the epithelium is an **ulcer** (Fig. 2.6),
with fibrinopurulent exudate in the floor. In a skin ulcer, the exudate will dry,
forming the **scab**.

Acute inflammation has important local beneficial effects

One minor result of inflammation occurs at a conscious level. The pain and
swelling discourage the use of an affected part. If the lesion is infected, active
movement would tend to spread the exudate, and hence the infection, through
the tissues.

The other local effects are of profound defensive importance and presumably
explain the evolution of inflammation. First, the increased blood flow improves
the local supply of oxygen and nutrients. Second, the exudate has the effect
of diluting any harmful chemicals in the area and also carries within it
vital plasma constituents such as the antibodies which can help to neutralize
infections.

Third, it encourages the emigration of the neutrophils and monocytes, the
professional **phagocytes** of the body, capable of moving about in amoeboid
fashion and engulfing debris and bacteria. Once monocytes reach the tissues
they enlarge and become more active, and are called **macrophages**.[3] Both
neutrophils and macrophages can not only phagocytose bacteria but also kill
them. The importance of this function is revealed by the fact that patients
with deficiencies of number or function of their phagocytes inevitably die of
bacterial infections.

Fourth, the fibrin meshwork acts as a sort of scaffolding along which the
phagocytes crawl in pursuit of bacteria. It also seems to help phagocytosis by
providing an anchorage for the phagocytes, which then trap the bacteria
against the fibrin.

In addition, the increased tissue pressure caused by the exudate actually
dilates local lymph vessels (Fig. 2.7), causing increased drainage of the fluid to
local lymph nodes. This not only delivers dead cells and debris to a large
population of macrophages resident in the lymph node, stationed there for this
very purpose, but also helps the immune response, as we shall see. So, in acute
inflammation there is a greatly increased flow of fluid through the tissue
towards the lymph nodes, flushing the tissue (Fig. 2.8).

3 Macrophage means 'big eater',
in contrast to the smaller
neutrophils, which used to be
called microphages, a term that
has now been abandoned.

19

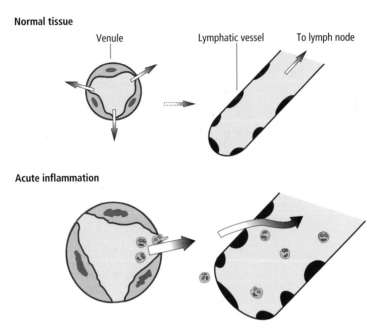

Figure 2.8 Increased lymph drainage in acute inflammation.

Finally, the increased flow of secretions from exocrine glands increases the rate of movement of the contents of hollow organs, helping to expel harmful chemicals or microbes.

All of these useful results of acute inflammation suggest that it evolved primarily as a defence against bacterial infection, although it is to some extent beneficial as a response to physical and chemical injury to tissues. Even animals lacking a vascular system, such as sponges, have primitive macrophage-like cells capable of phagocytosis; obviously the vascular elements of the response evolved later.

Acute inflammation, although local, also has general effects

Inflammation is usually accompanied by **fever**, because the function of neurons that regulate temperature is affected. The increased temperature may be of some slight significance in accelerating the local cellular processes of the inflammatory response. It may also be detrimental to some pathogenic bacteria,[4] whose optimum temperature for replication is usually 37 °C. Severe fevers are often accompanied by muscle pains and even mental disturbances, such as delirium. Most of these general effects, including fever, are due to release of a substance called interleukin-1 from leukocytes.

Another general effect is **neutrophil leukocytosis**. This refers to the increased numbers of neutrophils circulating in the blood. This results from both the release of less mature neutrophils from the bone marrow and also their increased production. The potential supply of neutrophils to the local lesion is obviously improved as a result.

4 In years gone by, syphilis was actually treated by infecting the patients with malaria; the high fevers were reputedly harmful to the causative bacterium of syphilis, *Treponema pallidum*.

Acute-phase proteins are produced by the liver, in patients with acute inflammation, including some, like complement components, that directly assist the inflammatory process (see below).

Summary

Acute inflammation is the early local response of living tissue to substantial injury of cells. It consists of vasodilatation, fluid exudation and phagocyte recruitment, localizing defensive components at the site of injury. It appears to have evolved primarily as a defence against infections but can be at least partially effective against other forms of injury.

Mechanisms of acute inflammation

Vasodilatation and increased permeability are caused by chemical mediators

It has gradually emerged that most of the events of acute inflammation are **controlled by chemicals** in the extracellular fluid, some of which are secreted by cells. The discovery of these molecules has resulted from gradual improvements in experimental techniques.

The light microscopy of the early days was supplemented by the use of improved **chemical analytical techniques** in experimental animals, the development of drugs that block certain steps in the process and the detection of increased vascular permeability, by injecting into the blood such things as carbon particles or marker molecules such as Evans blue.[5] The **electron microscope** led to improved visual analysis of the process, including the fact that exudation of large molecules occurs through gaps that appear between endothelial cells (see Fig. 2.2). Finally, the technique of **cell culture** has enabled the contributions of different cell types to be investigated.

Acute inflammation has proved to be much more complicated than expected. Nevertheless, from experimental findings, a number of important **chemical mediators** of acute inflammation have been identified. All these chemicals are labile, some lasting for only a few seconds. This accounts for the fact that acute inflammation is localized because, as they diffuse through the tissue, the mediators break down or are destroyed.

Complement is a good candidate for the final common pathway by which all cell disruption causes acute inflammation

Complement is the name given to an important system of proteins, present in the plasma and extracellular fluid, which can be activated to have several biological effects. It comprises a **cascade mechanism**, in which activation of one component leads to activation of another. The pivotal, central molecule is a large protein called C3 which can be **split by proteases to trigger the cascade**. This cleavage can be initiated in three ways (Fig. 2.9). The simplest, which

5 Evans blue is a small molecule that attaches to plasma albumin and therefore only leaks from blood vessels in visible amounts at sites of increased permeability.

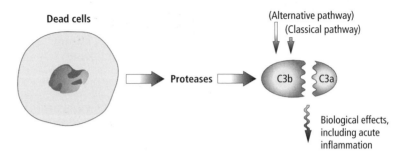

Figure 2.9 Complement activation.

probably evolved first, is the direct **cleavage of the C3 molecule by various proteases spilled from all necrotic cells, whatever the cause of injury**. The second is called the alternate or **alternative pathway**, and is stimulated by a variety of substances including bacterial components. The third is only triggered after the immune response, and is called the classical pathway, simply because it was discovered first. In fact it was probably the last to evolve.

Most of the biological activities of the complement cascade result inevitably from the splitting of C3. The activity that mainly concerns us here is due to two fragments[6] called **C3a and C5a**, which both have the important effect of causing degranulation of mast cells. **Mast cells** are found in all tissues of the body, especially near blood vessels, and contain membrane-bound granules which are stores of chemicals. In this context it is the **histamine** that they discharge when stimulated that is important. Histamine was the first chemical mediator of inflammation to be described. It causes both dilatation and increased permeability of small blood vessels, the latter due to the retraction of endothelial cells with widening of the intercellular gaps between them (see Fig. 2.2).

Histamine has a short life in the tissues (only about 30 seconds) because it is broken down by the enzyme **histaminase**. Drugs that interfere with the actions of histamine (antihistamines) are anti-inflammatory.

Other important events are caused by the complement activation, as we shall see, including chemotaxis, assistance with phagocytosis and sometimes lysis of microbes.

Some eicosanoids are chemical mediators of inflammation

Eicosanoids are cell-derived enzymatic oxidation products of **arachidonic acid** (a fatty acid with 20 carbon atoms and four double bonds) which is normally found incorporated in the phospholipids of cell membranes. The production of eicosanoids depends on the release of arachidonic acid from the phospholipids by the enzyme **phospholipase**,[7] followed by one of two enzymatic oxidation steps to give rise to the two types of eicosanoids (Fig. 2.10). Thus the action of the enzyme **lipoxygenase** leads to production of the **leukotrienes**, and of **cyclo-oxygenase** to **prostaglandins**.

There are a whole variety of leukotrienes and prostaglandins, all having differing biological effects. Different cell types produce varying proportions of these various molecules. It is sufficient for now to note that certain leukotrienes

6 C3a and C5a represent what used to be called **anaphylatoxin**. This old name is still used, but is now really redundant.

7 Phospholipase activity is stimulated by C5a.

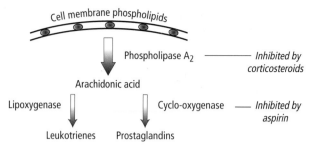

Figure 2.10 Eicosanoid production.

such as leukotriene E_4 (LTE_4) and prostaglandins such as PGE, PGD_2 and $PGF_{2\alpha}$ can cause vasodilatation and increased permeability. **Corticosteroids** and **aspirin** are drugs that inhibit eicosanoid production, which explains their usefulness as anti-inflammatory drugs (Fig. 2.10).

In some experimental models of inflammation, the increased permeability appears to be biphasic, a transient increase being followed after an hour or so by a delayed, longer-lasting increase. The evidence suggests that histamine may be responsible for the former, eicosanoids for the latter.

Many other inflammatory mediators have been described, and more are being discovered all the time.

Polypeptides called **kinins** (e.g. bradykinin) are produced from plasma precursors (kininogens) during acute inflammation and can cause vasodilatation and increased permeability. Among many other molecules that have been identified are **interleukin-1** and products spilled from phagocytes. It is therefore impossible as yet to understand the whole inflammatory process. It is, in fact, tempting to wonder why the response is so chemically complicated — perhaps it confers versatility on the reaction, so that different forms of injury stimulate one pathway more than another, but all have essentially the same result.

The abundance of chemical mediators prompts the question: why does acute inflammation ever stop when the injury ceases? There is no single answer to this question: most mediators are labile molecules; antagonists, such as histaminase and antiproteases, are present in tissues; and some mediators may become exhausted locally.

Summary

Vasodilatation and increased permeability are due to labile chemical mediators, generated from cells or from inactive plasma precursors, as a result of tissue injury. The mechanisms are complex and only partly understood.

Neutrophil function in inflammation

Polymorphonuclear neutrophil leukocytes are derived from a family of cells in the marrow, called the myeloid series. The parent cell is a myeloblast, whose offspring develop granules and are called myelocytes. Up to this point these cells have a large oval nucleus. The end-stage cell, the neutrophil granulocyte, or polymorphonuclear neutrophil leukocyte, has an elongated nucleus which gradually fragments into up to five lobes during its short lifetime of probably less than 2 days. Part of its life is spent in the marrow but, usually at the two-lobed stage, it leaves to enter the blood. It has now become a cell with few remaining functions and is unable to divide, but those functions that do remain are quite exciting.

Neutrophils emigrate from the blood and are attracted chemotactically to sites of injury

To understand adhesion and emigration, we need first to consider **cell movement**.

Cell movement has mainly been studied in fibroblasts, but the mechanisms are probably the same in other cells. First it is important to know that cells can't swim. They can only **crawl along surfaces**, by adhering at certain points and then dragging the cell body along by assembling contractile microfilaments in the cytoplasm, extending from the attachment sites. This caterpillar-like traction is greatly enhanced if the underlying surface has molecules on it for which the cell has receptors; if those molecules are more concentrated in one direction, **chemotaxis** results (Fig. 2.11).

There are two experimental techniques for investigating chemotaxis. One is the Boyden chamber (Fig. 2.12), in which the cells are separated from the candidate chemoattractant by a filter with pores about 4 μm in diameter. The number of cells crawling through the filter in a given time is a measure of chemotaxis. The other method is to put the cells and a candidate chemoattractant into separate wells in an agarose plate (Fig. 2.13). This is a solid medium containing cell nutrients (like the solid media used for bacterial culture). The cells crawl from the bottom of their well, underneath the medium, towards the chemoattractant. Using these methods, molecules that have been shown to be positively chemotactic for neutrophils include certain bacterial products, leukotriene B_4 and, of central importance in inflammation, the **complement component, C5a**.

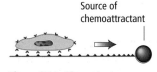

Source of chemoattractant

Figure 2.11 Chemotaxis.

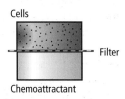

Cells

Filter

Chemoattractant

Remove filter after incubation
Count cells on bottom side of filter

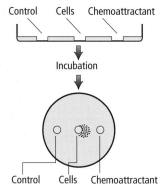

Control   Cells   Chemoattractant

Incubation

Control   Cells   Chemoattractant

Figure 2.12 Boyden chamber (left).

Figure 2.13 Agarose plate technique for chemotaxis (right).

Chemotactic molecules might also be responsible for adhesion (pavementing) of neutrophils and for their emigration, if the molecules were able to penetrate endothelial cell junctions and be presented on the endothelial surface (Fig. 2.13). There is experimental evidence supporting this idea. However, other mechanisms might also be at work. A number of **adhesion molecules** have been described which probably play a part in neutrophil adhesion and emigration. They are all molecules, expressed on the endothelial cell surface, for which the neutrophils have receptors. Their expression on endothelium is enhanced in inflammation. This is an interesting subject of great current research interest.

The process of emigration of a neutrophil from the blood into the tissues takes about 15 min. Adhesion and emigration of leukocytes tend to be diminished by one of the prostaglandins (PGI_2, or prostacyclin) which is secreted by normal endothelial cells, but PGI_2 production is probably diminished at sites of injury.

Phagocytosis is preceded by firm adhesion of the neutrophil membrane to a bacterium

The uptake of bacteria and other particles by neutrophils may be quite non-specific, but the process is greatly enhanced if the organism has molecules on its surface for which the neutrophil membrane has receptors. Molecules enhancing adhesion and phagocytosis may be a natural part of the organism's structure. For instance, phagocytes have lectin-like receptors for saccharides on the bacterial surface. However, other molecules have evolved which are manufactured by the host animal and attach to the bacterium within the tissues. Such molecules are called **opsonins**,[8] and a bacterium coated with them is said to be **opsonized**. Opsonins include both the **complement component C3b**, which is produced during inflammation and can attach to the cell wall of microbes, and also, as we shall see later, the antibodies.

For opsonins to work, the phagocyte has to have surface receptors that combine with the opsonins. It is easy to see how opsonins would therefore help phagocytosis by a sort of zipper mechanism which results in the bacterium entering the cell within a membrane-bound vesicle, called a **phagosome** (Fig. 2.14).

Neutrophils have two main mechanisms for killing and digestion of bacteria

All cells produce toxic oxygen radicals as an unavoidable side-product of oxidative metabolism, and scavenger mechanisms have evolved to minimize their harmful effects. These oxygen radicals are groups of atoms, including oxygen, that have an unpaired electron, signified by a dot. They include superoxide ($O_2^-\cdot$), the hydroxyl radical ($OH\cdot$) and singlet oxygen ($O\cdot$). Most are highly labile and tend to pass on a spare electron to other molecules, which can be damaged as a result. Dietary antioxidants such as vitamin E can damp down the process. Cytoplasmic scavenger molecules that detoxify the radicals include enzymes such as superoxide dismutase. In phagocytes, evolution has

8 From the Greek *opson*, meaning a sauce or relish.

25

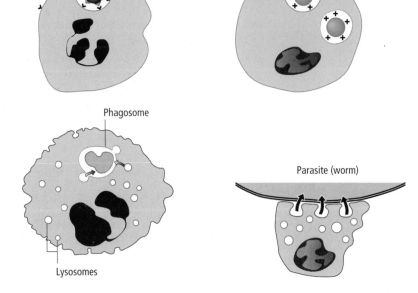

Figure 2.14 Phagocytosis of bacteria (left).

Figure 2.15 Sites of oxygen radical production (+) (right).

Figure 2.16 Lysosomal fusion with phagosome (left).

Figure 2.17 Lysosomal exocytosis on large parasite (right).

developed this potentially dangerous phenomenon to the animal's advantage. In phagocytes, the balance of radical production and scavenger processes has been tipped in favour of the radicals, which the phagocyte uses to kill the microbes. The oxygen radicals are produced at the cell surface and therefore also on the inner side of the phagosome (Fig. 2.15), very close to the surface of the bacterium, and are highly toxic to most bacteria. The radicals form more rapidly as a result of a **respiratory burst** which is triggered by phagocytosis.

The next event after phagosome formation is **lysosomal fusion**. The characteristic **granules** of neutrophils are in fact **lysosomes**, membrane-bound organelles containing degradative enzymes. The enzymes have an acidic optimum pH of about 4, which is the prevailing pH in lysosomes. Lysosomes are not all identical, but all types contain enzymes that are bactericidal and others that break down the bacterial constituents after killing. The **lysosomes fuse with the phagosome** soon after it forms and discharge their acid and enzymes into the phagosome (Fig. 2.16). The acid pH is itself harmful to the bacteria and also stimulates **more oxygen radical production**. The enzymes also contribute to bacterial killing and degradation. Examples are known of sequential fusion, first with lysosomes degrading the exterior of the bacterium, then later with those attacking the inner parts. How this phenomenon is controlled is unknown.

9 Eosinophils are more effective, because they also exocytose other molecules, including **major basic protein**, particularly toxic for parasites.

Larger organisms are attacked by exocytosis

Clearly a neutrophil is no match for a **parasitic worm**, which is relatively huge. What macrophages and eosinophils[9] do in these circumstances is to flatten against the surface of the worm, followed by **fusion of the lysosomes with the surface membrane** of the cell, on the side of the cell facing the worm (Fig. 2.17). Like phagocytosis, this process is enhanced if the parasite is **opsonized**. Neutrophils probably also participate in this activity. Their motto appears to be, if you can't eat it, spit at it! This process of **exocytosis** of radicals and enzymes is sometimes successful in killing the parasite, sometimes not.

At this point, we must introduce another cell type that also kills by exocytosis, but in a very different way. **Natural killer cells** (NK cells) are large lymphocytes with lysosomes that contain a molecule called **perforin**. NK cells attach, probably via lectins, to the surface of virus-infected cells and exocytose perforin on to the cell surface. This leads to a puncture of the target cell membrane, admitting other NK cell components that cause **apoptosis** in the infected cell.

Neutrophil death causes tissue damage

The neutrophils have a life-span of only a few hours in an inflammatory lesion, sometimes less. A severe local infection quickly becomes a graveyard of thousands of neutrophils. Their contents, especially enzymes, spill out and may damage cells and fibres, thus prolonging the local damage, and leading in the worst cases to liquefaction and **pus formation**. This vicious circle leads to more neutrophil recruitment, which only comes to a stop if the causative agent is eliminated; then naturally occurring antagonists in the extracellular fluid, such as **antiproteases**, damp down the enzyme activity, and the tissue damage ceases.

Neutrophils can spread bacteria

If neutrophils containing viable bacteria die outside the site of original infection, they may actually assist the spread of that infection. Normally, neutrophils appear to be confined within the fibrin meshwork through which they crawl but some bacteria secrete enzymes (fibrinolysins) that dissolve the fibrin. The neutrophils may then be dispersed passively through movements of the extracellular fluid. Sometimes they die before they have killed the bacteria they contain, so they are unwittingly spreading the bacteria.

Defects of neutrophil function lead to more persistent infections

Defects of neutrophil function may be hereditary or acquired, and studying them is an excellent way to make us appreciate their normal role. **Chédiak–Higashi disease** is a rare genetic disorder of humans, cattle, mice and other mammals, in which both chemotaxis and lysosome–phagosome fusion are defective, apparently due to **inadequate microtubule formation**.[10] Amongst the other rare hereditary diseases is **chronic granulomatous disease**, a condition in which the production of oxygen radicals is defective. All such genetic defects in neutrophil function lead to serious and persistent infections and often death in childhood.

10 Microtubules are assembled from the protein **tubulin** and are involved in movements of the cell, such as phagocytosis and lysosome–phagosome fusion.

Acquired defects may occur simply as a result of **decreased neutrophil numbers**, due to bone-marrow diseases such as leukaemia, to irradiation or certain chemicals. Defective neutrophil chemotaxis may occur in diabetes mellitus or during corticosteroid therapy. Other drugs can impair phagocytosis or lysosome fusion. All such conditions worsen infections greatly, showing how important neutrophils are as a defence against bacteria.

Bacteria have ways of evading phagocytic activity

Many bacteria have evolved strategies to avoid phagocytosis and killing. Some inhibit chemotaxis; others resist phagocytosis because of their polysaccharide capsules; many are resistant to the killing mechanisms inside the cell; some can even kill the neutrophils. These evasive tricks are an important part of bacterial pathogenicity and bacteria that lack such mechanisms are usually the least pathogenic.

The bacteria that live inside cells, usually macrophages, are, like other intracellular parasites such as viruses, particularly difficult to kill. They are often only eradicated with the help of the immune response.

The outcome of acute inflammation

The acute inflammatory focus is obviously a highly complex battleground. Putting it at its simplest, it is a contest between the causative agent tending to enlarge the area of damage and the inflammation tending to counteract the injury. Table 2.1 shows a few of the factors that can influence the battle, in the case of bacterial infection. Some of the factors also apply to inflammation caused by injuries other than bacteria.

Table 2.1 The balances of an acute bacterial infection.

Probacterial factors	Antibacterial factors
Bacterial factors	
High dose	Low dose
Virulence	Low virulence
Evasive strategies	
Host factors	
Malnutrition	Fever
Neutrophil defects	Good nutrition
Poor blood supply	Good blood supply
Other diseases	Immunity (see Chapter 4)
Stress (corticosteroids)	
Exogenous factors	
Anti-inflammatory drugs	Antibiotics
(e.g. aspirin, corticosteroids)	Surgical drainage of pus
	Hot applications (poultices)
	Immobilization

Failure of inflammation may be fatal

If the harmful agent cannot be confined by the inflammatory response, the injury spreads to involve a wider area and the causative agent may travel to distant sites via lymphatics or blood vessels. Entry of some bacteria into the blood (**bacteraemia**) can be relatively harmless, but if pathogenic bacteria are present in the blood in sufficient numbers to cause infection at distant sites (**septicaemia**, or **sepsis**), this almost invariably causes death, if not treated quickly by appropriate antibiotics.

Injury of a tissue by one agent often renders it more vulnerable to others

A simple skin wound such as a cut provides no great threat unless it is complicated by secondary bacterial infection, which will prolong the injury. Similarly virus infections, such as influenza, damage epithelial surfaces and are often followed by secondary bacterial infections.

Inflammation may become prolonged

We have hitherto been considering only injuries of short duration. If the injurious agent persists, however, the process of inflammation will be prolonged. It then becomes a more complicated process altogether, as we shall see in Chapter 6.

Acute inflammation is usually entirely successful

If all the petty injuries and transient infections are taken into account, including those we are not aware of, we are probably only rarely completely free of disease. Obviously acute inflammation usually comes out on top. When it does, what follows is the process of **healing**.

Summary

The outcome of acute inflammation depends on many variables, affecting the harmful agent and the host. The result may be failure, interrupted success, prolongation into chronic inflammation or, most commonly, healing.

Healing

Whatever the injury, if there has been tissue damage, one is left with disorganized junk—a mass of dead tissue and remnants of inflammatory cells. What happens to replace this disorganized material is the process of healing. Healing consists of three processes—**scavenging** of damaged material, **regeneration** of lost tissue and **repair**, which leads to formation of a scar. Sometimes only scavenging is required, in which case the result is **resolution**.

Resolution

Resolution is the most favourable outcome of the healing process, because it refers to the complete **restoration of the tissue to its original state**. It can only occur if tissue damage is slight, followed by rapid removal of debris. **This important scavenging process has to occur after every episode of tissue damage**, including those accompanied by repair and regeneration. The responsible cell is the macrophage.

Macrophages are ubiquitous scavenger cells

Up to now we have mentioned macrophages only briefly, as phagocytic and bactericidal cells that develop from blood monocytes which emigrate into acute inflammatory lesions, in smaller numbers than neutrophils. Macrophages are in fact most remarkable cells, with an astonishing range of activities, which will gradually emerge in the chapters that follow. They play a central role in many biological processes, including healing.

The blood monocyte derives from monoblasts in the bone marrow, cells which share a common parent cell type with the myeloblasts, from which the polymorphonuclear cells develop (Fig. 2.18). Circulating monocytes, like circulating neutrophils, probably cannot phagocytose, because contact with particles is presumably very brief in flowing blood. After circulating in the blood for a day or two, monocytes do one of two things. Whichever of the two roles they play, they become bigger and more active than monocytes, and are now called **macrophages**.

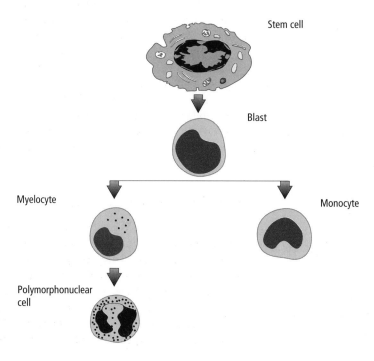

Figure 2.18 Origin of polymorphonuclear leukocytes and monocytes.

Some macrophages settle down amongst the endothelial cells lining **blood sinusoids** and probably remain there for the rest of their lives. Sinusoids are capillary vessels that are unusually **broad**, and blood flow through them is therefore relatively **slow**. Sinusoids are found in many places, but especially in the bone marrow, liver and spleen. The macrophages that form part of the lining of these sinusoids are called stationary or **sessile macrophages**.[11] They act as a sort of **filter** for the blood, because they can now phagocytose any abnormal large molecules or particles which may be present in the blood, such as toxins or bacteria. They are also responsible for phagocytosis and destruction of aged red blood cells and platelets, eventually releasing their component molecules into the blood for reuse elsewhere in the body (**recycling**).

The second major activity of blood monocytes is emigration from the blood into the tissues. This is most likely to happen at sites of injury, as we have already seen, probably as a result of mechanisms similar (but not identical) to those responsible for neutrophil emigration. Like neutrophils, macrophages phagocytose and kill bacteria; their lysosomes do not stain so obviously as those of neutrophils, but their bactericidal mechanisms are similar. Macrophages show chemotaxis, like neutrophils, but unlike neutrophils they are also attracted by various abnormal or degraded large molecules, such as fragments of collagen or elastin. However, all normal tissues and body cavities contain populations of macrophages, so presumably continuous random emigration occurs from normal blood vessels. These tissue macrophages are often referred to as **wandering macrophages** to distinguish them from the sessile macrophages of sinusoids.

Macrophages are highly adaptable to their environment and often behave slightly differently in different tissues, so they have often been given different names. All of them retain some common properties, however, and collectively are referred to as the **macrophage system**.[12] Their adaptability extends to **enzyme induction**. Exposure to particular microbes induces the macrophage to increase production of enzymes that will damage them.

Some tissue macrophages find their way into lymphatic vessels and hence to lymph nodes. There they settle down on the walls of the lymph sinusoids (where they are called **littoral cells**[13]) or attach to fine collagen fibres crossing the sinusoids. These sessile macrophages confer on lymph nodes the function of a filter for the lymph (Fig. 2.19), because they remain actively phagocytic, like those in blood sinusoids.

Macrophages are highly activated cells

The conversion of a monocyte into a macrophage appears to be due simply to contact with the tissues. The transformation is momentous. The cell becomes bigger—a process called hypertrophy—with more organelles and increased enzyme content. The cell is also more active and capable of more diverse functions. Scanning electron microscopy (Fig. 2.20) shows that it is constantly throwing out pseudopods, cell processes that protrude and often fuse with each other, effectively constantly endocytosing[14] tissue fluid and the molecules it contains. This non-specific 'drinking' is called **fluid-phase pinocytosis**. It was

11 In the liver they are referred to as Kupffer cells, after the pathologist who described them.

12 Also occasionally called the mononuclear phagocyte system. The old name, 'reticuloendothelial system', is misleading and should be abandoned.

13 Littoral refers to the fact that they sit 'on the shore' of the sinusoids.

14 Endocytosis is a term including both phagocytosis (uptake of particles) and pinocytosis ('cell drinking'). *Pinos* (Greek) = beer!

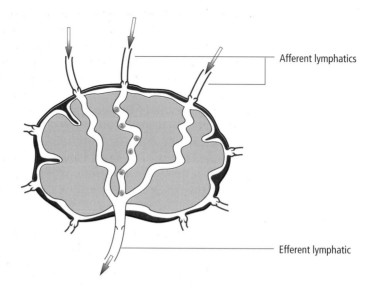

Afferent lymphatics

Efferent lymphatic

Figure 2.19 Filter function of a lymph node. Macrophages shown in only one sinusoid.

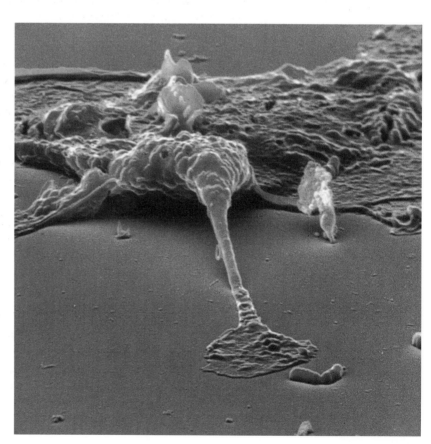

Figure 2.20 Macrophage reaching out to catch bacteria.

known long ago that macrophages would take up colloidal dyes *in vivo* by this process. Non-specific uptake of particles can also occur. For example, we all inhale carbon particles, especially in towns, and the particles are taken up by macrophages, which are normally resident in the alveoli of the lung. Carbon-laden macrophages that are not coughed up wander about the lung tissue and end up either in the less mobile parts of the lung, such as the fibrous tissue, or travel in the lymph to local lymph nodes. As a result, the lungs of an adult town dweller are patterned in black, and the thoracic lymph nodes are usually also black in colour.[15]

This continuous non-specific sampling of the macrophage's environment goes on at an astonishing rate. It has been calculated that 3% of the macrophage's surface membrane is internalized every minute!

The macrophage, once activated, develops receptors specific for abnormal molecules

Although neutrophils can only manage to phagocytose particles up to the size of bacteria, **macrophages can also phagocytose bigger cells** such as red blood cells (7 μm in diameter). However, they will not phagocytose living self cells, but only foreign cells, dead cells or cells that have abnormal molecules on their surface. This selectivity is very striking; they will not phagocytose living neutrophils, but avidly take up dead or damaged ones. Moreover, in the blood sinusoids, they are capable of distinguishing a red blood cell that is old, and has reached the end of its life, from those that are younger.

Presumably, this selective recognition of abnormal cells depends on the macrophages having receptors for abnormal molecules on the target cell-surface. It can equally well be presumed that toxic foreign molecules, such as bacterial toxins, are endocytosed and degraded by phagocytes to some extent, although they are probably not very good at this without the help of the immune response. In the case of certain large molecules like albumin, macrophages have no receptors for the normal (self) molecule, but do show receptor-mediated uptake of albumin that has been chemically altered in some way. This avidity for the uptake of damaged, abnormal and non-self molecules and cells means that macrophages are ideal **scavenger cells**, and this is one of their most important functions.

Cell division is uncommon in tissue macrophages

Almost all macrophages in the tissues began life in the bone marrow. They are probably nearly always committed to their way of life once they have entered the tissues, because it is believed that only in exceptional circumstances do they ever return to the blood stream.[16] Macrophages can certainly live for months, perhaps longer, but they die somewhere in the tissues, and their remnants are then phagocytosed by other macrophages.

15 This carbon, incidentally, does no harm at all, unlike some other dusts.

16 Possible exceptions are in the brain and the arterial wall.

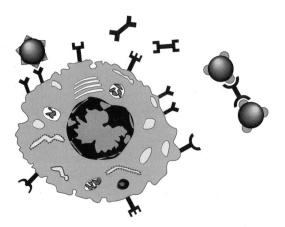

Figure 2.21 Various lectin-like receptors on macrophages; and secretion of lectins.

Macrophages are a primitive, conserved cell type which have evolved lectin-like recognition systems

Mononuclear cells resembling macrophages were the first phagocytes to evolve. Even in those primitive animals, the sponges, there are macrophage-like cells called **amoebocytes** which are capable of phagocytosing foreign particles. One recognition system that evolved even in such primitive forms of life is the presence of **lectin-like** receptors.[17] These are glycoproteins on the cell membrane that have recognition sites for various sugars on the surface of microorganisms.

Lectins are abundant in plants and important in many and various cell–cell interactions[18] in both plants and animals. Macrophages use them to enhance adhesion to and phagocytosis of bacteria. One can visualize the macrophage surface as having a wide variety of these lectin-like receptors enhancing defence against different microbes (Fig. 2.21). Macrophages also secrete bivalent versions of these molecules, true lectins, which can cause agglutination of foreign cells into clumps (Fig. 2.21). At least one lectin can activate complement by the alternative pathway. Repeated exposure to bacteria carrying particular sugars causes increased presentation of the appropriate lectins on the macrophage surface. This might be regarded, in fact, as nature's first tentative experiment in the development of an immune response.

Lectins and lectin-like molecules can be responsible also for other cell interactions and they are among the molecules involved in events such as leukocyte emigration from blood vessels.

Scavenger receptors are not highly specific

The so-called **scavenger receptors** are those which are responsible for the self/non-self discrimination by macrophages, mentioned previously. They merit closer examination. The most-studied scavenger receptor is the so-called **modified low-density lipoprotein (LDL) receptor**.[19] Most cells are supplied with essential cholesterol, from the blood, by means of high-affinity receptors on the cell membrane for a carrier protein (apolipoprotein B). In the plasma this

17 Lectins are by definition bivalent but some of the macrophage lectin-like receptors are univalent.

18 These include symbiotic plant–bacterium adhesion such as between plant roots and nitrogen-fixing bacteria.

19 It has emerged that this is not one receptor, but at least two; however, this is not important in this context.

34

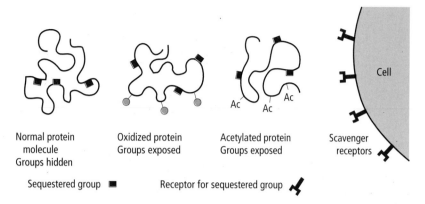

Figure 2.22 Scavenger receptors for hidden (sequestered) parts of protein.

protein transports cholesterol and other lipids, in particles known as LDL. However, although monocytes have these receptors for normal LDL, when they become macrophages they quickly lose them and develop receptors that will only recognize LDL that has been chemically altered (modified) in some way.

This scavenger receptor is interesting for two reasons. First, the number of receptors for normal LDL on other cells decreases when the cell contains sufficient cholesterol for its needs. However, the scavenger receptor for **modified LDL** is not so down-regulated, so the macrophage continues to take up the abnormal LDL until it is bloated with lipid droplets—a **foamy macrophage**. Foamy macrophages are often seen in areas of tissue damage.

The second feature of interest is that the modified LDL receptor is not specific for any particular chemical modification. Thus it will take up, almost equally well, acetylated, maleylated or oxidized LDL and so on. Not only that, but it also takes up maleylated **albumin**. A possible explanation is that this receptor, and probably other scavenger receptors as well, does not recognize the parts of the protein molecule that have been chemically altered but some hidden part of the molecule which is exposed by a common shape change, caused by all the various different modifications (Fig. 2.22). That newly exposed group may be the one recognized by the receptor.

It would be highly economical if this were a general property of other scavenger receptors, because macrophages would be able to recognize and endocytose a wide variety of damaged molecules and cells using only a small number of receptor types.

Macrophages scavenge the remains of inflammatory damage

Although macrophages are heavily outnumbered by neutrophils in the early stages of acute inflammation, as the hours go by the neutrophils die and monocyte emigration accelerates until, once the cause of the inflammation has been neutralized, macrophages are the predominant viable cell. The macrophages then commence the scavenging process of phagocytosis and pinocytosis of the dead and abnormal material.

A good example of the process of resolution is a **bruise**. As you know from your own expericence, a bruise at first looks **purple–red**. This is because it results from bleeding from damaged blood vessels beneath the skin. Over the course of a few days, however, the bruise gradually becomes **yellowish-brown**. This is because macrophages have entered the bruise; when they have phagocytosed the spilled blood cells, the haemoglobin of the red blood cells is converted within the macrophage to a golden-yellow iron-containing pigment called **haemosiderin**.[20]

But then **the yellow bruise gradually disappears** over the next few days. Where does it go? The answer is that one by one the macrophages, together with their burden of cell debris and haemosiderin, enter the local lymphatics and are carried in the lymph to the **local lymph node**. There they settle down in the sinusoids to digest their meal. The large molecules are broken down within the macrophage to small ones, which are then released into the lymph to be recycled elsewhere in the body. Very little, in the end, is wasted. A good example of this conservation is **iron**. The iron remaining in the haemosiderin is eventually released into the lymph and carried into the blood, on a transport protein called transferrin, to be used again eventually in the manufacture of haemoglobin, by the red cell precursors in the marrow.

Macrophages in the tissues are easiest to identify when they contain phagocytosed material. Examples of ingested material include red cells, lipid droplets, haemosiderin or carbon, as we have seen. Other recognizable contents may include bacteria, dusts, nuclear debris and pigments of various sorts, depending on the circumstances.

So, in a bruise, or a similar small lesion, the end result is **resolution**— complete restoration to normal.

Larger lesions, as we shall see, cause additional reactions, but **the basic process of scavenging by macrophages always occurs as the first step of healing**.

Regeneration

Many lower animals can regenerate tails, limbs or even heads, but mammals have lost that useful facility and regeneration can only occur in certain tissues.

Regeneration in mammals is confined to the **replacement of lost cells by the multiplication of their neighbours**. Different tissues vary greatly in their capacity for regeneration and can be roughly divided into three categories in this respect—labile, stable and inert.

Labile tissues are normally regenerative and have a very high capacity for cell division

In tissues like the skin or bone marrow, normal function demands that regeneration occurs constantly. The multilayered stratified squamous epithelium of the epidermis is constantly shedding its superficial cornified layers and cell division, evidenced by mitoses, can always be found in the basal layer. The bone marrow is analogous in that all the cells it produces are disposable, with

20 Whenever haemosiderin-laden macrophages are seen in tissues, it usually indicates that haemorrhage has previously occurred there.

a varied but limited life-span, and constantly need replacement by division of their precursors in the marrow. Such **labile tissues** are particularly quick to regenerate if cells are lost due to disease processes such as abrasion of the skin or haemorrhage.

Stable tissues normally undergo a slow rate of cell division which can be accelerated by damage

Stable tissues include the liver, kidney and many epithelial and glandular tissues. Here the constituent cells have a long but limited life-span and single cells are one by one expiring, usually by apoptosis, and being shed or disposed of by phagocytosis.

Stable tissues therefore normally have a low rate of cell division, and small numbers of mitoses can usually be found in histological sections. When such tissues lose cells as a result of injury they are capable of gradual restoration of normal cell numbers, although the arrangement or architecture of the regenerated cells is not always exactly the same as before.

Inert tissues are incapable of cell division

Myocardial muscle fibres and neurons are incapable of cell division. During fetal development, these cells arise from myoblasts or neuroblasts, which obviously divide, but at around birth this activity ceases, and the mature tissue cells lose the ability to divide so that regeneration after injury cannot occur.

The mechanism of regeneration is unknown

In some tissues, cell division is influenced by **hormones**. For instance, the cells of the adrenal cortex are stimulated not only to increased activity but also to divide, by adrenocorticotrophic hormone (ACTH) secreted by the pituitary. If ACTH secretion is excessive for some reason,[21] the adrenal cortex becomes bigger because of excessive cell division (**hyperplasia**). If that stimulus is removed, and ACTH secretion goes back to normal, cell division decreases and the adrenal cortex reverts to normal size. If ACTH is diminished for any reason the cortex becomes smaller due to decreased cell division (hypoplasia). Although there are a number of other examples of hormones acting in this way, for most tissues hormonal control of division has not yet been found.

Growth factors[22] are molecules secreted by certain cells that can be shown to stimulate cell division in other cells. **Epidermal growth factor**, for example, is a polypeptide, first found in the salivary glands of mice, which can increase division of epidermal cells, other epithelial cells and fibroblasts. Blood platelets can produce **platelet-derived growth factor**, which is now known to be produced also by various other cell types, including macrophages and vascular endothelial cells, and therefore badly needs a new name! It causes cell division in fibroblasts and smooth-muscle cells. Many other growth factors have been discovered in recent years, mainly because of the increased use of cell culture techniques and improved analytical techniques.

21 For example, if there is a tumour of ACTH-producing pituitary cells.

22 This is another ghastly misnomer, caused by the fact that these molecules were discovered in cell cultures. They cause **cell division**, not cell growth.

In labile and stable tissues, cell division is balanced by cell loss

The cells that are continuously lost, in many stable and labile tissues, undergo an apparently regulated form of cell death, which we have previously referred to, called **apoptosis**. This mode of cell death also occurs during the essential remodelling of tissues during embryogenesis, which requires cell loss at various stages. An analogy is cell death during the loss of the tadpole's tail. This normal process of cell deletion is called **programmed cell death**.

Apoptosis is different from necrosis in several ways. It is triggered by the activation of genes that lead to enzymatic splitting of DNA, and can be considered to be a sort of **cell suicide**. It leads to characteristic chemical and morphological changes in the affected cell (see Fig. 1.5), which then breaks up and is shed, or is phagocytosed and disposed of by neighbouring cells, including macrophages.

Unlike necrosis, apoptosis does not cause acute inflammation, so it is an exception to the general rule that cell death always causes inflammation.

This curious process has not yet been completely explained, and is being actively investigated. It has already emerged that some toxic substances can also somehow cause apoptosis rather than necrosis. One reason why it merits careful study is that it is a factor in the control of the numbers of cells in any tissue, and therefore might be important in cancer.

Cell cultures show some additional features of regeneration

Mammalian cell culture is now widely used for a variety of investigations. Some cells, like fibroblasts, grow more easily than others in culture. Essentially scraps of tissue or cell suspensions are incubated in plastic or glass dishes, containing fluid medium composed of all the necessary nutrients for cell survival and division.

The technique has some major advantages. One particular cell type can be studied in isolation and the effects on the cells of single chemicals or cell products can be observed without the complications of *in vivo* experiments. In some cases human cells can be used, thus avoiding one criticism of animal experimentation, the possibility of interspecies variation. Unfortunately, the major disadvantage is that there is no guarantee that cells will behave in exactly the same ways in these artificial conditions as they do *in vivo*.

With that proviso, cell culture work has revealed two essential features of regeneration. One is that many cell types, such as fibroblasts and endothelial cells, show **contact inhibition**. This term refers to the fact that the cells multiply until they form a complete (**confluent**) monolayer of cells (one cell thick) all over the floor of the culture dish. Then they stop multiplying. The mechanism is unknown, but it tallies with the behaviour of some cells *in vivo*. Epidermis will regenerate to cover a skin wound, but **when the wound is covered, the regeneration stops**. The same is true of other epithelia and of vascular endothelium.

The second feature of regeneration seen in culture is that, if a monolayer is wounded by scraping some of the cells off, neighbouring cells not only divide but also **migrate** into the denuded area. This migration accompanying regeneration can sometimes be observed *in vivo*, for instance in epidermis growing over a wound.

Chalones are inhibitors of cell division

Much evidence has been presented to suggest that particular cell types produce molecules (**chalones**) that inhibit multiplication of their neighbours. This suggests that regeneration might be due to decreased chalone concentration. Although there are certainly molecules, such as heparin, which seem to have a general inhibitory effect on cell division, the evidence for true chalones was inconclusive until the discovery of a molecule called **transforming growth factor β_1**, which acts as a chalone in mammary gland.

Some cell types can become bigger although they cannot divide

Although regeneration, in the sense of true cell division, does not occur in damaged cardiac and skeletal muscle, the fibres can enlarge individually to improve total contractile performance. This is referred to as compensatory hypertrophy.

The so-called regeneration of severed axons of neurons is only regrowth of part of the damaged cell, not regeneration in the usual sense.

Repair

If the processes of macrophage scavenging and regeneration have not eliminated the damaged area in 2 days or so, then a third process begins—**repair**. This consists of the growth into the damaged area of newly formed loose connective tissue, rich in capillary buds and fibroblasts. Fibroblasts are elongated cells, capable of secreting collagen and elastin fibres and mucopolysaccharide ground substance; they arise from resting mesenchymal cells that are present in all tissues. Macrophages and other inflammatory cells are also present. This new young tissue is called **granulation tissue**.[23] It is instantly recognizable in histological sections because no other tissue has so many capillary buds lined by plump young endothelial cells. Because granulation tissue replaces a disorganized mess by orderly new fibrous tissue, the process is called **organization**.

The nature of the damage is irrelevant—granulation tissue will almost always grow into areas of haemorrhage, necrosis or exudates, however caused.

Granulation tissue has a characteristic orientation in relation to the injured area

Figure 2.23 shows that the granulation tissue grows, at about 0.2 mm/day, from the neighbouring viable tissue directly towards the centre of the wound. The reason for this brings us to yet another function of macrophages.

23 So called because of the red granular appearance, like red Morocco leather, in the base of an open wound if the scab is knocked off. The 'granules' are in fact the capillary buds.

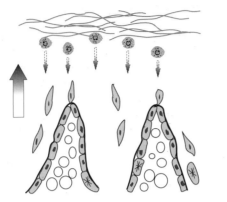

Disorganized area

Macrophages scavenging and secreting

Zone of fibroblast collagen production

Capillary buds

Zone of fibroblast and endothelial cell division

Figure 2.23 Granulation tissue.

Macrophages can survive better than any other cell in very low oxygen concentrations, even retaining their oxidative microbicidal mechanisms. Therefore they are the first cells to invade the edges of a necrotic zone and there of course they actively scavenge the debris. But in addition to their scavenging, they synthesize and secrete factors that stimulate the growth of granulation tissue and control its orientation (Fig. 2.23). These substances include **macrophage-derived growth factor**. This is a protein that **stimulates cell division** in both fibroblasts and endothelial cells, and is **positively chemotactic** for both cell types. Macrophages also secrete substances that stimulate the fibroblasts to begin their main function, that of secreting collagen, elastin and ground substance.

The **zone of maximum cell division** in fibroblasts and endothelial cells is about 0.5 mm behind the tip of the capillary buds. The fibroblasts migrate towards the wound, secreting their fibres and ground substance in a zone near the capillary tips. The endothelial cells extend from pre-existing surviving capillaries and migrate in the same direction, first as flat elongated cells which then curl upon themselves, creating the capillary lumen. As the capillaries grow, they join up with each other[24] to create little arches round which the blood flows. In bigger wounds, the new capillaries nearer the arterial end often become encircled by smooth-muscle cells to become arterioles. These smooth-muscle cells probably arise from those of the nearest arteriole and extend along the new vessel.

Oxygen concentration in tissues can be measured using special microelectrodes and shows, predictably, a gradient in granulation tissue between the properly vascularized area and the dead material. It seems likely that this may be a factor in explaining the orderly behaviour of the cells in the different zones of granulation tissue, but this has proved difficult to investigate. The same is true of various molecules produced in damaged areas, such as lactate, which may have a concentration gradient in the opposite direction.

Severe damage to small blood vessels causes blood platelets to release **platelet-derived growth factor**, which is virtually identical to macrophage-derived growth factor. This may be involved in stimulating the early stages of granulation tissue, as well as of regeneration.

24 A term often used for 'joining up' is **anastomosing**; the junction is an **anastomosis**.

40

Wounds shrink during repair

Over the first few days of the process of organization described above, the edges of the injured area become somewhat indrawn, because **granulation tissue has a tendency to shrink slowly**. The cause of this may be partly reabsorption of fluid, but another possibility is raised by one unexpected feature of fibroblasts. Electron microscopy shows that the cytoplasm of fibroblasts in granulation tissue contains long myofibrils, so the cells can contract—they are **contractile**. It is thought that they may anchor their two ends to collagen fibres and, by contracting, lead to shrinkage of the tissue. This shrinkage actively draws the edges of a damaged area together, thus diminishing the distance that the granulation tissue has to travel and therefore accelerating repair.

The result of repair is a scar

Once the granulation tissue has completed organization of the damaged zone, the new tissue undergoes further changes. Over the course of weeks, the tissue becomes less vascular and less cellular. Inflammatory cells mostly disappear, the fibroblasts cease to secrete and then shrink to become very thin **fibrocytes**. Much of the tissue fluid is reabsorbed into the shrinking vasculature. The result is fibrous tissue, rich in collagen, but requiring very little vascular supply and cellular support. This is the **scar**. A scar always therefore **occupies less volume than the tissue it has replaced**. A synonym for scar formation is **fibrosis**.

The gradual loss of size and vascularity of a scar is noticeable in surgical wounds, which remain red and slightly swollen for weeks, gradually shrinking and becoming paler until they eventually become white, often months later.

Elastin is only found in scars if there is repeated movement of the area during the repair process. How the movements so affect the fibroblast's secretions is unknown.

The outcome of healing in any lesion depends on a race between the three component mechanisms. Therefore the size of the lesion is important

We have seen that complete resolution is only possible if the macrophages have time to remove all the debris before repair begins. This can only happen in very small lesions or in areas where the damage is slight and diffusely spread amongst surviving blood vessels. Examples of the former include a bruise, or thin layers of exudate in a natural cavity; another example is pneumonia. In acute inflammation of the lung, although there may be exudate in quite large areas, the alveolar walls often survive. Each alveolus can be considered as an individual lesion, small enough to permit scavenging of the exudate so quickly that organization does not occur. Many episodes of acute pneumonia therefore heal by resolution and the lung is restored completely to normal. More severe or prolonged damage, however, leads to fibrosis.

If a scar does form, the size of the lesion governs the size of the scar. In most cases, the size of the lesion is solely dependent on the severity of the

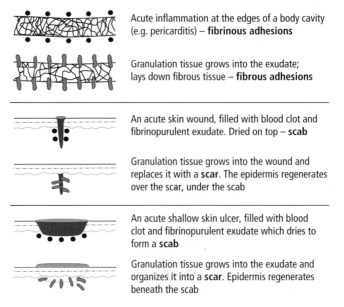

Acute inflammation at the edges of a body cavity (e.g. pericarditis) – **fibrinous adhesions**

Granulation tissue grows into the exudate; lays down fibrous tissue – **fibrous adhesions**

An acute skin wound, filled with blood clot and fibrinopurulent exudate. Dried on top – **scab**

Granulation tissue grows into the wound and replaces it with a **scar**. The epidermis regenerates over the scar, under the scab

An acute shallow skin ulcer, filled with blood clot and fibrinopurulent exudate which dries to form a **scab**

Granulation tissue grows into the exudate and organizes it into a **scar**. Epidermis regenerates beneath the scab

Figure 2.24 Examples of healing.

injury, but in some cases scar formation can be minimized by surgical intervention. This might be, for instance, the opening of a pus-filled cavity (an abscess) to allow the pus to drain and the cavity to collapse. Another example is the stitching (suturing) of wounds to immobilize the wound and bring the edges closer together.[25] Such measures shorten the distance that the granulation tissue has to travel. This means that the wound heals more quickly and the eventual scar is smaller. Some examples of healing wounds are shown in Figure 2.24.

The outcome of healing depends on the type of tissue involved

Here the crucial difference is between tissues with different regeneration potential. Death of myocardial muscle fibres inevitably results in a scar. This is also true even in stable tissues like the liver if the lesion is large enough; the regeneration that occurs in a tissue like the liver is not necessarily in the same place as the lost cells.

In two particular tissues, repair occurs in a different way altogether. Fracture of a bone (Fig. 2.25) leads to the formation of granulation tissue which is just as described above, except that it also contains **osteoblasts**, probably derived from division and migration of those in the nearby bone. These cells secrete bone matrix, little pieces of which are initially found throughout the granulation tissue. This granulation tissue containing spicules of new bone is called **callus** and is frequently bulkier than the original bone. When the fracture line has been repaired, callus is gradually remodelled until the resulting bone approximates to the original shape.[26] Like elastin formation, this is an example of mechanical factors governing connective tissue structure. The healing is again greatly assisted by surgical immobilization and apposition.

25 An example of the surgical principle of **immobilization** and **apposition**, the immobilization also helping organization to be completed.

26 This assumes the fractured bone is in the correct alignment. Immobilization and apposition are obviously also important for fractures.

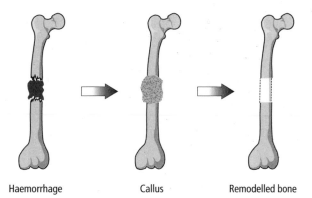

Figure 2.25 Healing of a bone fracture.

Haemorrhage   Callus   Remodelled bone

The other tissue that is unusual in this respect is the central nervous system, where fibrosis does not occur. Instead the damaged tissue is removed by **microglia** (the local representatives of the macrophage system) and the area becomes surrounded by **astrocytes**, whose fine elongated cell processes form a living mat of fibres enclosing what is now a fluid-filled cavity.[27] The central nervous system is different in another way, too. Because it has no lymphatic vessels, the macrophages cannot take the tissue debris to local lymph nodes, as they usually do elsewhere in the body. They may simply digest their contents locally and then die, but it is conceivable that they might actually re-enter small blood vessels and lodge in the spleen or elsewhere.

Healing is affected by various other factors

As well as all the above considerations, all the processes of healing are energy-consuming. Therefore good healing requires adequate nutrition and a good blood supply, and healing will be slow if either is defective. **Vitamin C** is of particular importance in repair, because it is necessary for collagen formation. Scar formation is therefore poor in vitamin C deficiency (scurvy). In some species, temperature has an effect. Wound-healing is very slow in hibernating animals, and wounded reptiles are said to seek warmer places.

Glucocorticoids tend to inhibit not only inflammation but also repair. Therefore healing may be impaired by stress, when glucocorticoid secretion is increased; and it is seriously hampered in patients receiving large doses of therapeutic glucocorticoids.

Inflammation can do harm

In many conditions, the patient perceives only the less pleasant symptoms of inflammation such as pain or excessive secretion, and could be forgiven for considering inflammation as a disease. We now know that these symptoms are the price we pay for what is in fact a protective mechanism. However, there are a number of circumstances in which inflammation appears to be harmful.

27 An abnormal cavity filled with fluid is called a **cyst**.

43

Fibrosis can do harm

As we have seen, although scar formation is second-best to resolution or regeneration, at least the fibrosis repairs the damage, and fibrous tissue is certainly resilient. It is no substitute for the damaged tissue, however, and can be cosmetically undesirable. In two circumstances it is demonstrably harmful. One is that occasionally the existence of fibrosis, or its shrinkage, can lead to blockage of hollow organs, such as the biliary tract or the bowel, after abdominal operations. Another is that scarring in the region of joints may lead to fixed deformities or contractures that impair the joint's function.

Neutrophils can do harm

Neutrophils live for only a few hours in the tissues, especially if they have phagocytosed something or been injured by certain bacteria, so dead neutrophils and their noxious contents are a common disadvantage of acute inflammation, especially purulent inflammation. Until there is release of pus, or until macrophages have had time to dispose of them, these dead cells are a nuisance in several ways. Their spilled enzymes and oxygen radicals probably cause additional tissue damage; this is especially true when the inflammation has not been elicited by microbes. For instance, in myocardial infarction the dead cells elicit an acute inflammatory response. The neutrophil component of the resulting inflammatory exudate is useless, since they cannot contribute significantly to removal of the dead muscle and there are no bacteria to kill. In fact, their death and spillage of enzymes actually do more harm than good. In an experimental animal pretreated to deplete complement and hence inhibit the inflammation, the infarct produced by tying off a coronary artery is actually smaller than that in untreated animals.

If the neutrophils have phagocytosed bacteria and failed to kill them, they may spill living organisms when they die. If in the meantime the neutrophils have wandered some distance, this may continue the spread of the bacteria through the tissues. This is thought to be one reason why streptococci so often cause rapidly spreading damage.

There are also a number of circumstances in which living neutrophils may spill their toxic contents and damage tissues. Minor spillages occur all the time as neutrophils crawl about, but especially during phagocytosis. Neutrophils are messy eaters. This is because lysosomes may fuse with the phagosome before the phagosome is completely closed off—so-called 'regurgitation during feeding' (Fig. 2.26). Similarly, stimulation of release of neutrophil contents seems to be one important way that bacterial endotoxins cause injury.

Certain crystals, on being taken up by neutrophils, cause disruption of lysosomes, cell death and spillage of contents. This occurs, for instance, after uptake of monosodium urate crystals; this is the way that tissue damage is caused in **gout**. In this disease, for various reasons the blood urate levels are abnormally high; monosodium urate crystals are deposited in connective tissue and joints. The exquisitely painful lesions that result are due to this neutrophil disruption, not to the crystals themselves.

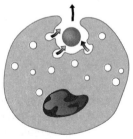

Figure 2.26 Regurgitation during feeding.

44

Macrophages can do harm

Similarly, in various lung diseases that can be caused by inhalation of dusts, called the pneumoconioses,[28] the damage is due not to the dusts themselves but to the fact that when they are ingested by alveolar macrophages, the cells spill their noxious contents.

Inflammation and healing — the advantages and disadvantages

Any serious defects in inflammation lead to death from infections, so the process is literally vital. It has evolved from the crude beginnings of amoebocytes in sponges until in vertebrates it is so complicated that we do not yet completely understand it.

Clearly the first line of defence of an animal is the instinctive and learned avoidance of dangers. The second is the inbuilt defensive armament of skin, evacuation of secretions and the like. Inflammation and healing are only necessary when these fail.

The inflammatory process has two most important attributes. The first is its **speed**; it starts within minutes, whatever part of the body is affected. The second advantage is its **non-specificity**. No matter what the injurious agent, if it damages cells the inflammatory mechanisms are triggered off. The main value of this is in infections, because inflammation can defend against, or at least greatly hinder, pathogens that have never been encountered before, even if they have only recently evolved, which must have happened many times over millions of years.

However, inflammation and healing are by no means always effective on their own; and they do not learn much, from experience of particular injuries. What has evolved in vertebrates, subsequently, is a system that boosts the inflammatory response to microbial damage after a few days and moreover, amazingly, that memorizes that particular microbe, so that if it is encountered again the inflammatory response to it will be even stronger. This system is the **immune response**.

28 Examples include silicosis in coal miners inhaling silica, and asbestosis from inhaling asbestos fibres.

3   The immune response: antibodies

The immune system consists of cells and cell products that provide additional protection against pathogenic microbes. One important thing about it is that it can recognize and damage these microbes without inflicting much damage on oneself. In other words, it can detect the difference between **self** and **non-self**. Usually, therefore, its role is clearly one of protection. What the system recognizes is **foreign large molecules**, which are referred to as **antigens**.

The immune response can be regarded in three phases (Fig. 3.1)

First, there has to be a recognition system for antigens, the most important of which are carried on microorganisms. This is often called the **afferent loop** of the immune response and consists of conveying the antigen, from the site of its entry into the body, to the sites at which cells can react to it. This job is done mainly by macrophages and similar cells (**antigen-presenting cells**).

Second, the immune system's central task is to **react to the antigen**, to produce the tools of immunity. **The cells that do this are lymphocytes.** Lymphocytes create immunity in several ways. They can kill infected cells and stimulate macrophages (**cell-mediated immunity**); but in this chapter we shall consider only the **antibodies** that they produce. For the moment, the central mechanism of lymphocyte activity can be a black box. We shall discuss it later.

Third, the **effects of the immune response** need to be examined. This **efferent loop** of the response consists of a range of mechanisms that boost the inflammatory response.

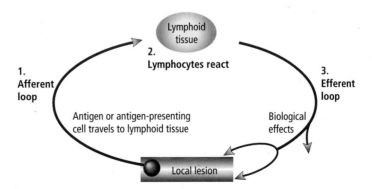

Figure 3.1 The three phases of the immune response.

The immune response boosts the inflammatory reaction

We have seen that acute inflammation is a rapid reaction, whatever causes the injury. However it has the disadvantage that it never learns. On its own, its reaction to a second invasion by the same microorganism would be no different from the first. The immune response, on the other hand, is **specific to the antigens on the particular microbe** and, although slower to respond, when it does so (after a few days) it increases the intensity of the inflammatory response already mounted to the infection. Most importantly, it also has a **memory**, which boosts both the speed and effectiveness of the inflammatory reaction to a second infection by the same organism. Indeed, this response to the second infection can now be so quick and effective that the patient does not notice the infection at all—this is what is meant by immunity. **In their protective role, the immune response and inflammation work hand in hand**.

We now know quite a lot about how the immune system works, but we should first consider those basic facts about immunity and its medical applications that were the first to be discovered.

The immune response is caused by antigens

Unlike the inflammatory response, which is caused by any disruption of host cells, the immune response can only be triggered, as we have said, by the presence in the tissues of **foreign, or abnormal large molecules**, which are called **antigens**. Large, in this context, usually means a molecular weight of over about 2500 Da. Antigens are most commonly proteins, but carbohydrates and even lipids can also be antigenic. Microorganisms and other foreign cells always carry surface antigens. Presumably the **immune response evolved because of its effectiveness against pathogenic microbes**, but other foreign large molecules, even if unassociated with cells, are also antigenic. So, for example, injections of sheep red blood cells or sheep serum albumin would always be antigenic in humans. Equally, human cells or human serum albumin are antigenic in sheep and other species.

The immune response is protective, and specific to the antigen that causes it

An early demonstration of this principle was provided by Ehrlich.[1] He was interested in the effect of **bacterial exotoxins** on animals. Exotoxins are proteins that are produced by some bacteria, and have toxic effects on animal cells. Ehrlich found that large doses of tetanus toxin, isolated from the bacterium, *Clostridium tetani*, injected into a group of mice, would kill every animal in the group; small doses killed none and an intermediate dose would kill 50% of the animals. He then asked the question—were the survivors of this experiment affected by it? He therefore tested the survivors again, days later, and found that they could now survive 100 times the original dose of tetanus toxin!

However, the survivors of exposure to tetanus toxin were just as susceptible to a different exotoxin, diphtheria toxin, as those animals which had never

1 Paul Ehrlich (1854–1915), one of the great German pioneers of immunology.

48

experienced tetanus toxin. Therefore **the response, and the protective effect, were specific**.

In the same way, in humans, one attack of chickenpox confers immunity to a second attack of chickenpox but not to measles.

The immune system is usually tolerant to antigens encountered before and just after birth

There is a critical time in life, which differs from species to species, before which exposure to a large molecule confers **tolerance** to that molecule (i.e. lack of immune response). After that time, any different large molecules encountered are treated as non-self and do elicit an immune response. In humans, this critical time occurs a few days after birth. This is one mechanism that ensures that the immune system does not destroy the cells of the host.

There are two main mechanisms of immunity — humoral and cellular

Humoral immunity is due to the presence in the plasma of antibodies. **Antibodies are plasma protein molecules** that are produced in response to an antigen. They can combine with their specific antigen, like a key in a lock, and confer protection against it. The protection is partly due to the fact that phagocytes have receptors on their surface that recognize antibodies, so anything the antibody is attached to, such as bacteria, or the exotoxins mentioned above, is rapidly endocytosed and destroyed. This is a good example of **opsonization**, which we have mentioned previously. Temporary immunity can therefore be transferred artificially from one individual to another by transferring serum, which contains antibodies. However, the memory is not transferred. The half-life of antibodies is only about 30 days. Clearly it is not the antibody itself that provides the memory.

Cellular immunity cannot be transferred by serum at all. In general, antibodies are effective against extracellular microbes and toxins, cellular immunity against intracellular organisms. Let us look at antibodies first.

Amounts of serum antibodies can be measured in the laboratory

One simple way to measure antibody depends on their ability to cross-link antigens. Antibodies are always at least bivalent (Fig. 3.2). Therefore, in the laboratory, in the absence of cells, they can form a lattice-work (**immune complexes**) with their particular antigens to form a visible **precipitate** (Fig. 3.3). To measure antibodies in the laboratory it is necessary first to allow a blood sample to clot, discard the clot, and use the fluid **serum** which is left over. The serum contains the antibodies, the amount of which can be roughly measured by testing the ability of the serum to precipitate known amounts of antigen, in test-tubes.

Antibodies against antigens on the surface of cells, such as bacteria, cause

49

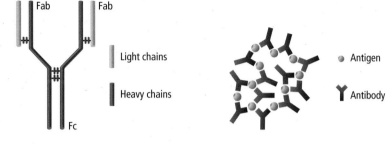

Figure 3.2 Antibody (immunoglobulin G) (left).

Figure 3.3 Immune complex (right).

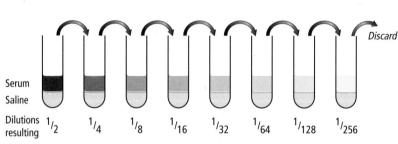

Figure 3.4 Doubling dilutions. A volume of saline is mixed with the same volume of serum in the first tube. One volume is removed and mixed with saline in the second tube, and so on.

them to **agglutinate** in test-tubes; this is the same as precipitation except that larger, fluffy particles appear in the tube.

One example of an agglutination test is that used in the diagnosis of typhoid fever, which is caused by the bacterium *Salmonella typhi*. Serum from the patient is serially diluted in a row of test-tubes so that each successive tube has half the concentration of serum of its predecessor (Fig. 3.4). This technique is called **doubling dilutions**. Then an equal amount of a suspension of killed *S. typhi* is added to each of the tubes, which are then incubated for an hour. The tube containing the least amount of antibody to produce visible agglutination is noted and the dilution of serum in that tube is called the **titre** of antibody in that serum. Thus a serum with a titre of 1/64 has a **greater** amount of antibody than one with 1/32.

By testing samples of serum taken on successive days, changes in the antibody titre can be monitored.

The production of antibodies is quicker on the second introduction of an antigen

Figure 3.5 shows the result of an experiment measuring antibody in the serum of an animal in the days following the first and second injections of the same antigen. After the first injection there is a delay of some days before antibody is detected in the serum. Then there is a gradual increase in titre of antibody, reaching a peak and declining fairly quickly, nearly to the baseline. This is the **primary response**.

Subsequent injections of the same antigen have a different effect, which is

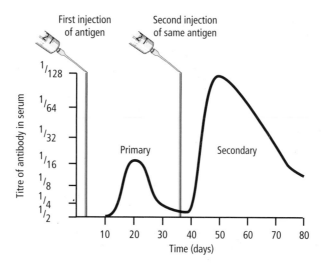

Figure 3.5 Primary and secondary responses.

called the **secondary response**. The time lag is shorter, the rise in titre more rapid, the peak titre higher, the decline slower and the residual resting level slightly higher.

Therefore, when a patient encounters a microorganism for the second time there is already some circulating antibody present and the amounts are rapidly increased, which helps to explain immunity.

Of course, some of the antibody being produced is being mopped up by the antigen in the body, so what is detected in the serum is only what is left over from that. Therefore the start of antibody production must be occurring well before threshold amounts can be detected in the serum.

Serological diagnosis depends upon finding a rising titre of antibody

The presence of antibody in a patient's serum is one way of diagnosing a particular infection. However, if for example a patient is suspected of suffering from typhoid, to find a raised titre of antibody to the typhoid bacillus (*S. typhi*) is not in itself diagnostic. As Fig. 3.5 shows, a raised titre might be due to a previous episode of typhoid. However, if a further sample taken later in the illness shows a titre that has risen significantly, that is diagnostic.[2]

Haptens are small molecules that cannot elicit an immune response themselves, but when incorporated into a large molecule can do so

Although small molecules cannot be antigens, if they attach themselves to large molecules, even host (self) large molecules, they may convert it into an antigen. Such small molecules are called **haptens**. Although they need to be attached to a large carrier molecule to elicit antibodies, they can then be shown to be capable of combining with the antibody, even when on their own (Fig. 3.6).

2 A fourfold rise in titre is significant, because this is 'two tubes difference', which is beyond experimental error.

51

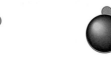

Hapten
(not antigenic)

Hapten attached
to large molecule
(antigenic)

Antibodies react with hapten
and with hapten/large molecule
complex

Figure 3.6 Haptens.

Complement was discovered because of its participation in antigen–antibody reactions

Early in the history of immunology it was discovered[3] that if red blood cells were added to fresh serum containing antibodies to them, the result was red cell disruption or **lysis**. However, if the serum was old, or had been heated to 56 °C for half an hour, the result was not lysis, but agglutination. This heat-labile agent which had caused lysis was called **complement**, because its activity complemented the process of antigen–antibody combination. The lysis could not be caused by antibody alone, nor by complement alone, but only by the presence of complement, antigen and antibody together. This, then, was the discovery of the **classical pathway** of complement activation by immune complexes. This complement activity is not species-specific, and fresh guinea-pig serum was the traditional source used in laboratories.

We have seen in Chapter 2 that the cleavage of C3, the crucial event in complement activation, can be brought about by cell proteases and by other agents (the alternative pathway). **Complement therefore probably evolved before the immune response and can be thought of as an essential part of the inflammatory response.** The pathway by which antigen–antibody complexes activate complement probably evolved later and is called the classical pathway only because it was discovered first (Fig. 3.7).

Complement activation can be used to assay antibodies

At first, complement was thought of simply as a single substance, capable of causing lysis of cells in the presence of the appropriate antibody. It was then found that complement was fixed, or used up, by a wide variety of antigen–antibody combinations and this formed the basis of another serological test for the presence of antibodies to microorganisms.

This test, the **complement fixation text** (Fig. 3.8) again begins with making doubling dilutions of the patient's serum and then adding a small constant amount of the suspected antigen. But in addition, a small measured amount of complement is included; after incubation, we need to find out whether the complement has been used up, or fixed. The way this is done is to add to each tube some red blood cells already coated with antibody against them. If the complement has not been fixed by the first reaction, the red cells will lyse. Thus if the red cells do not lyse, this means the complement was used up. The titre is expressed as the highest dilution at which lysis is prevented.

3 By Jules Bordet and Octave Gengou, in 1900–1902.

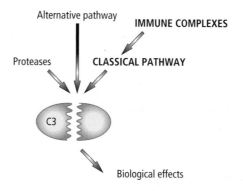

Figure 3.7 Complement activation.

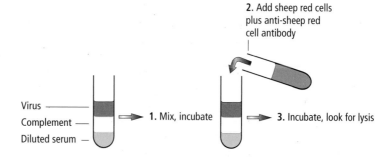

Figure 3.8 Complement fixation text. If antibody is present in the serum, complement is used up and there will be no lysis of the red cells at stage 3.

The advantage of this test is that it can be made very sensitive—the large numbers of organisms necessary to form a visible agglutinate are not needed. Therefore for practical reasons the complement fixation test tends to be used to detect serum antibodies in the diagnosis of diseases whose causative agent is difficult to culture in the laboratory, especially virus diseases and venereal diseases.

The discovery of antibodies led to the development of artificial immunization

Natural immunization refers to the active production of antibodies on encountering the antigen naturally, as in infections, or the passive receipt of maternal antibodies by the fetus, across the placenta, and the newborn, in breast milk. Artificial immunization is the deliberate induction of immunity by introducing, into an individual, either antibodies or antigens.

Diseases caused by exotoxins can be prevented or treated with antibodies

This was an early and highly successful application of the discovery of antibodies. Tiny doses of diphtheria exotoxin were injected into a horse, which then became immune to higher and higher further doses. Serum from this horse, now rich in antibody (**antitoxin**) was then used to inject into patients with diphtheria, or known to be at imminent risk of developing diphtheria. The horse antibody within the patient's blood neutralized the toxin as soon as it was formed, with the saving of many lives as a result. The same principle is of course applicable to other exotoxins such as tetanus, and is referred to as **serum therapy** or **passive immunization**.[4]

It was soon found to have the disadvantage that the human patient developed antibodies against the horse antibodies, which are of course foreign proteins, antigenic in humans, and therefore they only lasted a few days. This difficulty, which will be further explained later, did not prevent horse serum therapy being a great boon in the first half of the 20th century. Nowadays passive immunization is even more successful because human antitoxin is used, but even human antibodies only have a half-life of about a month in the circulation. Therefore passive immunization has the advantage of having a rapid effect, but the disadvantage of not lasting very long, and not providing memory.

Active immunization is better than passive, for most purposes

The father of active immunization was Edward Jenner (1749–1823), an English country physician. Jenner obviously had an eye for the ladies, because he was struck by the fine complexion of milkmaids. He wondered if their frequent exposure to the virus of cowpox, which causes only a trivial infection in humans, might have prevented them catching the disfiguring disease, smallpox. He subsequently demonstrated that deliberate inoculation of cowpox virus in humans is virtually harmless and results in immunity to smallpox. We now know that is due to the fact that the two viruses possess some shared antigens. The cowpox virus elicits antibodies (and cellular immunity) that also react with, and confer immunity to, the smallpox virus. Sadly such natural coincidences are rare and the production of vaccines against some other diseases has proved difficult or impossible.[5]

One type of active vaccine that does work efficiently, however, is **toxoid**. The principle behind active vaccines is to introduce into a normal person a preparation to elicit antibody formation and thereby diminish the chance of suffering from a particular disease. In the case of exotoxin-mediated disease it was discovered that there were ways of treating an exotoxin molecule that retained its antigenicity but destroyed the toxic part of the molecule (Fig. 3.9). This is virtually 100% effective in preventing diseases, such as diphtheria and tetanus, that are caused by exotoxins. When toxoid is inoculated, that individual produces his or her own antibodies; this is called **active immunization**, to distinguish it from **passive immunization** by introducing ready-made antibody.

Active immunization is much longer-lasting because it elicits a response similar to a natural infection. The immunized person now has a 'memory' and will react to subsequent exposure to the antigen by a secondary response. It does, however, take some days for the initial immunization to provide protection, so there are still some urgent circumstances in which passive immunization is necessary.

Other forms of vaccines used for active immunization against various infections by bacteria and viruses use **killed microbes** (e.g. typhoid), **attenuated**

4 Passive, because the doctor (or more accurately, the horse) provides the antibody, rather than the patient.

5 Cowpox virus is called vaccinia (*vacca* (Latin) = cow)–hence the terms vaccine and vaccination.

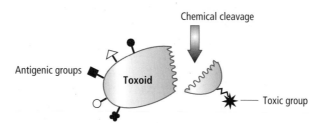

Figure 3.9 Production of toxoid by cleavage of an exotoxin molecule.

microbes[6] (e.g. polio), or sometimes **fragments of microbes**, to elicit the antibody response.[7] The design of vaccines is a complex subject. Most vaccines have some disadvantages and for many diseases suitable vaccines do not yet exist.

One disease, however, has apparently been eradicated from the world by immunization. That is smallpox. Here we had the advantage of the naturally occurring cowpox vaccine, discovered long before antibodies had been described. In addition, smallpox virus has no other source but human sufferers from the disease; there is no animal reservoir and no silent carrier state, as in many diseases. Moreover it is easily recognizable by the characteristic rash. Thus it was possible to seek out residual cases wherever they occurred, and to vaccinate all those who might come in contact with the patients. The last recorded natural case was in Bangladesh, in 1977.

Antibodies are immunoglobulins

By separating plasma proteins into various fractions and testing them for antibody activity, it was found that this resided in the globulin fraction. With the great improvements in protein chemistry, we know a good deal about the responsible molecules, now called **immunoglobulins**. Not all immunoglobulins are alike—several **classes** exist, but the simplest to visualize is immunoglobulin G (IgG; see Fig. 3.2), which typifies the basic unit structure.

IgG is a Y-shaped molecule. **The two arms of the Y are the two reacting-sites for antigen** (Fab) and are therefore different (**variable**) according to the antigen that stimulated their production. The other end (Fc) is **constant** (or almost so) for all IgG molecules. The details of the structure need not detain us here but, in terms of function, it is clear that the two Fab ends ensure the IgG is both specific to the antigen and bivalent; **the Fc end is responsible for the biological consequences of antigen–immunoglobulin binding**. For example, the Fc end contributes to the activation of complement, and can also react with Fc receptors on phagocytes, thus acting as an **opsonin** (Fig. 3.10). The results of antigen–immunoglobulin reactions (the efferent loop of the immune response) are described in more detail in Chapter 5.

IgM is much larger and rather like a bunch of five IgG molecules, with 10 antigen combining sites. IgA is usually a dimer, resembling two IgG molecules. IgE is superficially similar to IgG, **but each different class of antibody has a different Fc region**. These differences in the Fc region are of great importance in determining the function of the different classes of immunoglobulins.

6 Attenuated organisms have been cultured in adverse conditions, which leads to mutations. These mutations can remove their ability to cause disease while retaining their antigenicity.

7 Immunization can also elicit cell-mediated immunity, which will be considered later.

55

The different classes of immunoglobulin serve different functions

IgG is the most abundant class,[8] and makes up about 75% of the immunoglobulins in the plasma. At a molecular weight of 150 kDa, it is small enough to be **normally present in extracellular fluid** as well as in plasma. It is the only class that is **actively transported across the placenta**, thus affording temporary protection for the newborn baby against antigens that the mother has experienced. It is also present in milk, and is taken up in some species through gut epithelial cells.[9]

IgM is always the first class of immunoglobulin to be produced after antigenic stimulus, followed later by IgG. Its **large size** (900 kDa) confines it to the plasma, except that, importantly, the increased vascular permeability at a site of acute inflammation allows IgM **access to areas of injury and infection**. It is not itself an opsonin, because phagocytes do not possess IgM receptors, but it is **particularly good at activating complement**, which results in opsonization (see Fig. 5.3b).

IgA is present in the plasma but its principal characteristic is that it is **transported across epithelium** to be secreted into the gut, bronchi and other cavities, including into the milk. Therefore it encounters microbes before they have the chance to invade the tissues. Its other peculiarity is that it activates complement by the alternative, rather than the classical pathway. Like IgG, it is present in milk.

IgE is mainly characterized by its **avid attachment to mast cells** by its Fc end. If two nearby IgE molecules on the mast cell surface are encountered by their antigen and are linked by it, there is mast cell degranulation. Thus IgE's function is mainly to boost the early stages of the inflammatory response, in this way. IgE does not activate complement. Eosinophils have receptors for the Fc end of IgE, which we shall find is important in resistance to parasites.

The immunoglobulin classes offer a comprehensive defence system

The fact that IgM is produced first—an emergency reaction—has the effect of providing priority protection for the blood stream itself and the actual site of injury where the microbes may still be present. The later and long-lasting IgG response means that representative IgG molecules with that particular specificity will guard all tissue fluids against subsequent invasion. The presence of IgE on mast cells ensures a more rapid inflammatory response if the same microbe is encountered again. IgM, IgG and IgE therefore provide some protection against second infections **wherever they occur in the body**. IgA, of course, specializes in the protection of epithelial surfaces.

Exactly how the production of immunoglobulins of different classes is governed is not entirely clear. However, it is known that antigens administered into the gut provide the best IgA response. This is why poliomyelitis vaccines are most effective when given orally. The portal of entry of the poliovirus is the alimentary tract, so the best protection against it is IgA.

[8] There are four subclasses of IgG with varying properties. This account summarizes approximately the collective properties of all four.

[9] In cattle and sheep this is the only way IgG is transferred to the offspring, because IgG does not cross the placenta in those animals.

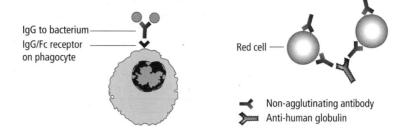

IgG to bacterium

IgG/Fc receptor on phagocyte

Red cell

Non-agglutinating antibody

Anti-human globulin

Figure 3.10 Opsonization by immunoglobulin G (left).

Figure 3.11 Coombs test (right).

Animal cells carry molecules that are antigenic to other individuals of the same species

One example of this is **blood groups**. This refers to antigens on the surface of red blood cells, the nature of which is genetically determined by simple Mendelian rules. The best-known are the **ABO groups**.[10] Individual humans may have antigens A, B, AB or O on their red cells. Those who are A have anti-B antibodies in their plasma, those who are B have anti-A; AB individuals have neither antibody; those who are O have both.

At first sight this seems to contradict what we have learned—that antibodies are only produced when the antigen has been encountered. The explanation is that A and B antigens are encountered very early in life, because they are carbohydrates that are very widespread in nature, including on the surface of plant and bacterial cells. The bacteria that enter the hitherto sterile alimentary tract of newborn babies carry both A and B. The neonate will be tolerant to whichever of the two is present on its own cells, but will produce antibody throughout life to whichever is not.

In contrast, all the other blood group antigens—and there are many, including **Rhesus antigens**—do follow the rules and antibodies to them are only produced if the individual encounters red cells bearing them.

In blood transfusion, therefore, the main thing is to ensure that the recipient is given blood from a donor with the **same ABO group**. If A blood were given to a B patient, for example, the transfused cells would rapidly become coated with anti-A (of the IgM class), and complement-mediated lysis of donor cells would occur in the blood stream, with severe complications including kidney damage.

ABO incompatibility can therefore occur the first time an individual is given a blood transfusion. Second or subsequent transfusions may be complicated by other antibodies elicited by earlier transfusions or pregnancies. A patient who is Rhesus-negative has an antigen (d) on his or her red cells. If given a transfusion of Rhesus-positive cells (carrying a different antigen, D), he will produce anti-D antibodies and a subsequent transfusion of D blood might be fatal. Given that there are many other blood-group antigens as well, this seems an insurmountable problem. In practice it is solved by doing a **cross-match** before every transfusion. The patient's serum is incubated with a sample of the donor red cells in the laboratory; if the patient's serum contains antibodies to any

10 Described by the Austrian scientist, Karl Landsteiner (1868–1943).

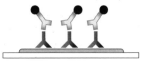
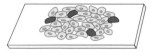

Section of tissue on glass slide

Only muscle cells 'stain red'

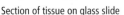

Rat anti-human muscle cell
Red dye on rabbit anti-rat Ig

Figure 3.12
Immunocytochemistry
(example).

antigen on the donor's cells, there will be red cell agglutination. If there is no agglutination, it is usually safe to transfuse that bottle of blood.

However, not all blood-group antibodies that attach to red cells cause agglutination, because they are the small IgG molecules. You might think, therefore, that they wouldn't cause trouble after the transfusion; but they would, because *in vivo* there would be opsonization of the donor cells and red cell destruction. Originally described as incomplete, these antibodies were difficult to detect until Coombs[11] hit upon the idea that antibodies raised in animals against human globulins would reveal whether the red cells were coated with antibody —the **Coombs test** (Fig. 3.11).

Real problems only occur when a particular patient has to receive many transfusions over a long period, because or she he may develop antibodies to many incompatible groups. When one reads that someone 'has a rare blood group' this is wrong—we all have rare blood groups—what it means is that this patient has many antibodies, and compatible donors are difficult to find.

Blood transfusion is possible only because red cells have relatively limited antigenicity and a relatively short life. Tissue cells are much more of a problem because they have, in addition, **histocompatibility antigens**, which means that tissue or organ grafts (except between identical twins) are usually rejected by the host's immune system.

Antibodies can be useful laboratory tools

Obviously the biological importance of antibodies is their contribution to immunity. But we have already seen examples of their use in the clinical laboratory in the serological diagnosis of infective disease and they have many other uses. Antibodies can easily be produced on demand by injecting an antigen into an experimental animal (e.g. a rabbit). After repeated injections, the serum will have a high titre of the specific antibody which can then be used to identify that same antigen in the laboratory. Examples of the usefulness of this principle include the accurate identification and classification of unknown bacteria isolated from patients, the distinction between blood stains from different species or different human individuals, assays of various biological molecules and the identification of cell types in histological sections.

The use of antibodies on sections of tissues has been particularly helpful in investigating disease processes. Ordinary histological sections are interpreted by identifying cells and other tissue components using various stains. Sometimes cells are difficult to distinguish from one another in this way. Artificially

11 Robin R.A. Coombs, of
Cambridge (1921–   ).

raised antibodies, however, can be prepared to react only with antigens characteristic of a particular cell type. There are ways of combining the antibodies with fluorescent or coloured compounds to permit accurate identification of cell types, or indeed any large molecule in the tissue. This technique is known as **immunocytochemistry** (Fig. 3.12). In recent years it has been made even more accurate, because new techniques, to be explained later, allow absolutely pure antibody of a single specificity to be prepared (**monoclonal antibodies**).

Summary

Antibodies are the major component of the immune response. They are easily detected in the serum as immunoglobulins of various classes. Their protective effects are demonstrable both in the laboratory and as a result of immunization. Antibodies are of use in many laboratory procedures. Their main effects *in vivo* will be discussed in Chapter 5, but first we must examine how they are produced in the body by the **cells of the immune response**.

4 The immune response: cells

We must now approach the questions: **how are the antibodies produced?** and **what is cell-mediated immunity?** The answers to these questions may be summarized briefly.

Lymphocytes are the cells which provide the immune response, both humoral (antibody-mediated) and cell-mediated immunity. These are the two major activities of the immune system and the cells responsible for both are the lymphocytes. Although lymphocytes all look the same, in fact they perform several different functions. Antibodies are made by one type which are known as **B lymphocytes** or **B cells**. The other major type are the **T lymphocytes** or **T cells**. Some T cells help the B cells to make antibodies in response to antigen and this combined activity is known as **humoral immunity**.

Antibodies are effective against antigens which are either extracellular or on the surface of cells but cannot recognize or react with any **intracellular antigens**. Reactions which are known as **cellular immunity** are mounted against cells which hide antigens within them or are abnormal in some other way. Certain of the T lymphocytes are able to carry out these activities. The cells most likely to contain foreign antigens are macrophages because they are both phagocytic and survive for a long time. Some of the T cells can **help macrophages to destroy foreign antigens**, particularly those on microorganisms which they have ingested.

Viruses can infect and hide within almost any kind of cell and T-cell help cannot bring about their destruction. In these cases, the entire cell is destroyed, removing all the replicating machinery that the virus is exploiting. This **destruction of entire cells** is brought about by a special type of T cell, the **cytotoxic T cell**.

We will return to cell-mediated immunity later, but we will begin by examining how antibodies are produced.

The immune response occurs in lymph nodes or other lymphoid tissue

This is a fundamental difference between the inflammatory and immune responses. **The inflammatory response is local**, in the tissue that is injured. **The immune response begins in the nearest lymphoid tissue.**

This was established many years ago by a simple experiment in a horse. After local injection of antigen, antibody could be found some days later, in the lymph leaving the nearest lymph node in its efferent lymphatic vessels, but not in the afferent lymphatics between the site of injection and the lymph node (Fig. 4.1).

61

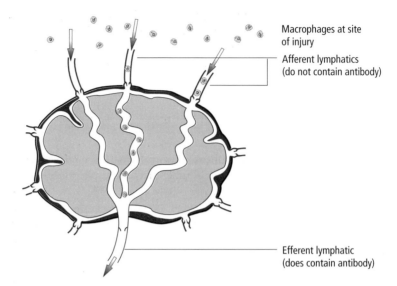

Macrophages at site of injury

Afferent lymphatics (do not contain antibody)

Efferent lymphatic (does contain antibody)

Figure 4.1 Macrophages are carried to draining lymph nodes.

We now know that other lymphoid tissues serve more or less the same function as lymph nodes. Nearly all the tissues of the body contain lymphatic vessels, which carry tissue fluid and antigen-presenting cells to the nearest lymph node, but there are also functional collections of lymphocytes at other sites which are not within an encapsulated structure like a node. These include massive accumulations in the throat (**tonsils**) and nasopharynx (**adenoids**) as well as smaller collections dispersed along the **alimentary canal** and, to a lesser extent, the **respiratory tract**. Every likely site of entry of antigens seems to be guarded by lymphoid tissue (Fig. 4.2). Exit routes for fluid, such as the biliary

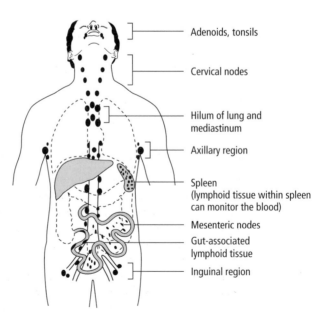

Adenoids, tonsils

Cervical nodes

Hilum of lung and mediastinum

Axillary region

Spleen (lymphoid tissue within spleen can monitor the blood)

Mesenteric nodes

Gut-associated lymphoid tissue

Inguinal region

Figure 4.2 Lymph nodes and other lymphoid tissue are strategically sited so that lymphocytes can be brought into contact with antigens which cross physical barriers.

or urinary tracts, have little or no lymphoid tissue. Nodules of lymphoid tissue are also found in the **spleen**; this monitors blood-borne antigens.

The cellular events of the immune response will be outlined as they take place in lymph nodes, but the same events take place in all other lymphoid tissues.

Lymphocytes make the antibodies

Since the vast majority of the cells in the lymph nodes are lymphocytes, it was likely that they were the cells actually making the antibodies, but this was not established until years after antibodies had been shown to exist. This was in the 1960s, when Gowans, in Oxford, demonstrated that rats, depleted of their lymphocytes by chronic drainage of the thoracic duct,[1] showed decreased antibody production but that the response could be restored by returning the lymphocytes to the animals.

Antigen has to be delivered to the lymphoid tissue

Molecular antigens, and antigens on cells such as microbes, can be carried passively in the lymph to the lymph node but more often they are **carried by cells such as macrophages**. This delivery service is speeded up by the **increased rate of lymphatic drainage** of tissues in acute inflammation.

The role that macrophages and similar cells play, as a primary link between the inflammatory and immune responses, can be explained if we return again to consider a **bruise** (p. 36). Macrophages phagocytose the spilled blood cells and debris. After a day or two, the bruise turns yellowish, because the phagocytosed haemoglobin is converted into haemosiderin. But **then the bruise disappears, because the macrophages have departed to the local lymph node** (Fig. 4.1). There they settle and degrade (break down) the larger molecules into smaller ones.

Suppose now, that instead of a bruise, you had a small injection of sheep red blood cells. The events would follow exactly as above, **until the macrophages reached the lymph node**. There the presence of **foreign** red cells would trigger lymphocytes into making antibodies. The only difference between the bruise and the injection of sheep red cells is that the sheep cells carry foreign antigens, unlike your own red cells.

Antigen has to be presented to the immune system

Except in a few rare instances, an immune response cannot take place as a result of a simple encounter between the antigen and the lymphocytes. A rather formal introduction must be made and this is the role of **antigen-presenting cells**. Macrophages can act as antigen-presenting cells, particularly when they have been activated by ingesting bacteria. However, there are other cells that specialize in this function.

Macrophages frequently scavenge debris, but do not always alert the lymphocytes to what they are doing, especially if they are not being activated during the process of scavenging. For instance macrophages, such as the

1 The thoracic duct is the main lymph vessel, which collects lymph and returns it to the blood.

63

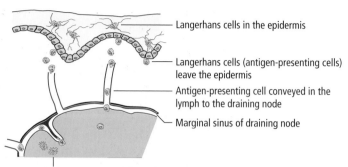

Langerhans cells in the epidermis

Langerhans cells (antigen-presenting cells) leave the epidermis

Antigen-presenting cell conveyed in the lymph to the draining node

Marginal sinus of draining node

Antigen-presenting cells settle in the **paracortex** as interdigitating cells

Figure 4.3 Antigen-presenting cells convey antigens to lymph nodes.

Kupffer cells in the liver and macrophages in the lung, are constantly scavenging but, at those sites, they are not normally brought into contact with lymphocytes, so they just continue with their normal functions, like destroying old red blood cells or inhaled particles, undisturbed.

The large mononuclear cells that are particularly good at antigen presentation are of uncertain lineage, but resemble macrophages with unusually abundant elongated cell processes, almost like the dendrites on a neuron. They are said to have dendritic morphology and in some sites are just called **dendritic cells**.

One well-characterized example of what we might call these 'professional' antigen-presenting cells are the **Langerhans cells,** found scattered among the cells of the **epidermis.** They take up any antigen that they encounter and then migrate through the tissues to the local lymphatics and hence to the nearest lymph node (Fig. 4.3). Cells with similar function are found in the epithelial linings of the respiratory and alimentary tracts.

Lymph nodes themselves contain antigen-presenting cells. We have already met the sessile macrophages in the lymph sinusoids but other specialized antigen-presenting cells are present, some actually derived from the dendritic cells in tissues and epithelia, which have migrated to settle in the nodes.

Now we must turn to where the action is—the lymph node.

Lymphoid tissue is populated by two main types of lymphocytes—T cells and B cells

2 The thymus is a bi-lobed structure in the front of the upper part of the chest. Like other lymphoid organs, it is largest in early life and becomes much smaller in adults.

3 In birds, B cells undergo their major development in a special organ, the bursa of Fabricius. This was the origin of the term 'B' cells.

Although all lymphocytes look alike by conventional methods, they are found to vary in respect of the different large molecules which are inserted into their surface membranes. These **cell markers** have been demonstrated by immunocytochemistry, as explained on p. 58. This ability to identify the different lymphocytes, together with many experimental studies, has to some extent clarified how the immune system works.

All lymphocytes originate from the bone marrow but, before entering the peripheral lymphoid tissue, some of them (T cells) **spend some time in the thymus.**[2] Others (the B cells) proceed directly from the bone marrow to the lymphoid tissue.[3] The structure of lymph nodes is important (Fig. 4.4). **Lymph**

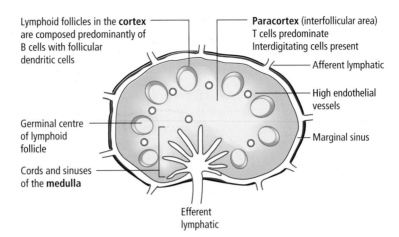

Lymphoid follicles in the **cortex** are composed predominantly of B cells with follicular dendritic cells

Paracortex (interfollicular area) T cells predominate Interdigitating cells present

Afferent lymphatic

High endothelial vessels

Germinal centre of lymphoid follicle

Marginal sinus

Cords and sinuses of the **medulla**

Efferent lymphatic

Figure 4.4 Diagram of a lymph node.

from the tissues or other nodes is brought by the afferent lymphatics and enters the periphery of the node; it passes through sinusoids towards the hilum and then leaves in just one or two efferent lymphatics. The sinusoids and larger sinuses contain sessile macrophages. **The efferent lymph may pass to at least one more node** before it joins most of the rest of the lymph in the **thoracic duct,** which returns to the blood by draining into the left subclavian vein in the neck.

The T and B cells enter the lymph node from the blood and then migrate mainly to particular areas of the node. The B cells form aggregates, **lymphoid follicles,** towards the periphery (**cortex**) of the node and, when antigenic stimulation occurs, a paler staining core called a **germinal centre** develops within each aggregate. The lymphoid follicles form in the vicinity of cells with long dendritic processes, **follicular dendritic cells**. The T cells are more diffusely distributed in the node, roughly in the interfollicular areas and more towards the hilum. The area is often called the **paracortex** and the T cells are found in association with the special **antigen-presenting cells** formed from the dendritic cells which have migrated to the node and settled down there. Their surface membranes can interlock with those of the T cells, and they are now known as **interdigitating cells**.

Summary

Antigen, either free or within cells, can pass in the lymph from the periphery to the draining lymph node. It can be carried by macrophages or cells which begin by being dendritic but mature to special antigen-presenting cells once they reach the node. When they become activated, macrophages can also present antigen to lymphocytes. Two kinds of lymphocyte, B and T, enter the lymph nodes, where they can encounter antigens. The two types tend to localize to different areas of the lymphoid tissue. In those areas they associate with particular cells which are accessory to their function.

Lymphocytes recirculate

Gowans' experiments, mentioned above, also revealed that, when the thoracic duct was cannulated and the cells removed, not only did the blood become depleted of lymphocytes but so too did the lymphoid tissue and lymphatic vessels. This was a practical demonstration of the fact that the **lymphocytes circulate** around the body.

Naïve lymphocytes, after their maturation in either the bone marrow or the thymus, are **carried in the blood and enter lymphoid tissues**. The details of B-cell circulation are not well-known but, in the case of T lymphocytes, some enter lymph nodes and others are more likely to enter lymphoid tissue which is associated with the intestine. **Once in the lymphoid tissues, the lymphocytes traverse them slowly**, making intimate contacts with other cells and thus maximizing the chances that they may **encounter their specific antigen** which may have been brought there from a nearby site of inflammation.

If specific antigen is encountered, then the lymphocytes are arrested, but if not, they leave in the afferent lymph and thus return to the blood, possibly passing through other nodes on the way. Having reached the blood the whole process may be repeated.

The endothelial cells lining venules in lymph nodes are seen to be enlarged when many lymphocytes are adherent and passing through them. This probably represents an activated state in which surface molecules are being expressed which cause the lymphocytes to adhere. They are usually referred to as **high endothelial vessels** (Fig. 4.4).

A histological section of a lymph node suggests a monotonous, stationary population of lymphocytes, but in real life they are mostly on the move.

B-cell stimulation leads to the secretion of antibodies

We can postpone for the present the question of how B-cell stimulation by antigen is brought about, and simply look at the results of the encounter. When a B cell is stimulated, it begins to divide rapidly to form a **clone of B cells**, all of which are dedicated to the production of one antibody. **One clone, one antibody**. The rapidly dividing daughter cells of the clone are much bigger than lymphocytes and are called **immunoblasts**.

Later, two types of B cell will arise from the clone. One type are the **memory cells** which are highly specific against the antigen and long-lived. They leave the lymph node to circulate in the blood to all parts of the body, where they can react with antigen whenever they meet it again. They are small cells and resemble the naïve B cells which first left the marrow.

Daughter cells of the second type are the **effector** B cells and differentiate into end cells which are factories for making antibodies. Many migrate to the medulla of the lymph node and are the source of the antibody which can be detected in the efferent lymph leaving the node. B cells which have differentiated to antibody-producing cells are called **plasma cells** (Fig. 4.5) and can release antibody molecules at a rate reckoned to be 2000 molecules per second!

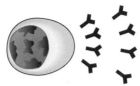

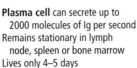

Plasma cell can secrete up to
2000 molecules of Ig per second
Remains stationary in lymph
node, spleen or bone marrow
Lives only 4–5 days

B lymphocyte has surface Ig
molecules to detect antigen

Figure 4.5 A plasma cell (left).

Figure 4.6 A B lymphocyte
(right).

Notice that, although the immunoglobulin molecules are released and circulate through the blood and tissue fluids, the plasma cells themselves do not. However, some effector B cells migrate to the spleen before they give rise to plasma cell clones.

The B-cell receptors which recognize antigen are immunoglobulin molecules inserted in the cell membrane

Each B cell develops its own specific immunoglobulin as it matures in the marrow. When inserted into the B-cell membrane, the same immunoglobulins become the receptors that receive the antigenic stimulus (Fig. 4.6). At this point, however, it is important to note that each single immunoglobulin does not recognize a whole antigen molecule, but only a part of it, called an **antigenic determinant**, or **epitope**. Thus any large antigenic molecule can stimulate a variety of B cells, that are reactive to different epitopes of the antigen (Fig. 4.7). These B cells between them make a variety of antibodies that can react with the different antigenic determinants on the antigen molecules.

How could B lymphocytes give rise to such a wide variety of antibodies?

As it began to be realized that more than a million different **epitopes** or **antigenic determinants** could be recognized by a corresponding number of

Figure 4.7 Most antigens have several different epitopes which can react with B cells bearing different immunoglobulin receptors.

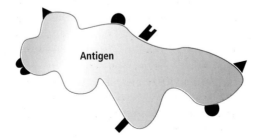

Antigen

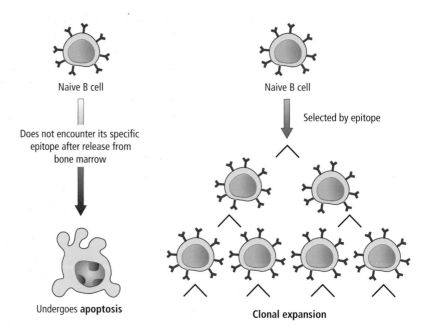

Figure 4.8 Selection of B-lymphocyte repertoire.

different antibodies, there was controversy over how it happened. It was unlike any other phenomenon already described in the field of biology. One early idea was that **antigenic determinants** could act as **templates** and somehow instruct the B lymphocytes to secrete antibodies which would fit around them. It was difficult to explain how this could occur, and it is now known to be completely wrong.

Burnet[4] however, proposed a revolutionary **clonal selection theory** to explain the findings. He suggested that there had to be **more than a million different kinds of B cell, each cell already dedicated to the synthesis and secretion of a single antibody**, before even meeting the antigen with which its antibody would react. It would then only be as a result of encounter with the specific antigen that the cell capable of making the appropriate antibody would be chosen, or **selected** (Fig. 4.8). Thus selection would be restricted to those B cells able to make antibodies against antigens present in the lymphoid environment at any particular time, for example during an attack of measles, and as a result the appropriate B cells would produce clones.

What then happens to all the other B lymphocytes, equipped to make anti-tetanus toxin, or antibodies to yellow fever, or to a million other things, not actually required at the time? They **survive for a short time**, exactly how long is not known, but eventually, if they do not encounter their antigen, they **undergo apoptosis.** The whole immune repertoire is regenerated continuously through life from the lymphocyte precursors in the marrow, so that it is always ready for anything; but at any one point in time, relatively few of the newly produced B cells may actually be required and the rest eliminate themselves. It

4 Frank MacFarlane Burnet (1898–1985).

68

was this apparent wastage in the theory that seemed doubtful at first but, eventually, Burnet's theory was shown to be the correct one and the mechanisms responsible for antibody diversity elucidated. It is now thought that there are at least 100 million different antigenic specificities amongst B lymphocytes. It follows from Burnet's theory that the specialization of B cells, to produce their different antibodies, occurs in developing B cells, long before they actually have the chance to meet their antigen.

How is the huge variety of antibodies generated?

The part of the antibody which binds to the epitope is a three-dimensional structure (FAb) made up of the variable or V regions of **one light chain** and **one heavy chain**. The whole antibody has two separate but identical binding sites, because it is made up of two heavy and two light chains. The variations between binding sites depend entirely upon differences in the structure of their variable regions. Their amino acid structure is determined by the genes which code for them and RNA is used to carry the message from the DNA to the machinery where the proteins are made.

Every B lymphocyte starts out with exactly the same genes for making heavy and light chains, but these genes are arranged quite differently from any others (except some of those in the T cells, as mentioned below). Instead of being a single sequence determining a protein, the **antibody genes** are made up of a **large number of alternative pieces or segments** (Fig. 4.9). A small selection of these can be fitted together with excision of the DNA in between them. The result is a more or less conventional gene but with enormous variation between those of different B cells, because of the random selection process. RNA is now made in the usual way, leading to each B cell making its own individual antibody chains.

Gene segments on chromosome 14 from which heavy chains are encoded

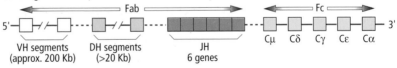

Gene segments for kappa light chains on chromosome 2

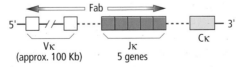

Figure 4.9 Simplified diagrams to indicate the numerous gene segments available to B cells for the generation of immunoglobulin molecules.

Gene segments for lambda light chains on chromosome 22

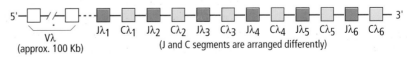

The gene segments coding for the variable end of the heavy chain are rearranged first. Sometimes, the juggling of segments produces sequences which cannot be transcribed into an RNA message. After such an unsuccessful attempt at rearrangement, there is a second chance to try the same thing with the heavy chain variable gene segments on the second chromosome of the pair. If, after this, an RNA message still cannot be made, the B cell dies in the bone marrow.

As soon as an RNA message has been made, the B cell can now make a complete heavy chain. The Fc or constant region of the heavy chain must be added and to make it, Cμ (see Fig. 4.9), which codes for the μ heavy chain, specific for immunoglobulin M (IgM), is always used first.

Successful synthesis of heavy chains is followed by a similar process to make the light chains. There are two kinds of light chains which B cells can make; these are called κ and λ. The genes for each kind are on different pairs of chromosomes. Every B cell tries to rearrange the κ **gene segments first** and, only if the process is unsuccessful, as explained above, on both chromosomes of the pair, does it try to rearrange the λ gene segments. This means that there is a greater chance of B cells making κ than λ light chains and this is why more κ chain antibody is normally present. **No B cell makes both types of light chain.**

As soon as the B cell can synthesize **both heavy and light chains**, whole antibody molecules can be made and are inserted into the cell membrane to become the antigen receptor.

The eventual **class of the antibody** secreted by the B cell will depend upon the structure of the constant region (Fc) of the heavy chain. It is called **constant** because it is the same for all antibodies of a particular class, even though their specificities for antigen vary. However, the structure of the Fc region can be altered by using different gene segments of the C region (see Fig. 4.9) and this is how **the class of an antibody can be changed**. At first, every B cell synthesizes and inserts IgM into its membrane and most also insert another class, IgD, which they make at the same time.

IgD was not mentioned in the previous chapter because it is not secreted in any significant amount. Its function is not completely understood but it seems to be important as a signalling molecule during the early life of B lymphocytes. It disappears later on.

Although, when first stimulated, B lymphocytes secrete IgM, as antibody responses mature, the daughter cells of the clones may switch to using a different gene segment coding for the constant region of the heavy chain, as explained above. In this way, antibodies of the IgG, IgA or IgE classes can be secreted instead.

B cells nearly always need T-cell help to respond to their epitope

In almost all cases, it is not enough for the antibody molecules on the surface of a B lymphocyte simply to encounter the appropriate epitope for the cell to be stimulated.

When the immune response began to be investigated, it was found that if the thymus was removed from a newborn animal, the animal's subsequent ability to make antibodies was impaired. Similarly, if mice deprived of lymphocytes by irradiation were given lymphocytes from another mouse of the same strain, it was discovered that reconstitution by **B** lymphocytes **alone** could not restore antibody production when challenged with antigen. However, **antibodies could be made when T cells from the thymus were also added**. These experiments showed that B cells and T cells had to **cooperate** with each other before there could be an antibody response, an activity which came to be called **T-cell help** for the B cells.

Further experiments showed that, usually, **both types of lymphocyte, B and T, had to recognize the same antigen independently** for cooperation to be possible. Once naïve lymphocytes have responded to antigen, they and their daughter cells are **primed** or sensitized.

How do the T cells help the B cells?

They do it in two ways, by secreting factors which can affect B cells and also by surface molecular interactions with the B cells. There must be an antigen-dependent intimate contact between the two cell types, which is explained below, and then a molecule called **CD40** on the B-cell surface, quite separate from the antibody molecules which recognize antigen, can interact with **CD40 ligand** which is present on the surface of activated T cells.

Another reciprocal pair of surface molecules also have to interact; these are B7 on the B cell and CD28 on the T cell. In this way, **the T cell is encouraged to help** because it is itself activated by the B cell.

When these complex interactions between pairs of surface molecules take place, the T cell responds by secreting **lymphokines**, soluble factors with a short half-life, which promote the growth and development of the B cells. T cells also control changes in the **class** of antibody secreted by the B cells. They can induce the synthesis of the Fc portion of the heavy chain to be switched from one C segment to another. This alters the structure and hence the antibody class. Thus, the T and B cells work together to bring about the humoral response (Fig. 4.10).

We shall see later how specific antigens are responded to independently by the B and T cells and how these cells cooperate with each other to produce antibodies.

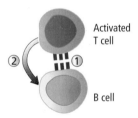

Activated
T cell

B cell

Figure 4.10 Two mechanisms for helping B cells: 1, molecular interactions; 2, lymphokines.

There are a few special exceptions to the need for T-cell help

One exception to the need for cooperation is when the immunoglobulin molecules over the B-cell surface are cross-linked by regularly spaced epitopes carried by certain polysaccharides. Because stimulation of B cells can be achieved in this case without T-cell help, these polysaccharides are called **T-independent antigens**. The effect can be shown experimentally using synthetic molecules, but arrays of such epitopes occur naturally as part of some bacterial cell walls. In such circumstances, direct activation of an antibody response by a pathogen, without the need for T-cell help, is an advantage.

There are also other bacterial products, mainly lipopolysaccharides, that can stimulate B lymphocytes directly and indiscriminately in the absence of T-cell help. Often referred to as **mitogens**, because they stimulate B cells by a direct effect, quite independently of their surface immunoglobulin molecules and therefore of their antigen specificity, they bring about **polyclonal B-cell activation**. Again, this non-specific but rapid response may help in defences against bacteria.

These particular examples are exceptions to the general rule that **B-cell stimulation needs T-cell help**.

The humoral immune response occurs when B-cell receptors recognize their specific antigenic determinants and T cells help them to develop into antibody-secreting clones.

But for T cells to help B cells, they must be stimulated too. How does this happen?

Whereas B cells use their surface immunoglobulins to recognize their specific epitopes, for T cells it is not so simple. They too have antigen receptors at their surfaces but these can only react with stretches of peptides which form part of the **internal structure of antigens**. It is the job of macrophages and other antigen-presenting cells to isolate these peptide sequences and then display them at their surfaces, held by **antigen-presenting molecules**.

The T-cell receptor can only react with the antigenic peptide when it is displayed in this way because **it has to bind to the antigen-presenting molecule at the same time as the antigen** (Fig. 4.11). This specialized interaction with antigen is not only important for the help which T cells give B cells, but for all their other activities as well. We must now explain the antigen-presenting molecules.

MHC 'table' presents
a meal of peptide

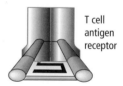

T cell
antigen
receptor

T cell receptor
1. recognizes the sides of the 'table'
2. reaches and recognizes the peptide

Figure 4.11 Peptide presentation to T cells.

All nucleated mammalian cells except neurons advertise their identity by presenting their own characteristic peptides on the cell surface

Within each cell, proteins called MHC Class I are secreted into the endoplasmic reticulum. Their structure includes a cleft within which short peptide segments can bind. Under normal circumstances, only self peptides are in the endoplasmic reticulum and become bound. They are then carried to the cell surface by the MHC Class I, where they can be displayed.

When tissue is grafted from one individual to another, it is the presence of these peptide **presenting molecules** on the surface of donor antigen-presenting cells within the graft which is a major cause of graft rejection. The cells of the graft all express MHC molecules which are different from those of the recipient cells.

This effect, **causing rejection,** led to the name **major histocompatibility complex** for the set of genes responsible for the molecules, and hence the abbreviation MHC.

A second kind of antigen-presenting molecule is normally found only on professional antigen-presenting cells

MHC Class II molecules are analogous to Class I, but undergo a different sequence of events. Within the endoplasmic reticulum, **when the Class II molecules are assembled, their cleft is occupied temporarily by a chaperone protein**. This prevents binding of self peptides as happens with MHC Class I. MHC Class II molecules are then **transported to a phagolysosome,** where the chaperone protein is destroyed. Here the MHC Class II may encounter **peptide fragments from microbes** or other foreign material being degraded. These foreign fragments can be picked up, transported to the cell surface and, sitting in the MHC Class II cleft, they can be presented in the correct way for T-cell recognition (Fig. 4.12). In this way, cells present peptide from inside them-selves on MHC Class I and, if they have MHC Class II, also peptides from

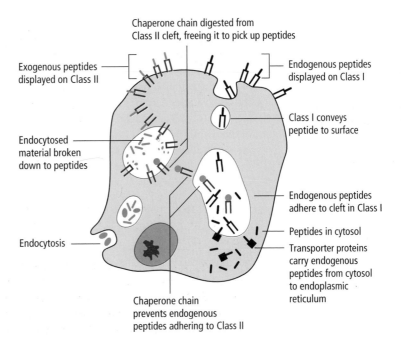

Figure 4.12 Two pathways for peptide presentation in antigen-presenting cells.

Chaperone chain digested from Class II cleft, freeing it to pick up peptides

Exogenous peptides displayed on Class II

Endogenous peptides displayed on Class I

Class I conveys peptide to surface

Endocytosed material broken down to peptides

Endogenous peptides adhere to cleft in Class I

Peptides in cytosol

Endocytosis

Transporter proteins carry endogenous peptides from cytosol to endoplasmic reticulum

Chaperone chain prevents endogenous peptides adhering to Class II outside the cell. This mechanism enables the T cells to 'see' where the antigenic peptides come from when they react with the MHC molecules as described below.

T cells have receptors for antigen recognition and other surface molecules for activation

An enormous variety of antigen receptor molecules are present on the surface of T cells, each individual cell expressing its own receptor which recognizes a single antigenic peptide. The function of the T-cell antigen receptor (TCR) is different from that of immunoglobulin receptors. For one thing, it is not destined to be secreted. It is used to make a specific bridge between the T cell and the antigen-presenting cell and is helped to do this by special co-stimulatory molecules which at the same time recognize the base of the antigen-presenting structure, the MHC (Fig. 4.13).

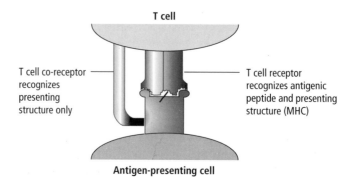

Figure 4.13 T-cell receptor and co-receptor.

As a result of the TCR combining with specific peptide and the MHC, a signal can be transmitted to the T cell but, by itself, the signal is insufficient to stimulate it. (Imagine that at this point the T cell and antigen-presenting cell have shaken hands but that the T cell will only be **activated** if the antigen-presenting cell also pats it on the back!) Other connections must also be made between interlocking pairs of molecules on the T cells and the antigen-presenting cells (for instance CD28 of T cells and B7 on the antigen-presenting cell). Without the stimulation these non-specific interactions bring about, the T cell cannot be activated. In addition, when macrophages are the antigen-presenting cells, they secrete a factor celled **interleukin-1** (IL-1) which helps in T-cell activation (Fig. 4.14).

Thus, we can see that the recruitment of the naïve T cells into immune responses is quite a complex matter, and far from a chance encounter between the cell surface and specific antigen.

Let us now look in more detail at the TCR molecules and the process of antigen presentation. **Each TCR is made up of two protein chains. The majority are composed of α and β chains.** Variation in the structure of these chains is brought about by rearranging gene segments on chromosomes, as the T cells develop. The process is similar to that which takes place in B cells when they generate their diverse FAb regions.

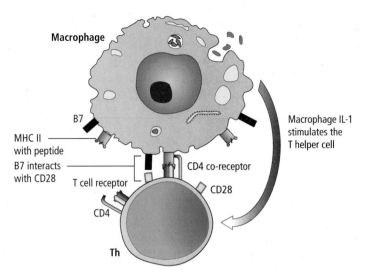

Macrophage

B7

MHC II
with peptide

B7 interacts
with CD28

T cell receptor

CD4

Th

Macrophage IL-1
stimulates the
T helper cell

CD4 co-receptor

CD28

1. Macrophage presents peptide in MHC Class II cleft
2. Macrophage expresses B7 which interacts with CD28
3. Macrophage secretes cytokines, especially IL-1

Figure 4.14 Activation of T-helper cell by macrophage.

As indicated in Fig. 4.13, these two TCR chains interact with the MHC, if the peptide in the cleft is the one specifically recognized by the TCR. The co-stimulator molecules which help the attachment by bonding with the base of the MHC can be of two different kinds, called CD4 and CD8, and the major function of the T cell is related to which kind of co-stimulator molecule it bears. This is because they guide the T cell on to the appropriate kind of MHC, either Class II or I (Fig. 4.15).

Those which carry **CD4 are the helper T cells**, a name which describes their activities in helping other cells to grow and function. Some are the cells which help antibody production. CD4 T cells are reduced in patients with acquired immunodeficiency syndrome (AIDS). You can now understand part of the reason why the immune responses of AIDS patients are abnormal.

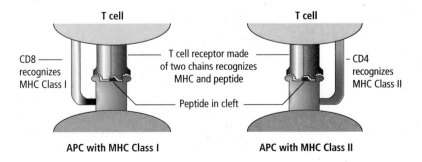

T cell

T cell

CD8
recognizes
MHC Class I

T cell receptor made
of two chains recognizes
MHC and peptide

Peptide in cleft

CD4
recognizes
MHC Class II

APC with MHC Class I

APC with MHC Class II

Figure 4.15 Co-receptor molecules help T cells react with the appropriate class of MHC.

The CD4 molecules recognize only MHC Class II molecules

Class II are the presenting molecules used mainly by cells participating in immune responses, to display peptides derived from exogenous material which has been broken down in phagolysosomes. Usually, such peptides are derived from cell membranes and extracellular proteins but, of course, if the cell has phagocytosed foreign material, such as bacteria, this too can be presented to the T-helper cells. Recognition of the foreign peptides, as long as it is accompanied by the other activation signals which the antigen-presenting cell can provide, results in **activation of the T helper**. It then enlarges, divides and goes on to secrete lymphokines.

First it is essential that a T cell which has recognized antigen **proliferates** to give a **clone of identical cells**; this is brought about by self-stimulation. The T cell and its progeny secrete interleukin-2 (IL-2) which is a powerful T-cell growth factor and at the same time they express **IL-2 receptors** so they can respond to it. The effect of IL-2 is not restricted to the cell which makes it but it also stimulates any other nearby activated T cells (including cytotoxic T cells, which are described below) carrying IL-2 receptors, thereby assisting specific responses, but not affecting resting T cells. Activated T cells produce **interferon-γ** which **increases the efficiency of antigen presentation** by other cells.

Just how do the B cells get T cells to help them?

Eventually it was realized that it was because **B cells themselves could present antigen to T cells**. The immunoglobulin molecules at the B-cell surface bind to antigen and then take it into the phagolysosomes, where it is digested to peptides and displayed on MHC Class II (Fig. 4.16).

A particular kind of T-helper cell, known as **Th2**, responds better to peptides presented by B cells than to those presented by other cells such as macrophages and it reacts by secreting the lymphokines which are particularly potent in their effects upon B cells. At the same time Th2 cells produce a lymphokine which tends to **suppress** the other kind of helper cell, Th1, and suppress antigen presentation by macrophages which cooperate particularly with Th1.

Th2 cells not only encourage the growth of, and immunoglobulin synthesis by, B cells, but they are also able to direct them to change the **class** of antibody they make, although the antigen specificity remains the same. This is done by switching to another gene segment for making the Fc part of the heavy chain, as explained above.

Naïve B cells are not able to stimulate T cells because they lack the necessary surface molecules. However, mature B cells can do so. However, when antigens are encountered for the **very first time**, the priming of naïve T cells is the job of the professional antigen-presenting cells. Often the priming is done by the interdigitating cells in the lymphoid tissues (Fig. 4.17). Later in immune responses, mature B and T cells have enough stimulatory molecules of their own to be able to cooperate independently of other cell types.

76

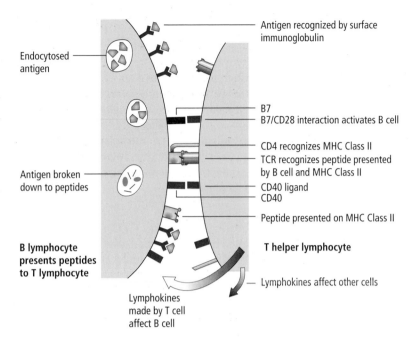

Antigen recognized by surface immunoglobulin

Endocytosed antigen

B7
B7/CD28 interaction activates B cell

CD4 recognizes MHC Class II
TCR recognizes peptide presented by B cell and MHC Class II
CD40 ligand
CD40

Antigen broken down to peptides

Peptide presented on MHC Class II

B lymphocyte presents peptides to T lymphocyte

T helper lymphocyte

Lymphokines affect other cells

Lymphokines made by T cell affect B cell

Figure 4.16 Interaction between B cell and T cell.

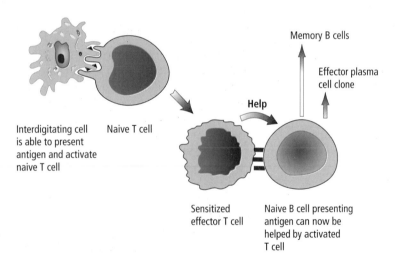

Memory B cells

Effector plasma cell clone

Help

Interdigitating cell is able to present antigen and activate naive T cell

Naive T cell

Sensitized effector T cell

Naive B cell presenting antigen can now be helped by activated T cell

Figure 4.17 Naïve T cell requires activation by professional antigen-presenting cell.

Cell-mediated immunity is the job of Th1 helper cells and cytotoxic T cells

When **Th1 cells become predominant**, help is being directed chiefly towards **macrophages**. That help consists of both IL-2 to recruit more T cells and interferon-γ which increases the amount of antigen macrophages can present and improves their ability to kill. This is important when macrophages have been invaded by microorganisms such as tubercle and leprosy bacilli or leishmania, which are able to grow inside them (thus escaping antibodies and neutrophil leukocytes). The macrophages return the compliment by secreting a factor which causes the Th1 cells to increase their numbers. It is this cooperation between the Th1 cells and the macrophages which underlies **cellular immunity**. When the two cell types are working together to overcome intracellular bacteria or protozoa or other foreign material, more macrophages are recruited to the site by lymphokines secreted by the Th1 and even stimulated to form aggregates which are recognized as granulomas. The Th1 cells also help in dealing with viral infections — another form of intracellular parasitism.

At first in an immune response, the T-cell help is non-specialized, but when it continues for some time, either the Th1 or Th2 helper cells may come to predominate.

T cells which carry CD8 co-stimulator molecules destroy the cell which presents antigen to them. These are cytotoxic T cells and do not have any helper activity

The other kind of co-stimulator molecules carried by T cells are **CD8**. They only recognize **MHC Class I**, the antigen-presenting molecule which is carried by all nucleated body cells except neurons. This means that if any cell displays a peptide on its MHC Class I which is recognized by a T cell, **it will be destroyed**, because **only cytotoxic T cells** will respond.[5] Usually, of course, only peptides from inside normal cells are present on their MHC Class I and these are ignored by the immune system, but if unusual peptides are displayed, this informs the immune system that something is **profoundly wrong** inside the cell, usually a virus infection. As a result, it is destroyed. The cytotoxic T cell has several mechanisms which cause the target cell to self-destruct, making it undergo apoptosis. The cytotoxic cell can then move on to destroy further cells.

Summary

By using more than one kind of molecule to present antigenic peptides to T cells, two completely different types of T cell can be activated, quite separately. The effect of one type is to destroy cells presenting antigen to them and the effect of the other is to initiate or increase the activity of other lymphocytes, both T and B, as well as macrophages and other cells (Fig. 4.18).

Th1 cells cooperate with macrophages in one arm of cellular immunity; another arm is the cytotoxic T cells. Th2 cells control and aid B cells in humoral immunity.

T cells complete their development in the thymus

T cells enter the thymus, proliferate and then move through it from the outside towards the interior. It is during their passage through it that the T cells synthesize and and express their specific antigen receptors and develop **both**

5 It may be easy to remember that cytotoxic T cells bite the hands that feed them!

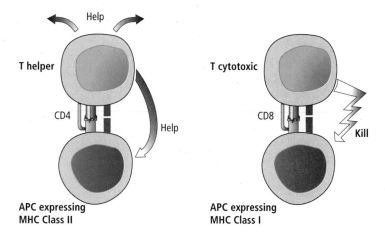

Figure 4.18 The effects of major histocompatibility complex restriction.

CD4 and CD8 co-receptors. Also during the passage, it must be established that the TCR expressed on every new T cell is able to react with one or other of the MHC molecules but not bind so strongly that contact with MHC alone would be enough to stimulate the T cell.

Epithelial cells of embryonic origin form much of the thymic environment. As the new receptors appear in the membranes of T cells they are tested against self MHC molecules in the surrounding environment, mainly on the epithelial cells, without any other stimulus. Those which **react strongly are eliminated** because they would be potentially harmful after the cells leave the thymus. Also eliminated are those **which fail to recognize MHC at all** because they would not combine sufficiently well to make contact with any peptides in the cleft. Those T cells whose TCRs establish the right relationship with **MHC Class I retain CD8** but cease to express the CD4 and will be the **cytotoxic T cells**. Those which similarly recognize **MHC Class II retain CD4** but lose CD8 and will be the **helper T cells**.

This arrangement, by which T lymphocytes are brought to respond to only one or other of the MHC classes, is called **MHC restriction**. We saw above how important it was in deciding which kind of T cell, **a helper or a killer**, responds to antigen presentation.

As the T cells migrate towards the central part of the thymus, their antigen receptors are shown a range of **self-peptides** by **efficient antigen-presenting cells.** This mimics a situation outside the thymus in which they would be expected to respond if their receptors recognized self-peptides and of course, **those that do react are eliminated**.

This thymic processing of the T lymphocytes (both positive and negative selection) is stringent because, of the total number of cells which begin the thymic journey, only about 2% actually emerge and circulate. When they do so, they have differentiated into **CD4-positive helper T cells and CD8-positive cytotoxic T cells.**

The normal state in which the immune system does not mount responses against self-antigens is known as tolerance

The main way tolerance is achieved is by the removal of strongly self-reacting lymphocytes, as they develop, in both the bone marrow (for the B cells) and the thymus (for the T cells). In fact, since B cells do not usually synthesize significant quantities of antibody without T-cell help, it is much more critical that self-reacting T cells are eliminated.

There are, though, some other mechanisms to prevent activation of any self-reacting cells which do escape from the thymus. This is where the elaborate process of antigen presentation is so important because, in the absence of the appropriate simultaneous second activation signals, the result of interaction between the TCR and antigenic peptide can be paralysis or death of the T cell. In addition, it is possible for some T cells to prevent the activity of others. Such an activity can be demonstrated experimentally and is called **suppression**. It probably helps prevent unwanted responses occurring.

Summary

Passage through the thymus ensures that T cells recognize the MHC molecules well enough to interact with them. This is positive selection and is combined with MHC restriction—either CD8 to MHC Class I or CD4 to MHC Class II. Finally, those that would recognize self-peptides as their 'specific' antigen are eliminated in the process of negative selection, which is the main basis of tolerance.

Immune memory relies mainly on having circulating lymphocytes specific for certain antigens

Prior to first exposure to antigen, the frequency of lymphocytes reacting specifically to it is very low indeed. After exposure and clonal expansion of lymphocytes able to recognize the antigen, populations of long-lived specific lymphocytes circulate. These are known as **memory cells**.

In the case of T memory cells, they may be easier to activate than the naïve cells. Also, as a result of changes in their surface molecules, they no longer simply pass through lymph nodes. They circulate more widely, with a bigger search area.

When B memory cells are compared with naïve B cells, it can be shown that their immunoglobulin receptors have a more refined specificity and higher affinity for the epitope. Once encountered by these sensitive receptors, the antigen can be rapidly endocytosed and broken down inside the B memory cell for presentation to T memory cells. The B memory cells also possess the surface molecules which are necessary to activate T cells.

B memory cells are formed within germinal centres

During an immune response, not only do small lymphocytes enlarge to

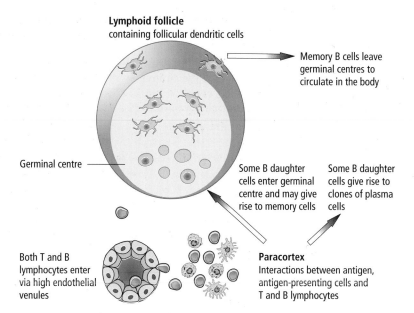

Lymphoid follicle
containing follicular dendritic cells

Memory B cells leave
germinal centres to
circulate in the body

Germinal centre

Some B daughter
cells enter germinal
centre and may give
rise to memory cells

Some B daughter
cells give rise to
clones of plasma
cells

Both T and B
lymphocytes enter
via high endothelial
venules

Paracortex
Interactions between antigen,
antigen-presenting cells and
T and B lymphocytes

Figure 4.19 Antigen recognition by B cells results in the production of effector cells and memory cells.

immunoblasts and plasma cells appear, but well-defined rounded collections of larger cells appear within the B lymphocyte follicles in the cortex of lymph nodes. There is considerable evidence of mitotic activity in these areas, which led to the name, **germinal centres**. It was also noted that many cells appeared to be dying there and, as a result, many macrophages are present, removing the dead cells. Most of the lymphocytes in germinal centres are B cells but there are also some T helpers. They are all within a network formed by the long cytoplasmic processes of the follicular dendritic cells.

A few of the daughters of B cells which have recognized antigen in a lymph node enter the germinal centre and once there, they proliferate (Fig. 4.19). As they do so, they make further minor random changes to the FAb ends of the heavy and light chains which are responsible for interaction with the epitope. As a result, some receptors are actually a worse fit, but some are better. Now, at the same time, within the germinal centres, the follicular dendritic cells are holding tiny fragments of antigen in the form of complexes with antibody, at the surface of their cytoplasmic processes. The B cells use their newly altered receptors to compete with each other for attachment to the antigen in the complexes. Those which are successful are selected to persist as memory cells; those whose changed receptors do not fit well with the antigen are the ones that can be seen undergoing apoptosis in the germinal centres.

In fact, it is now thought that antigen may be retained in the form of complexes for long periods of time by the follicular dendritic cells of the germinal centres and act as a reservoir to maintain the memory cell populations.

How long is immune memory?

We know that in some cases it is very long indeed. A childhood attack of most common viral infections confers lifelong immunity in the majority of individuals. One of the best examples was that of a remote island where the initial exposure of the inhabitants to Europeans caused a measles epidemic. The islanders were then isolated for 60 years before measles was reintroduced. At that date, the survivors of the first measles outbreak were still immune to the measles virus, whereas it was rampant amongst those born in the meantime.

We could perhaps explain long-lived immunity in populations where subclinical reinfections could boost it from time to time, but it is more difficult in the island example. When it was demonstrated that some human lymphocytes could survive for many years (the persistence of radiation-damaged cells, incapable of division) it was thought they might be memory cells.

However, studies using artificial immunization show that there is considerable variation in the time over which specific memory can be maintained. It varies with the physical nature of the antigen, its dose and the route of administration, whether the antigen persists *in vivo*, and of course, whether there are subsequent exposures to it. Current opinion, based on careful animal studies, has moved more towards the idea that **persistence of antigen** in the body is more likely to govern really long-term memory than persistent lymphocytes.

The site where this might take place was a mystery but it has now come to be thought that germinal centres may act as one reservoir for persistent antigen in the body.

Summary

Immunological memory depends largely on expanded populations of specific B and T cells continuing to circulate. These memory cells are different from the the naïve cells. In the case of B memory cells, they carry many highly specific receptors for antigen, whereas the T memory cells are more readily activated. The germinal centres which develop in B cell follicles play a crucial role in the development of memory.

It was a neoplastic disease, myeloma, which helped in the understanding of immunoglobulin structure

Myeloma is a neoplasm of plasma cells, which develops in the bone marrow. It arises from a single cell but consists of millions of cells all secreting **identical immunoglobulin**, so vast quantities of a particular **monoclonal antibody** can be obtained from the serum of patients. Once purified, these products of neoplastic cells provided the material for investigation of the detailed structure of immunoglobulins.

It is now possible to **make monoclonal antibodies *in vitro*** and they have become one of the most useful tools in immunological research and for therapy. Briefly, after antigenic stimulation of a laboratory animal has resulted in antibody formation, spleen cells which include B lymphocytes making antibodies against that antigen are obtained and induced to fuse with neoplastic myeloma cells, which can be maintained indefinitely in culture. Thus the **specificity** of the short-lived responding B lymphocyte is combined with the **potential**

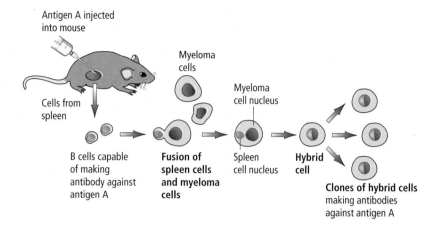

Antigen A injected
into mouse

Myeloma
cells

Myeloma
cell nucleus

Cells from
spleen

B cells capable
of making
antibody against
antigen A

**Fusion of
spleen cells
and myeloma
cells**

Spleen
cell nucleus

**Hybrid
cell**

Clones of hybrid cells
making antibodies
against antigen A

Figure 4.20 Outline of
technique used to make
monoclonal antibodies.

immortality of the neoplastic cells. Fusion is not always successful but in some
cases results in long-lived clones dedicated to the production of a single
antibody directed against the antigen used to immunize the original animal
(Fig. 4.20). This audacious technique was pioneered by Milstein[6] and his
collaborators.

Technological advances, often using monoclonal antibodies, have permitted
recognition of an enormous range of different surface molecules expressed by
human leukocytes and so many were separately described that it became
necessary to agree on a terminology for them. If a number of antibodies appeared to recognize the same component, it was designated a 'cluster of differentiation' and given a CD number. Examples we have referred to frequently are
CD4 and **CD8**, the co-receptors on T helpers and cytotoxic T cells, respectively.

Summary

It has emerged that lymphocytes are not all the same. The complex interactions of B cells with T cells are responsible for antibody production. T cells
are responsible for cell-mediated immunity. The huge repertoire of antigen-
specific receptor molecules is the result of gene rearrangements within
lymphocytes, in either the bone marrow or the thymus, long before the
antigens are encountered. The result is a defence mechanism of astonishing
versatility. We must now see how it does its job.

6 Cesar Milstein (1927–   ), in
Cambridge.

5 The immune response: the effects

The complex mechanisms of production of immunoglobulins and specifically sensitized cells evolved in vertebrates **to improve defence against pathogenic microbes**. To do this, evolution could have done one of two things: it could have devised a second, completely new form of defence; or it could have concentrated on improving the one that had already evolved in invertebrates—inflammation. Not surprisingly, perhaps, it chose the latter.

The immune response works by boosting the inflammatory response

We must now revisit the inflammatory response and, first, remember that it is a **local reaction to injury**. For the immune response to help it, the immunoglobulins or sensitized lymphocytes, or both, must reach the local inflammatory lesion. In fact, acute inflammation assists access of immunoglobulins by the locally increased vascular permeability. Longer-lasting inflammation encourages access of T and B cells from the blood to the local lesion. These are probably mainly circulating memory cells; their numbers can be quickly expanded within the lesion. Thus, the **afferent loop** takes the antigenic message **from its site of entry to the lymphoid tissue**. The **efferent loop** brings the antibodies and cells **from the lymphoid tissue to the local lesion. It is there, in the lesion, that the boosting effects of both humoral and cellular arms of the immune response take place.**

One way this is brought about is that **antigen–antibody complexes augment complement activation**. They do this by means of the classical pathway, thus increasing all the inflammatory activities of complement (Fig. 5.1). The other is that both immunoglobulins and sensitized T cells interact with inflammatory cells in various ways, and improve their efficiency. We shall find that every single component of inflammation can be assisted by the immune response.

We must remember that, **for the first few days of a first infection, the inflammatory response is acting alone. The immune response then begins to help**; and, importantly, if the host survives the first infection, the **immune memory** is ready to boost inflammation immediately on a second infection by the same organism.

We can think of the inflammatory response as having four components: (I) the initial production of chemical mediators of acute inflammation; (II) the killing of microbes by phagocytosis or exocytosis; (III) the endocytosis and destruction of toxins; and (IV) the difficult task of eliminating microorganisms that live inside cells. We can now re-examine these components of in-

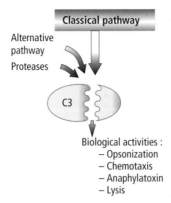

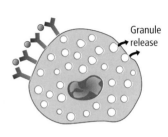

Figure 5.1 Boosting of complement activation by the classical pathway (left).

Figure 5.2 Activation of mast cells by antigen linking immunoglobulin E (right).

flammation one by one, and see how each is accentuated by the immune response.

I. Antibodies boost the production of chemical mediators of inflammation

The earliest events in inflammation are vasodilatation, increased permeability and recruitment of phagocytes, all mediated by local release or activation of chemical mediators. The role of **complement activation** in initiating these events is central. In the absence of an immune response, we have seen that complement is activated by proteases spilled from damaged host cells, or activation of the alternative pathway by certain organisms, or both (Chapter 2). Once antibodies arrive on the scene, however, and react with antigens, **complement can now be activated also by the immune complexes via the classical pathway**. This generates C3a and C5a which cause mast cell degranulation and release of inflammatory mediators. C5a also brings about release of prostaglandins and leukotrienes. C5a is also chemotactic for neutrophils and macrophages, which accelerates their encounter with any microorganisms that may be present.

Another important 'early warning system' also brings about rapid release of chemical mediators. This relies on immunoglobulin E (IgE), found in the blood at much lower levels than IgG or IgM, but having a very different role. **Mast cells have surface receptors with high avidity for the Fc end of IgE molecules**, which therefore become affixed in this way to mast cells all over the body. If a microbe, carrying antigen, contacts its corresponding IgE molecule (or rather cross-links a pair of IgE molecules) on the surface of a mast cell, this leads to degranulation and hence local boosting of inflammation (Fig. 5.2).

Because IgE of a particular specificity spreads throughout the body, mast cells in all tissues may be primed with it. Therefore, this mechanism is effective even if the second infection is at a different site from the first. It is also of importance to this early warning system that any one mast cell carries IgE molecules of varying specificity. So a single IgE-laden mast cell can boost the inflammatory response to many different reinfections.

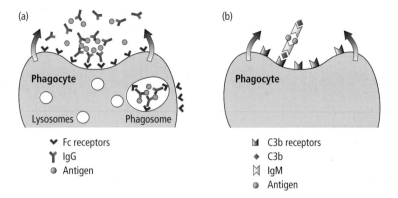

Figure 5.3 Opsonization by (a) immunoglobulin G (IgG) and by (b) IgM–C3b complexes.

The second infection therefore always elicits inflammation more efficiently than the first. This is because both IgG in the extracellular fluid and IgE on local mast cells are lying in wait, and the existence of B memory cells will cause a rapid increase in specific antibody production.

II. The humoral immune response boosts the killing of foreign cells

The usual way that the inflammatory response kills microbes (e.g. bacteria) is by phagocytosis and then attack by oxygen radicals and enzymes. The process of phagocytosis is assisted in the absence of immunity by lectins and by non-specific complement activation. It is improved further by the immune response, in two ways. **IgG opsonizes bacteria directly**, because both neutrophils and macrophages have IgG Fc receptors; and **IgM opsonizes bacteria indirectly by increasing the attachment of the opsonin C3b** (Fig. 5.3).

If this opsonization occurs in the tissue spaces, neutrophils and wandering tissue macrophages will normally take up the microbes; if in the lymph, the sessile macrophages of the lymph nodes; if in the blood, the sessile macrophages (e.g. in spleen or liver) will do so.

The result is more rapid uptake and exposure of bacteria to the phagocyte's toxic oxygen radicals and lysosomal enzymes. This usually leads to much more efficient **killing and degradation of the organisms**, so **opsonization contributes crucially to immunity**.

The discovery of this mechanism of opsonization of bacteria by antibodies played an important part in the history of pathology. At the beginning of the 20th century, there were two opposing camps in the field of infectious disease. One, led by the Russian, Elie Metchnikoff,[1] asserted that the phagocytes were the principal defence of the body against infection. The other, led by the German, Paul Ehrlich,[1] held that antibodies fulfilled that role. Then came the discovery, in 1906, by Almroth Wright in London, that antibodies could opsonize bacteria to enhance phagocytosis. The happy result was that, in 1908, the Nobel Prize for Medicine was awarded jointly to both Metchnikoff and Ehrlich.[2]

Another way of killing some pathogenic organisms is by **complement-medi-**

1 Metchnikoff, 1845–1916; Ehrlich, 1854–1915.

2 It not infrequently happens, in scientific controversies, that both sides are eventually proved to be right.

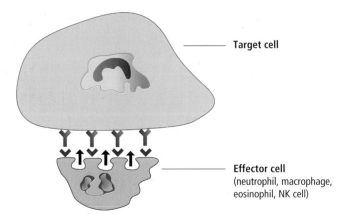

Target cell

Effector cell
(neutrophil, macrophage,
eosinophil, NK cell)

Figure 5.4 Exocytosis to kill cells coated with immunoglobulin.

ated lysis. Clearly any organisms with attached IgG and especially IgM are much more vulnerable to this, because the attachment leads to additional activation of complement by the classical pathway, close to the microbial surface. IgA in the various bodily secretions also participates in this function, thus protecting mucosal surfaces from invasion although, alone among the immunoglobulin classes, IgA–antigen complexes activate complement by the alternative pathway.

The third inflammatory mechanism for killing foreign cells is **exocytosis**. You will remember that neutrophils, macrophages, eosinophils and natural killer cells are all capable of exocytosing their toxic components when in close apposition to foreign cells. This is greatly boosted if the target cells are coated with immunoglobulin (Fig. 5.4), because it enhances the attachment to the receptors of the effector cell. This mechanism is probably particularly important in defence against metazoan parasites, which are too big to be phagocytosed. The usual general term for this antibody-mediated boosting of the exocytotic form of cell killing is **antibody-dependent cell-mediated cytotoxicity**.

III. The humoral immune response accelerates destruction of foreign large molecules

The macrophage scavenges foreign large molecules, as we have seen, probably partly by fluid-phase pinocytosis but mainly by scavenger receptors that recognize abnormal and non-self molecules. Other cells may well participate in this function, but it is only well-documented for macrophages. IgG or IgM attached to foreign large molecules would obviously assist this process, in exactly the same way as they lead to the opsonization of microbes. Thus the immune complexes formed when immunoglobulin attaches to the antigen would be recognized by the Fc or C3b receptors of phagocytes (Fig. 5.5). As a result they would be cleared more efficiently from the tissues by wandering macrophages, and from the blood by the sessile macrophages in the sinusoids of the spleen and liver. After endocytosis, the antigen will be degraded by lysosomal enzymes.

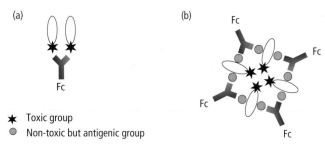

(a)

Fc

(b)

Fc

Fc

Fc

Fc

★ Toxic group

● Non-toxic but antigenic group

Figure 5.5 Alternative ways of neutralizing toxins: (a) immunoglobulin attaches to toxic group, neutralizing it; (b) immunoglobulin opsonizes toxic molecules for uptake and degradation by macrophages.

The defensive potential of this is seen when the foreign large molecules are potentially harmful, e.g. bacterial exotoxins. In the absence of immunity, the toxin causes disease. Clearly, the macrophages cannot cope alone. Their improved efficiency when antibodies have 'opsonized' the toxin explains the immunity to a second exposure to the same toxin (or after immunization by toxoid), in such diseases as diphtheria and tetanus.

Attachment of antibody to molecular antigens also activates complement by the classical pathway. The resultant boosting of local inflammation increases the numbers of phagocytes capable of endocytosing and destroying the toxin.

It is of course always possible that the toxic part of an exotoxin molecule might itself be an epitope and reaction site for antibody, in which case the attachment of antibody to it would render it innocuous (Fig. 5.5). If this does happen, it is probably the exception rather than the rule.

IV. Cellular immunity enhances killing of intracellular pathogens

One of the ways that some bacteria and protozoa evade host defences is by surviving and multiplying inside macrophages (e.g. *Mycobacterium tuberculosis*, *Leishmania* spp.). Often they achieve this by some sort of **inhibition of lysosomal fusion with the phagosome**. The organisms in the phagosome are exposed to toxic oxygen radicals, but not to the increased bactericidal effect of lysosomal fusion. This impediment enables the organisms to survive. However, specifically activated T cells (the Th1 subset) are recruited to the local lesion from the blood; once they reach the lesion, they can tip the balance in favour of the host by secreting **lymphokines**.

Lymphokines secreted by T cells that have encountered their specific antigen include **macrophage chemotactic protein**, recruiting more macrophages to the site of infection and, crucially, molecules such as **interferon-γ**, which can boost the production of oxygen radicals by the macrophage sufficiently to kill the resistant organisms (Fig. 5.6). Interferon-γ also helps cells to resist virus infections.

The other main role of cellular immunity is the generation of **cytotoxic T cells**. These are cells of the T-cell lineage which, when sensitized, can kill target cells carrying the appropriate antigen, in a similar way to the natural killer cells described previously and, like them, cause apoptosis of the target cell. The main strength of this arm of the immune response is that it can kill **cells**

89

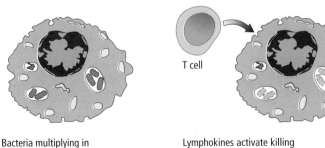

Figure 5.6 Activation of microbial killing by lymphokines.

T cell

Bacteria multiplying in phagosomes of macrophage

Lymphokines activate killing by macrophages

infected by viruses, which often present a virus antigen on the cell surface (Fig. 5.7). This reinforces the natural killer cell activity against virus-infected cells, by providing an additional population of cells available for this activity, and therefore accelerates the eradication of the viruses.

In summary, therefore, **the immune response is protective because it boosts the inflammatory response**, either by increasing the number of effector cells in the lesion or, more commonly, by enhancing their activity.

One additional effect of immunity which does not fall easily into this generalization concerns IgA. IgA in secretions **blocks the adhesion of bacteria and viruses to mucosal surfaces** – often an essential preliminary to their invasion of tissues.

Without the immune response, the inflammatory response is not capable of protecting mammals from infection

Just as we have seen that any major defects in inflammatory mechanisms can be fatal for the host, this is also true of defects in the immune response. A variety of **inherited specific defects in the immune response** have been described, and most of them render the patient so susceptible to infection that early death is almost inevitable. Similarly, **acquired defects in the immune response**, such as those seen in acquired immunodeficiency syndrome (AIDS), or in patients given immunosuppressive drugs, are life-threatening. Thus, in mammals, the inflammatory response seems unable to maintain life for long without the assistance of the immune response.

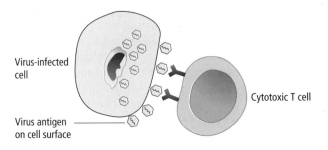

Virus-infected cell

Cytotoxic T cell

Figure 5.7 Reaction of cytotoxic T cell with virus-infected cell, leading to apoptosis.

Virus antigen on cell surface

Normal immune reactions can do harm

We saw in Chapter 2 that there are a number of circumstances in which **the inflammatory response can do harm**—sometimes more harm than good. The spilling of phagocyte contents in diseases like gout and the pneumoconioses are examples. **Because essentially all the immune response does is to boost the inflammatory response, it is not surprising to find that this boosting of inflammation can also do harm, in some circumstances.** The harmful effects of immunity are, as with inflammation itself, the exception rather than the rule, but can result in important disease. The harmful effects, it must be emphasized, are **produced by exactly the same mechanisms as the beneficial effects**. It is purely a matter of clinical judgement as to whether, in a particular circumstance, the effect is helpful or harmful; sometimes it is quite difficult to make this judgement, but the examples below are clearly detrimental to the host. The simplest way to explain them is to retrace our steps through the four elements of the inflammatory response.

I. Boosting production of chemical mediators of inflammation can do harm

The most striking example of harm arising in this way is **inappropriate IgE activity**. This is responsible for a number of diseases, collectively called **atopy**.

Atopy illustrates a phenomenon of general importance, to which we shall return again; it is that **inflammation caused by harmless agents is not only a waste of energy but also often positively harmful**.

Atopic diseases include **asthma** and **hayfever**. Both are due to inhalation into the respiratory tract of harmless particles bearing antigens to which IgE antibodies have previously been produced. Such inhaled particles include pollens, faecal pellets from housedust mites, and many others, **all of which would by themselves not cause disease**. Their antigens encounter the IgE molecules on mast cells in the lining of the nose, nasal sinuses or bronchi; as a result, inflammatory mediators are released (Fig. 5.2), and the damage is done. The most noticeable effects of the inflammation are the excessive secretions (fluor) —watery fluid from the upper respiratory tract in hayfever and excessive mucus in the bronchi in asthma. The inflammatory mediators also lead to the contraction of bronchial smooth muscle and therefore the characteristic difficulty in breathing in asthma.

It was experiments in guinea-pigs that first explained the mechanism of atopy, including the fact that it never occurs on the first exposure to antigen. The experiments also showed that, if the antigen was introduced subsequently into the skin, instead of the respiratory tract, local inflammation occurred at the injection site. This again demonstrates that the mast cells in any tissue can have specific IgE attached, regardless of the site of first exposure. The reaction also provides a means of finding out which antigens are responsible for a particular patient's atopy, because a tiny dose of the responsible antigen injected into the skin will cause inflammation. Indeed, some antigens are encountered more frequently by the skin, in which case there is no respiratory involvement but, instead, a **contact dermatitis**. **Food allergies** are due to the same mechanism, but the reaction takes place in the gut.

Injection of antigens into sensitized animals can result in generalized mast-cell degranulation, with severe bronchospasm and generalized dilatation of blood vessels, which can be fatal—**anaphylaxis**, or **anaphylactic shock**. Rarely, this can cause death in humans, for instance after bee- or wasp-stings.

The reason why some people develop atopic diseases and most do not is a complicated problem which has not been completely settled, but one factor is a hereditary predisposition to production of a high proportion of antibodies of the IgE class after antigen stimulation.

II. Humoral immune mechanisms of cell killing can cause harm

It was easy to see how IgG or IgM attached to microbes enhanced their killing, by opsonization, complement-mediated lysis or by cell-mediated cytotoxicity. It is just as easy to see that if by some mischance the same thing happened to host cells, it could be disastrous. Unfortunately, this does sometimes happen.

The simplest example arises only in the artificial circumstances of **incompatible blood transfusions**. Transfusion of blood to which the patient has antibodies should never happen these days, but when it does (usually due to human error or extreme urgency), the donor's red blood cells are quickly coated with antibody and destroyed in the blood, either by complement-mediated lysis or by phagocytosis of the opsonized red cells by sessile macrophages in sinusoids.

A similar but naturally occurring catastrophe occurs in **haemolytic disease of the newborn**. The fetus is not, of course, genetically the same as the mother and therefore always has some different blood group antigens. This only causes trouble if a strong blood group antigen (usually the **Rhesus antigen** called D) is present on the fetal red cells and not the mother's. The mother is stimulated to produce antibodies to D, because fetal red cells spill into the maternal circulation at around the time of birth (Fig. 5.8). These antibodies do not affect the first baby, but they persist and, during a subsequent pregnancy, the maternal **anti-D** IgG is transferred across the placenta (Fig. 5.8). The red cells in the fetal circulation, if again D-positive, are therefore opsonized by the maternal antibody, and destroyed by sessile macrophages in the fetal spleen and liver. Depending on the severity of the destruction of red cells, the fetus may not survive, or may be severely anaemic at birth.[3]

It seems at first sight unlikely that an individual would actually produce antibodies to his or her own cells, but it can happen in rare circumstances. One was the result of the use of a drug called Sedormid, which was introduced as a sleeping pill. A few patients developed haemorrhages (purpura) after taking the drug. It was found that Sedormid was acting as a hapten, attaching to a large molecule on the surface of blood platelets[4] and thereby eliciting antibodies that led to opsonization and destruction of the platelets. Lack of platelets causes haemorrhages. So **haptens on cell surfaces can lead to cell-killing by antibody-mediated mechanisms**. Examples affecting other cell types will be found in Chapter 6.

3 The disease can now be prevented by injecting anti-D into the mother at the birth of the first child; the antibodies destroy any fetal red cells in the maternal circulation and prevent the immune response.

4 Blood platelets are tiny anucleate cells involved in blood-clotting, as explained in Chapter 14.

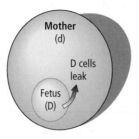

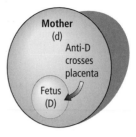

First pregnancy with
incompatible fetus

Second pregnancy with
incompatible fetus

Figure 5.8 Haemolytic disease of the newborn.

III. Immune complexes can cause damage

Although the endocytosis and degradation of toxic large molecules is obviously protective, the complexes formed by harmless molecules and antibodies to them are not always entirely innocuous. We have already noted that endocytosis is often accompanied by **spillage of phagocyte contents**—phagocytes are, in fact, messy eaters. It is certainly possible for tissue damage to result.

The best example of damage of this sort was first shown by a simple experiment. A rabbit is immunized by injection of a harmless antigen, say bovine serum albumin (BSA). After the rabbit has developed circulating antibodies to it, if a further injection of BSA is given into the dermis, there is **rapidly developing local inflammation**. The way this happens is as follows. The antigen is diffusing away from the site of injection; antibody in the blood diffuses in small quantities through the walls of small vessels; and the two meet, in and around these vessels. Immune complexes then form and activate complement. Thus, neutrophils are attracted chemotactically to the site and begin to endocytose the complexes. The endocytosis of the complexes is often incomplete, and lysosomes fuse with the plasma membrane before it has closed off to form an endosome. As a result, oxygen radicals and enzymes are released, causing local tissue damage and more inflammation. This is made more likely because the complexes are forming in antigen excess, which hinders closure of the endocytotic vesicle (Fig. 5.9). This purely experimental example was first demonstrated by Arthus,[5] and known as the **Arthus phenomenon** (Fig. 5.10). It can be prevented if the animals are first artificially depleted of complement or of neutrophils.

However, this same phenomenon, localized to the site of antigen introduction, is the cause of some important spontaneous human diseases, not usually of the skin, but the lung. Various occupations involve inhalation of dusts that are antigenic; antibodies are formed, and subsequent inhalations therefore cause inflammation in the lung exactly as in the Arthus reaction. One example is **farmer's lung**, due to inhalation of non-pathogenic microorganisms in mouldy hay; but there are many others,[6] all due to a variety of antigens inhaled in different occupations.

5 Nicholas Maurice Arthus (1862–1945) was a French bacteriologist.

6 Examples include pigeon-fanciers' disease and maple bark strippers' disease.

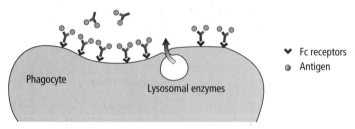

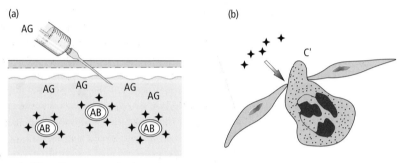

Figure 5.9 Leakage of lysosomal enzymes during immune complex endocytosis, especially in antigen excess.

Figure 5.10 The Arthus phenomenon. (a) Intradermal injection of antigen (AG); antibodies (AB) already present in blood vessels. (b) Immune complexes activate complement (C′), which attracts neutrophils to the site. They then exocytose toxic contents, as in Fig. 5.9.

A related process can take place in the circulation, leading to **serum sickness**. In the early days of serum therapy (passive immunization), the antitoxin (serum) used was from a horse. Three weeks or so after this single injection of horse serum, a proportion of patients developed fever, joint pains and sometimes a rash. Subsequently, it was shown that this **serum sickness** was due to the patient's antibody response to the foreign (horse) protein. The reaction was occurring during the time that the antibody titre was rising, but **the antigen was still present in excess in the blood** (Fig. 5.11). It is now known that serum sickness is due to inadequate uptake of immune complexes, formed in antigen excess, by the sessile macrophages, because the complexes have few available Fc ends (Fig. 5.9). As a result of this inadequate clearance mechanism, **the immune complexes are deposited in small blood vessels**, particularly in kidney, joints and skin. This leads to precisely the same sequence of events as in the Arthus phenomenon, with resultant tissue damage and inflammation. In this case, however, the damage is not confined to the local injection site, because the reaction occurs wherever the immune complexes have been deposited from the blood.

The so-called **vasculitis** (inflammation of blood vessels) that results from deposition of immune complexes in small vessels can also occur naturally. Sometimes the responsible antigen can be identified, but often it is unknown.

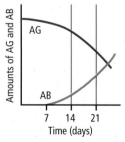

Figure 5.11 Period of danger of serum sickness.

Capillaries and venules are usually worst affected in the various types of vasculitis, but an example involving arteries is a disease known as **polyarteritis nodosa**.[7]

IV. T-cell-mediated reactions can do damage

We have seen repeatedly that the activities of phagocytes can cause tissue damage. This is usually only a minor disadvantage of inflammation, but in some of the diseases where inflammation is boosted by T-cell-mediated reactions, the amount of tissue damage can be quite severe. This is true, for instance, of diseases such as tuberculosis, where there may sometimes be difficulty in interpreting whether the immune response is being helpful or harmful. On balance, however, it must be helpful, because such destructive diseases are most life-threatening in immunosuppressed patients.

A demonstration of the activity of T cells in tuberculosis is seen in the **tuberculin test**, used to test for previous exposure to tuberculosis. A protein extract of *M. tuberculosis* injected into the skin of a normal volunteer elicits no reaction. However, if the subject is suffering from tuberculosis, or has done so in the past, after 48h or so a skin reaction occurs which is quite unlike the **immediate reaction** seen when skin-testing patients with atopic diseases. This **delayed reaction** is due to the slow local accumulation of specific T cells in the skin, followed by macrophage infiltration prompted by lymphokines. Since the tuberculin itself is harmless, the local inflammation is entirely due to the T-cell recruitment and reactivity.

An identical train of events occurs naturally in skin rashes due to exposure to certain chemicals in the environment. Some of the initiating chemicals are naturally occurring (e.g. poison ivy, some insect bites); others are of industrial origin (e.g. certain dyes and chemicals). These conditions certainly represent harmful effects of T-cell-mediated reactions.

Importantly, although it is an unnatural situation, T-cell-mediated reactions contribute to rejection of transplanted organs. This was first shown in experiments on skin grafts in mice.[8] Unless the two mice were genetically identical, skin from one mouse transferred to a wound in the other survived only about 10 days. The graft first became infiltrated with lymphocytes and macrophages and then became necrotic. A second graft from a different mouse led to the same outcome, but **a second graft from the first donor was rejected more rapidly**, suggesting an immune reaction. This memory of a particular graft donor was transferable to another mouse by transfusion of lymphocytes from the first recipient to the second. Mice who had had the thymus removed soon after birth were unable to reject grafts. All of this adds up to a T-cell-mediated reaction, although antibodies are also involved.

Organ transplantation between genetically different humans is of course bedevilled by the problem of rejection, and the recipients therefore have to be given immunosuppressive drugs. It is much more complicated than blood transfusion because tissue cells all carry, in addition to the blood group antigens, large groups of antigens called **histocompatibility antigens**, products of the **major histocompatibility complex**, whose role in the immune response was discussed in the previous chapter.

7 So called because many arteries are involved and the lesions sometimes look nodular.

8 Grafts between members of the same species are **allografts**.

Immune reactions that do harm are usually called hypersensitivity

As we have seen, it is often difficult to judge, but some immune responses are clearly harmful, and these are commonly called **hypersensitivity**, or **clinical hypersensitivity**. This is really an inappropriate term, implying there is something overactive about the reactions. In truth, the reactions are usually perfectly normal; but, because they elicit inflammation in response to a harmless antigen, they are certainly unfortunate.

Equally unfortunate is the common tendency to talk and write about 'immunity' and 'hypersensitivity' as if they were different reactions. You now know that they are not. **They are the same reactions, with varying results**.

You will need to know that in most books, **hypersensitivity is classified into four types** (I–IV), described some years ago by Gell and Coombs. Luckily, these tally with the harmful effects of the immune response mediated through the four components of inflammation (I–IV), as described above, so they are not too difficult to remember.

Therefore: **type I hypersensitivity** refers to harmful results of IgE-mediated mechanisms, including atopy and anaphylaxis; **type II hypersensitivity** refers to killing of host cells by immune mechanisms; **type III hypersensitivity** is damage caused by immune complexes; and **type IV hypersensitivity** is damage due to T-cell-mediated reactions.

You will often find the word **allergy** (literally, 'altered reactivity') used in the same sense as hypersensitivity. It was originally used to mean both immunity and hypersensitivity and would be a useful word with that definition. Unfortunately, usage has now resulted in 'allergic' being taken to mean the same as 'hypersensitive'.

Damage to tissues inflicted by immune reactions to self antigens is called autoimmune disease

Thus far, both the helpful and harmful effects of the immune response we have discussed have all been the result of an **immune response to exogenous antigens**. We have taken for granted that self molecules do not elicit immune responses because of specific tolerance to them.

It is therefore surprising, and not a little alarming, to find that **in some individuals antibody or T-cell-mediated responses can apparently occur to some self antigens**. When this happens, the reactions can lead to injury to tissues and therefore inflammation. This undoubtedly harmful effect is by definition a special example of hypersensitivity, but the important question is —how could it possibly happen? There is no single answer to this question.

One obvious explanation is provided by **sequestered antigens**. Tolerance is acquired during fetal life only if the self antigen is encountered by T lymphocytes. Thus, certain large molecules that are hidden within cells or inside a non-vascularized cavity, for example antigens on spermatozoa, do not elicit tolerance. If some injury allows spillage of such antigens into vascularized tissue, then an immune response will be mounted to them. Antibodies to spermatozoa are found when there is damage to the epididymis, for instance. Another example is seen when the normally sequestered protein, crystallin, in the lens of the eye becomes antigenic after injury to one eye. The antibodies produced can damage the other, uninjured lens, and target it for immune attack. This is sympathetic ophthalmia.

Large self molecules can also become antigenic because they are modified by attachment of a hapten, as we have seen. This is perhaps stretching a point but, because it can lead to disease, such as Sedormid purpura, it is sometimes included as an example of autoimmunity. A more natural example of the same thing occurs when a large self molecule becomes antigenic because it is altered in some way. There are many examples of this, including lipoproteins that become oxidized and proteins that are damaged by microbial enzymes. This mechanism might well have a beneficial part to play in improving scavenging of degraded tissue components, but it can probably also cause disease. For instance, autoantibodies to IgG modified by enzymatic activity probably play a part in the development of **rheumatoid arthritis**.

A third cause of autoimmunity is the occasional **coincidence of epitopes on microorganisms and host tissue**. Streptococci are bacteria, some of which share antigens with connective tissue components. An immune response provoked by the bacteria, when thus misdirected against connective tissue of the heart, is thought to cause the disease known as **rheumatic fever**.

Another way that self-reacting antibodies may arise is the activation of autoreactive clones of B cells as a result of **infection**. Both bacterial endotoxin and a virus called Epstein–Barr virus can do this.

There is still a lot to learn about how autoimmunity can be triggered. One certainty is that there is a genetic element, because particular histocompatibility antigens are associated with autoimmune diseases.

Examples of autoimmune diseases will be mentioned in later chapters.

Summary

The effects of the immune response are almost entirely due to its **ability to boost inflammation**. The result in mammals **is a partnership between the two responses that provides an efficient defence against most infections**. However, because inflammation inevitably does some harm, especially if excessive, so its boosting by the immune response may cause disease, particularly on exposure to harmless antigens. These unfortunate effects are called **hypersensitivity**. Diseases can also arise if an immune response is mounted against self antigens. This is **autoimmune disease**.

6 Chronic inflammation

Inflammation that continues for more than about two weeks is called **chronic**, which simply means **of long duration**. There is no sharp dividing line between acute and chronic inflammation, but most of the inflammatory diseases we call chronic last for months or years if untreated. It is important to note that the healing process occurring after a short-lived inflammatory episode is **not** chronic inflammation. To be chronic, the injury and the inflammation must be **continuing** over a longer period.

Persistent injury causes chronic inflammation

A common cause of persistent injury is **foreign bodies**. This term refers to inanimate indigestible objects that find their way into the tissues, such as bullets, splinters and the like. Anything that cannot be broken down by enzymes or phagocytes may persist in this way—even some self material. For instance, keratin squames from the surface of the skin, if driven into the tissues by accident or disease, are difficult to dispose of and therefore persist.[1]

Persistent injury is also seen in **peptic ulcers** of the stomach and duodenum. If the protective mucosal lining is breached as a result of injury, such as by some dietary indiscretion,[2] then the exposed submucosal tissues may be continuously damaged by the enzymes and, especially, the hydrochloric acid of the stomach contents.

Recurrent injury causes chronic inflammation

The repeated inhalation of noxious vapours, gases or dusts, usually in an industrial environment, causes chronic injury and inflammation in the respiratory tract. Probably the commonest example, though, is not industrial: **tobacco-smoking** leads to chronic chemical injury and inflammation of sinuses, larynx, trachea and, most importantly, to chronic bronchitis. The inflammation causes excessive mucus secretion—hence the chronic cough.

Some of the **industrial dusts**, such as silica or asbestos, also cause severe chronic inflammation in the lung. The general term for these dust diseases of the lung is **pneumoconioses**.

Other, usually much less serious (but memorable) examples include recurrent trauma as a result of repetitive occupational or recreational practices, e.g. tennis elbow, housemaid's knee and osteoarthritis in gardeners or athletes.

1 Another example was called 'jeep-driver's bottom' in the Second World War—hairs over the sacral area were pressed under the skin by repeated trauma.

2 There is also a school of thought that a bacterial infection may be responsible.

99

Some microorganisms cause chronic inflammation because they evade defence mechanisms

All pathogenic microbes have some trick of temporary evasion of the host responses, but there are ways in which microbes can be evasive, and therefore persistent, for longer periods.

An important one is that certain bacteria, including *Mycobacterium tuberculosis* and *M. leprae*, amazingly, can survive for long periods **inside macrophages**. As a result, **tuberculosis** and **leprosy** are diseases which can last for years. Certain protozoa such as *Leishmania* share this ability.

Another mechanism of microbial persistence is antigenic variation—eluding the immune response by changing the antigens expressed on the surface of the pathogen. The protozoa which are responsible for the diseases known as **trypanosomiasis** have this ability and are therefore able to persist in the blood of humans and animals they infect.

Persistent inflammation may be due to lowered host resistance

Worldwide, this is probably the most important cause of chronic inflammation because **malnutrition** leads to inadequacy of inflammatory and immune responses. In these circumstances, injuries that would normally be quickly healed can last for years, and trivial infections persist and even cause death.

Another essential for efficient inflammation and healing is a good **blood supply**. Elderly people frequently have arterial disease which diminishes the blood supply to the lower legs. As a result, trivial leg injuries may lead to chronic skin ulcerations and persistent secondary infection.

The most severe degrees of lowered host resistance, however, are seen in the **opportunist infections**. All pathogenic microorganisms are opportunists, but this term is commonly used only of certain extreme examples, in which organisms that are normally non-pathogenic or of very low pathogenicity cause serious chronic infections. This can only occur in patients whose resistance is drastically lowered by diseases such as **cancer**, where nutrients are being diverted away from defence mechanisms; or by **drugs**. The latter is really a problem created by modern medicine. In certain diseases, drugs such as **cytotoxic agents** or **corticosteroids** have to be given, and this unavoidably impairs host resistance to infection. The same is true of patients who have to receive **immunosuppressive drugs** after organ transplants. In all these circumstances, organisms of normally trivial pathogenicity create chronic life-threatening opportunist infection.

Examples of opportunist infections are varied. Cytomegalovirus, the fungus *Aspergillus fumigatus* and the protozoa, *Pneumocystis* and *Toxoplasma* are typical instances, but there are many others. All of these cause only very mild disease in normal humans, but devastating chronic infections in the immunosuppressed.

Chronic inflammation is sometimes caused by complications of the inflammatory response

The important group of lung diseases caused by industrial dusts, mentioned before (the pneumoconioses) are actually, you will remember, not due to a toxic effect of the dusts. What happens is that macrophages in the lungs are somehow damaged by the particles they have phagocytosed. The lung injury and chronic inflammation which follow are really due to spillage of toxic macrophage contents, including oxygen radicals and lysosomal enzymes, and not directly to the dust itself.

Many chronic inflammatory diseases are the result of hypersensitivity or autoimmunity

Diseases due to hypersensitivity become chronic if the exposure to antigen is recurrent. This is certainly true of **asthma**, in most patients; of **polyarteritis nodosa**, which is a disease due to arterial necrosis and inflammation caused by immune complex deposition; and of many diseases involving cell-mediated hypersensitivity, such as **sarcoidosis**, a granulomatous disease of unknown cause.

Most autoimmune disease is essentially chronic and inflammatory. Usually, the autoimmune damage is centred on a particular cell type, which is the target for the antibodies or T cells (Table 6.1). In a few cases, the autoantigens are not organ-specific and the damage can occur in many parts of the body. Examples include rheumatoid disease, which affects many other tissues as well as joints; this disease is accompanied by antibodies to IgG; and systemic lupus erythematosus, in which the target is DNA.

Some chronic inflammatory diseases are of unknown cause

Examples include Crohn's disease of the bowel and ulcerative colitis.

Histological patterns of chronic inflammation

Although acute inflammation shows similar features whatever the cause— namely, fibrinous exudate and a predominance of neutrophils—the histological pattern of chronic inflammation varies greatly depending upon its cause. This variation is mainly brought about by the different reactions of the host tissues, including some types of immune response, that have time to develop when the

Table 6.1 Examples of organ-specific autoimmune diseases.

Disease	Cell target
Hashimoto's thyroiditis	Thyroid epithelium
Autoimmune haemolytic anaemia	Red cells
Autoimmune thrombocytopenia	Platelets
Insulin-dependent diabetes mellitus	β Cells of the pancreatic islets
Myasthenia gravis	Muscle acetylcholine receptors

injury is chronic. As in healing, the macrophage has a central role in the development of chronic inflammation.

In the simplest form of chronic inflammation, continuing fibrinopurulent exudate is accompanied by persistent attempts at healing

A good example of this is the **chronic peptic ulcer** of the stomach or duodenum (Fig. 6.1). Here a breach in the mucosal lining has allowed continuing injury of the underlying tissue by the hydrochloric acid of the stomach contents. The base of the resulting ulcer consists of three layers. Nearest the stomach cavity, or lumen, there is a **layer of fibrinopurulent exudate**—the injury is continuing, so the processes of acute inflammation continue. But beneath this is a **layer of granulation tissue**, evidence that the inflammation has continued long enough for repair processes to have begun. Frequently beneath the granulation tissue there is **fibrosis**, the result of successful granulation tissue activity.

The exact histological pattern will depend upon the history of that particular ulcer. There is a **dynamic equilibrium** between the tendency of the acid to erode the stomach wall and enlarge the ulcer, on the one hand, and the tendency of the repair process to heal it, on the other. If the acid gets the upper hand, the stomach wall will be progressively eroded until it **perforates**, allowing catastrophic spilling of the stomach contents into the peritoneal cavity. Alternatively, enlargement of the ulcer may lead to erosion of an artery and severe **haemorrhage**. Both of these complications are life-threatening. If the healing process prevails, all the damaged tissue will be replaced by scar tissue, except that the mucosa itself is capable of regenerating over the surface of the scar, and then the threat has been removed.

This **delicate balance** can be influenced by a number of factors. A bland diet, especially accompanied by alkaline substances by mouth, will diminish the injury. Drugs that diminish acid secretion have a similar effect, leading to healing. However, lowered host resistance, especially anti-inflammatory drugs like corticosteroids, may have the opposite effect, and worsen the ulcer.

A similar example is a **chronic abscess**. An abscess may persist if the causative organism is not quickly eliminated. If so, the same three layers of inflammatory exudate and tissue may be found. The abscess cavity contains pus but outside this there will be granulation tissue and perhaps fibrosis (Fig. 6.1). Bacteria with a particular reputation for causing chronic abscesses include staphylococci and *Actinomyces*.

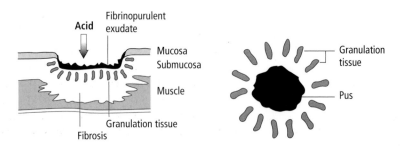

Figure 6.1 Simple chronic inflammation: peptic ulcer (left); chronic abscess (right).

Wherever granulation tissue is found, it contains not only capillary buds and fibroblasts but also a mixture of inflammatory cells, including lymphocytes and plasma cells. This implies that, even in the simplest forms of healing and chronic inflammation, some local immune reaction is involved.

In chronic inflammation the predominant cells may be lymphocytes

Most, but not all, chronic inflammatory lesions contain antigens, and therefore are accompanied by immune responses. Some of them, of course, are actually caused by these responses. In acute lesions, antigens must be conveyed to the local lymphoid tissues (usually lymph nodes) to encounter lymphocytes, but once the condition has become chronic, **lymphocytes can be recruited directly into the lesion, from the blood**. This is done by means of adhesion molecules and in response to cytokines produced by macrophages. The lymphocytes may then be stimulated by antigen presentation within the lesion. As a result, virtually all chronic inflammatory lesions contain some lymphocytes, and often they are the predominant cell type, e.g. in lymphocytic thyroiditis.

In fact, it has been shown in experimental animals that **the majority of lymphocytes in long-standing chronic inflammatory lesions are specific for the antigen that is present in the lesion**. So the majority of lymphocytes around a staphylococcal chronic abscess presumably carry antibodies for the antigens of staphylococci. This has usually been interpreted as meaning that lymphocytes emigrate from blood vessels into chronic lesions at random; those that do not have receptors for the local antigen then migrate onwards, into the lymph or the blood. It is however conceivable that a mechanism exists for selective recruitment of the appropriate lymphocytes. This would demand that the antigen, or fragments of it, were actually present on the surface of the endothelial cells of local venules.

It is interesting to find that the venules in chronic inflammatory lesions are frequently lined by **high endothelium**—the plump, active-looking endothelial cells that are normally found only in the venules of lymphoid tissue. This too hints at some active recruitment associated with this endothelial morphology, whether specific or non-specific.

The lymphocytes in chronic inflammatory lesions are a mixture of T cells and B cells. Either may predominate. Sometimes the B-cell population is made more obvious by the appearance of lymphoid follicles, complete with germinal centres. This is called a **lymphadenoid** infiltrate (meaning a resemblance to lymph node) and is seen in, for instance, Hashimoto's disease of the thyroid.

Plasma cells predominate in some forms of chronic inflammation

In lymph nodes, a B-cell response produces plasma cells that remain in the node and secrete immunoglobulin into the efferent lymph. It is therefore at first sight surprising that plasma cells are frequently found in granulation tissue and in chronic inflammation. Plasma cells do not emigrate from lymph nodes into the blood,[3] so how do they migrate into a chronic inflammatory lesion? The answer is that they don't. **Plasma cells in a lesion must be derived from B**

3 Indeed, normally they are not found in the blood, so the term 'plasma cells' is another ghastly misnomer.

lymphocytes that emigrate into the lesion and are stimulated there by the antigen to produce local clonal expansion, including plasma cell formation.

Considering that plasma cells normally only live a few days, it is astonishing that some forms of chronic inflammation are dominated by plasma cells. This must presumably reflect an immense continuing B-cell recruitment and/or local antigen-driven clonal expansion. Diseases in which plasma cells predominate include **syphilis**, a venereal disease caused by the spiral bacterium *Treponema pallidum*. Syphilis can persist in a patient for decades, so it is certainly chronic!

Eosinophils are frequent in certain chronic parasitic diseases and in some forms of hypersensitivity

Eosinophils are nearly always present in small numbers in any inflammatory exudate, be it acute or chronic.[4] In hypersensitivity, especially the **atopic diseases** like asthma, they are more numerous. They are also unusually frequent in **metazoan parasitic infestations**. This is probably because they are attracted chemotactically by certain molecules secreted by parasites and because mast cells release an eosinophil chemotactic factor, but the mechanisms involved are uncertain. What is certain is that they can contribute to defence against metazoans by attaching to them and exocytosing against them a **major basic protein**, which damages the parasite.

Macrophages are almost always a component of chronic inflammation

Some macrophages are almost always found in chronic lesions, sometimes demonstrably scavenging tissue debris or foreign material. In certain diseases, dense infiltrates of macrophages are the principal feature of the lesions. These include **typhoid and paratyphoid (enteric fever)**, some forms of **leprosy** and some protozoal diseases such as **leishmaniasis**. In these diseases, the macrophages are apparently randomly arranged. When suitably stained, they can usually be demonstrated to contain the microorganisms. In all chronic diseases of this pattern, the macrophages seem to be having difficulty in killing the organisms.

Bearing in mind their ability to present antigens and orchestrate granulation tissue formation, **macrophages seem to be central to the development of all forms of chronic inflammation** (Fig. 6.2).

Granulomas are a feature of certain chronic inflammatory diseases

The term **granuloma** is nowadays mainly restricted to a particular histological pattern of collections of macrophages.[5] It consists of a **tight collection of palely staining, elongated macrophages**, with indistinct cell boundaries. Electron microscopy shows that the macrophages have thrown out interdigitating pseudopods—'linking arms with each other'—because of a high degree of activation. They are sometimes called **epithelioid cells** due to a fancied vague resemblance to epithelium in some cases (Fig. 6.3).

4 They are also a conspicuous component of the leukocytes normally found in the mucosal lining of the gut. The reason is obscure.

5 Originally the term was a macroscopic description of any swelling (-oma) composed of chronic inflammatory tissue, or granulation tissue.

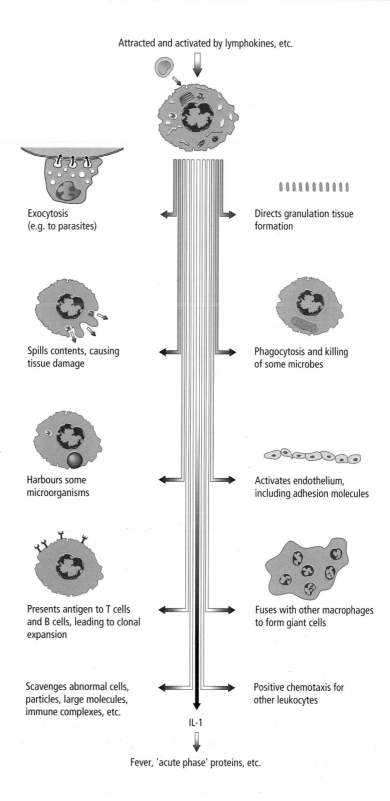

Figure 6.2 Some roles of the macrophage in chronic inflammation.

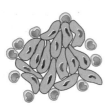 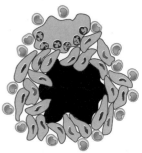

Small granuloma, consisting
of macrophages and some
lymphocytes

Larger granuloma, with
central necrosis and giant
cell formation

Figure 6.3 Granulomas.

Often the granulomas may show additional features (Fig. 6.3). Especially if they are large they may show **central necrosis**, perhaps partly because they have outgrown their blood supply. Frequently the granulomas are **surrounded by lymphocytes**. Not uncommonly some of the excited macrophages may fuse together to form occasional **multinucleate giant cells**. Their nuclei are often arranged around the periphery of the cell—a **Langhans giant cell**.[6]

The typical example of a granulomatous disease is **tuberculosis**, but similar (tuberculoid) granulomas are also seen in other infections such as **brucellosis**, one form of **leprosy** and some fungal and parasitic diseases. Several chronic inflammatory diseases of unknown cause also feature small granulomas, such as **sarcoidosis** and **Crohn's disease** of the bowel.

Most granulomas seem to be due to a T-cell-mediated immune response with lymphokine production. The lymphokines appear to be responsible for the chemotactic attraction, the activation and the retention of the macrophages. It is said that the characteristic high degree of macrophage excitement leading to the epithelioid appearance may be due to the additional factor that the cells have phagocytosed something they are unable to degrade. Perhaps they are not just **activated** (by lymphokines) but also **frustrated**.

There is one other context in which the term granuloma is used—the **foreign-body granuloma**. This is different from those described above, which are sometimes called epithelioid cell granulomas or tuberculoid granulomas. The foreign body granuloma is composed of macrophages, most of which have fused together to form **foreign-body giant cells**, which surround the foreign body (Fig. 6.4). Their nuclei are usually crowded together at the side of the cell nearer the foreign body. The lack of epithelioid collections, and the presence of the foreign body itself, distinguish these lesions from tuberculoid granulomas.

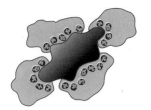

Mainly giant cells
applied to foreign body

Figure 6.4 Foreign-body
granuloma.

Some chronic inflammation is so slow that it appears only as progressive fibrosis

The best examples of this are the **pneumoconioses**, in which the recurrent injuries are almost imperceptible until they have induced areas of fibrosis

6 Theodore Langhans, German pathologist (1839–1915); not to be confused with his compatriot, Paul Langerhans (1849–1888), of greater fame.

which affect lung function. This usually takes many years, and at that stage all one finds is fibrosis of the lung. The patterns of fibrosis differ according to the nature of the dusts—silica seems to be carried into central parts of lung lobules, resulting in roughly spherical nodules of fibrosis (**silicosis**). In **asbestosis**, the asbestos fibres lead to diffuse fibrosis of alveolar walls, and also get carried to the pleural surface, causing massive patches of fibrous pleural thickening.

Chronic inflammation is often accompanied by chronic regeneration

Recurrent cell death leads to recurrent episodes of regeneration, if the affected tissue is capable of it. The regeneration is vital if the injury is at all severe; but sometimes regenerated tissue is not as functionally effective as the original tissue. Chronic injury of the liver by virus hepatitis or alcoholism, for example, leads to chronic inflammation and fibrosis of the liver. Repeated episodes of regeneration occur, but not in such a regular lobular pattern as normal liver; **regeneration nodules** of varying size grow between the bands of fibrosis. Liver function often suffers, because the fibrosis obstructs the blood supply and because the regeneration nodules do not have an orderly arrangement of blood supply and biliary drainage. This combination of repeated necrosis, regeneration and fibrosis of the liver is called **cirrhosis** (Fig. 6.5).

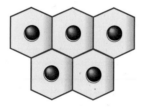

Regular lobular pattern

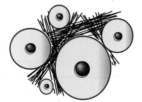

Irregular fibrosis and
regeneration nodules

Figure 6.5 Normal liver and cirrhosis.

Another variant of regeneration may be seen in chronic epithelial injury. Repeated injury to simple epithelia may lead to their eventual replacement by stratified squamous epithelium. Thus cigarette smoking may lead to patchy replacement of the respiratory epithelium of bronchi,[7] by multilayered stratified squamous epithelium. This **redifferentiation** of epithelia might be regarded as an attempt to provide increased protection, but is usually of dubious protective value. It is referred to as **metaplasia**. **Squamous metaplasia** (Fig. 6.6). is not the only example but is by far the commonest.

7 Normally pseudostratified, ciliated, columnar, mucus-secreting epithelium.

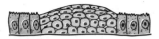

Figure 6.6 Squamous metaplasia in columnar epithelium.

The histological pattern of chronic inflammation is often mixed

Any combination of all the above patterns may occur. In tuberculosis of the adult lung, granulomas and fibrosis are found side by side; in other diseases, eosinophils are usually accompanied by lymphocytes, or plasma cells are mixed with lymphocytes, and so on.

The cause of chronic inflammation can often be suggested by biopsy

Because of all these variations, the diagnosis of chronic inflammatory conditions of uncertain cause can often be discovered if an experienced pathologist is sent a piece of the abnormal tissue for histological examination. Even if the causative agent is not recognizable, the pattern of the cellular reaction gives important clues.

Results of chronic inflammation

Diversion of nutrients can be a major problem

To sustain the long-continued reactions to chronic injury there are huge demands on nutrients, principally to keep up the cell division entailed in the inflammatory and immune responses and in regeneration. In time, this may lead to severe loss of weight and even inadequate production of blood cells, causing anaemia and decreased resistance to other forms of injury, especially infections. This is one main way in which extensive chronic inflammatory disease can cause death.

Fever and leukocytosis result from chronic inflammation

Fever is caused in just the same way as in acute inflammation, although it is usually less severe and often intermittent. The leukocytosis is not the same, however. Whereas in acute inflammation the leukocytes in excess in the blood are always neutrophils, the predominant white blood cell type in chronic inflammation is the same as that found in the lesions. Thus one may find **lymphocytosis, monocytosis, eosinophil leukocytosis or neutrophil leukocytosis** in the blood, in the various diseases.

Chronic inflammation can lead to secondary infection

Even if the cause is not originally infective, many forms of chronic inflammation predispose to secondary infection. The most obvious example is the chemical injury caused by tobacco-smoking. The whole respiratory tract is vulnerable because of the chronic epithelial injury. Amongst other things, the normal protective ciliary activity is grossly impaired, and bronchi become partically blocked by mucus. Smokers are therefore more likely to develop both bacterial and viral infections of the lungs (and nasal sinuses) and eventually these infections can be life-threatening.

A successful outcome is always accompanied by scarring

If the causative agent is eventually neutralized, some degree of fibrosis is always left behind. Patterns and severity of fibrosis obviously depend on the cause, location and severity of the disease, but sometimes scarring of internal tissues is found in which the cause is unknown. One scar looks very much like another.

Chronic inflammation often leads to arterial thickening

An inbuilt reaction of arteries to many forms of injury is that the lining layer (intima) is thickened by smooth-muscle cells laying down collagen and elastin fibres. They are just as capable of doing this as fibroblasts. This diffuse or concentric intimal thickening is frequently seen near chronic inflammatory lesions, whatever the cause, and is called **endarteritis obliterans** (Fig. 6.7). The mechanism is unknown but might be due to damage by immune mechanisms. Particularly good examples are often seen in tuberculosis, syphilis and at the base of chronic peptic ulcers.

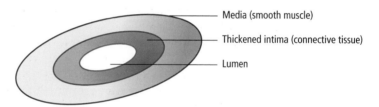

Media (smooth muscle)

Thickened intima (connective tissue)

Lumen

Figure 6.7 Endarteritis obliterans.

A small proportion of patients develop amyloidosis

Amyloidosis is a rather puzzling disease. It consists of the deposition of proteinaceous material (amyloid) in tissues, usually in the walls of arteries or between epithelial cells and their basement membranes. The liver, spleen and kidneys are the organs most frequently affected, but literally any organ or tissue may occasionally be involved.

Very rarely, amyloidosis can occur completely unexpectedly in otherwise normal individuals—**primary amyloidosis**. This has a slight familial tendency. In patients with various forms of chronic inflammation, such as tuberculosis or rheumatoid disease, amyloid deposition is more frequent, and 1–2% of such patients may develop **secondary amyloidosis**. The mechanisms leading to the protein deposition are complicated but there are a number of circumstances suggesting that in some cases it may be related to errors in immunoglobulin production. These include the fact that the highest frequency of the disease (about 5%) is in patients with the malignant tumour of plasma cells —**multiple myeloma**. Also, many years ago it was noted that laboratory animals being **hyperimmunized** for antibody production often developed amyloidosis. The other clue is that some amyloid consists partly of immunoglobulin light chains.

Local lymph nodes are usually abnormal in chronic inflammation

Lymph nodes draining sites of chronic inflammation not uncommonly show **reactive hyperplasia**. This is a broad term that means enlargement of lymph nodes due to stimulation. Histologically one may find hyperplasia of B-cell or T-cell areas, or an increase in the number of macrophages in the sinusoids. Which of these occurs depends on the nature of the chronic inflammatory reaction.

Sometimes the causative agent of the chronic inflammation may get carried to the local lymph nodes, often inside macrophages. If this happens, the nodes may contain lesions of exactly the same pattern as the primary site, for example, lymph nodes draining tuberculous lesions will contain typical granulomas. Therefore biopsy of lymph nodes may provide a histological diagnosis.

Summary

The complexities of chronic inflammation are mainly due to the longer duration giving time for many and varied patterns of immune and inflammatory mechanisms to come into play. Chronic inflammation can be difficult to diagnose, is sometimes of unknown cause, and can be hard to treat successfully. Its continuation and its complications frequently cause death.

7 Bacteria and disease

Bacteria cause many of the diseases that have been the greatest threat to humanity. Plague, tuberculosis, leprosy, diphtheria, cholera and typhoid are some well-known examples. Until recently it was thought that the discovery of antibiotics and vaccines had abolished this threat. Unfortunately, this view that bacterial diseases had run their course was premature.[1] The agents of bacterial disease have proved to be much more resourceful than anticipated. Strains of bacteria which are resistant to all commonly used antibiotics have appeared, new bacterial diseases have emerged, older diseases have returned, and the threat of untreatable bacterial disease–familiar to all our ancestors, but unthinkable a decade ago–is now being taken seriously.

These recent events have reminded us of a simple point which has been easy to ignore, which is that **fast-growing microorganisms can evolve more rapidly than their slowly reproducing hosts**. Changes in human lifestyle also create new opportunities for contact between people and microorganisms. For example, the origin of a virulent kind of pneumonia which came to be known as **Legionnaire's disease** was unidentified until it was recognized that the humidifiers of large air-conditioning systems provided a suitable medium for the growth of the causative bacteria.

This does not mean that it will never be possible to conquer bacterial disease. It has, however, become apparent that the **treatment of these diseases with antibiotics provides an insufficient basis for their long-term control**. More subtle and more varied approaches are needed to understand the mechanisms of bacterial disease in terms of modern molecular and cellular biology. The knowledge gained from these inquiries can be used to devise more sophisticated methods of preventing and treating bacterial diseases. If we cannot always cure a bacterial infection with an antibiotic, we may be able to enhance the body's natural killing mechanisms so that they can do the job for us.

We shall first describe the biological background to bacterial disease. In the following chapter we will take a look at some working examples of important bacterial diseases. Overall, our aim is to inquire into how bacteria are able to cause disease. When we do this we find that the answers are diverse–but they make fascinating stories!

1 Such a point of view ignored, for example, the fact that tuberculosis is one of the commonest infectious diseases, and the numbers have been on the increase for the past several years.

Bacteria are prokaryotes (Fig. 7.1)

This term indicates that the cell is small (0.5–2.0 μm), the bacterial chromosome is not bounded by a nuclear membrane, and organelles such as mitochondria are absent. The cell wall has a particularly complex structure, and is

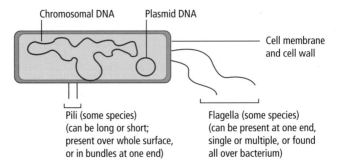

Figure 7.1 A prokaryote.

usually made up of peptidoglycan. The ribosomes are smaller than those of eukaryotes (nucleated cells). Some bacteria are motile, because they possess flagella. Prokaryotic flagella are made up of subunits, which associate to form a single protein fibre.

Disease-causing bacteria possess distinctive characteristics

Many bacterial species can digest and recycle organic compounds. Some of them have evolved further, to exploit the nutrient sources found in animals and human beings. For a microorganism in search of a niche to colonize, a mammal is an ideal hunting-ground. A range of different microenvironments are kept chemically and physically stable, plentifully supplied with nutrients and maintained at a constant temperature. The only catch is that these sites are all protected by defence mechanisms. If they weren't, the body would be in constant danger of microbial degradation.

Only a tiny proportion of the bacteria found in nature are capable of colonizing the body. Even fewer can cause disease. Those that do so are called **pathogenic bacteria**; these are the bacteria which are able to evade, at least temporarily, the body's defence mechanisms, and damage their hosts. **The majority of bacteria and other microbes in the environment are harmless to humans and animals, and fulfil useful functions by recycling a vast array of chemical substances, both organic and inorganic.**

Some harmless bacteria live in close association with animals or humans. The skin, nose, mouth, throat and particularly the large bowel are the home for huge numbers of bacteria that usually do no harm at all. In fact they are positively helpful in crowding out bacteria that could be harmful. These resident bacteria, the **normal flora**, are called **commensal** microbes, because they share the available nutrients with the host. These bacteria are first acquired from the mother and from the environment soon after birth. Distinctive communities of commensal species develop in the mouth, nose, pharynx, and different parts of the enteric and genital tracts (Table 7.1). However, some of these bacteria can live double lives, forming transient commensal associations with their hosts, but in certain circumstances also causing disease. The commensal bacteria also play an important role in providing the stimuli needed for the development of the immune system after birth.

Table 7.1 A few examples of typical normal flora.

Skin	Staphylococci
Nose and throat	Staphylococci Pneumococci
Intestine	*Bacteroides* *Escherichia coli* Clostridia
Vagina	Lactobacilli

What is bacterial infection?

One definition is 'the production of harmful effects by microbes in close contact with the body'. Because some stages of a bacterial infection can be difficult to detect, it is often best to indicate whether the term is intended to refer to overt infection accompanied by disease, or less active relationships such as periods of incubation, states of latency or carriage of bacteria.

Different groups of pathogenic bacteria can be characterized by their structural differences, especially those seen in their cell walls

Most bacteria can be cultured in the laboratory simply by introducing them into a suitable nutrient medium. Mixtures of bacteria can be separated if they are grown on a medium solidified with agar.[2] Individual bacteria then multiply, when they are incubated at 37 °C overnight, into **colonies** of identical organisms. The colonies can be individually sampled for further study (Fig. 7.2).

The two main groups of bacteria, the Gram-positive and Gram-negative bacteria, are so called because they can quickly be distinguished from each other by a staining procedure, known as Gram's stain.[3] These two groups contain the vast majority of all pathogenic bacteria. The stain also reveals, of course, the shape of the bacteria, under the microscope (shown in Fig. 1.3).

2 Agar is an extract of seaweed that can be mixed with a nutrient medium when warmed and solidifies the medium when cooled.

3 Hans Christian Joachim Gram (1853–1938), Copenhagen physician.

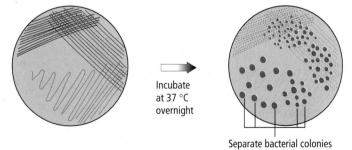

Incubate at 37 °C overnight

Separate bacterial colonies

Figure 7.2 Bacterial culture on agar medium. The bacteria are spread on one segment by means of a wire loop. The loop is flamed to sterilize it between spreading other segments, thus ensuring separate recognizable colonies somewhere on the plate.

In **Gram-positive bacteria**, the bacterial cell membrane is covered by a thick cell wall (Fig. 7.3) composed of numerous layers (approximately 10–20 in different species) of a basket-weave of sugars and amino acids, known as peptidoglycan. Gram-positive bacteria also commonly have protein molecules within the peptidoglycan, or present as crystalline-like arrays over their outer-most surface. Some of them—the streptococci, for example—also have hair-like fibrillae, each one comprising a large protein molecule, which protrudes through the peptidoglycan layer.

Gram-negative bacterial cells have a more complex surface structure, and appear to be a more highly evolved group of microbes (Fig. 7.4). The plasma membrane of the cell is bounded by a thin layer of peptidoglycan, having one or only a few layers. This is surrounded by an additional lipid-rich outer membrane with a complex structure. In general, Gram-negative bacteria have almost double the DNA content of Gram-positive bacteria. The processes of infection due to Gram-negative bacteria are also often more elaborate than those due to Gram-positive bacteria.

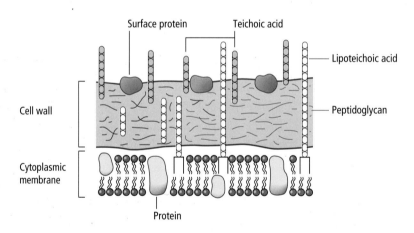

Figure 7.3 Cell wall of Gram-positive bacterium.

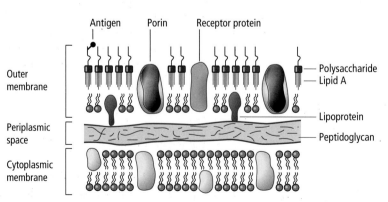

Figure 7.4 Cell wall of Gram-negative bacterium.

Most pathogenic bacteria fall into these groups of Gram-positive and Gram-negative, but there are others which do not

The mycoplasmas

These are small bacteria, unusual because they lack peptidoglycan cell walls. As a result they are variable in size and shape (pleomorphic). They have managed to overcome their potential osmotic fragility by reinforcing their plasma membranes with significant quantities of sterols. Genetically, they are closely related to Gram-positive bacteria. These organisms can cause pneumonia in humans and a variety of animal diseases; they should not be confused with the mycobacteria.

The mycobacteria

Typified by *Mycobacterium tuberculosis* and *M. leprae*, these bacteria have thick outer layers of different types of wax (long-chain hydrocarbons), and glycolipids. They can live inside tissue macrophages and lead to chronic infections—tuberculosis and leprosy, respectively. Their structure is that of a highly reinforced Gram-positive cell.

The spiral bacteria

The spiral bacteria include the bacteria which cause syphilis, *Treponema pallidum*. These organisms are capable of establishing chronic extracellular infections. It is possible that the outermost layers of the syphilis bacteria are composed of relatively non-antigenic lipids; other spiral bacteria survive the host's immune response by varying their surface antigens.

The rickettsiae

The rickettsiae, such as *Rickettsia prowazekii*, which causes the louse-borne disease, **typhus,** are **obligate intracellular parasites**, principally of **endothelial cells**. Several rickettsial diseases are **arthropod-borne zoonoses**—diseases of animals which are transmitted to humans by the bites of infected lice, ticks, fleas, etc. Because the rickettsiae destroy vascular endothelial cells, typhus is a severe haemorrhagic fever. It is one of the diseases which has influenced military balances of power by ravaging great armies. Its power to do this came to a dramatic end during the Second World War, when DDT was first used to kill lice.

The chlamydiae

The chlamydiae are obligate intracellular parasites of epithelial cells. Their cell walls are bilaminate and lack peptidoglycan, and their life cycle involves the differentiation of two cell types: the elementary body, which is transmissible, does not divide and can survive extracellularly; and the reticulate body, which is non-transmissible, and is the form in which the bacteria multiply within the host cell. Chlamydiae can cause pneumonia, urethritis and **trachoma**, which is one of the main causes of blindness worldwide.

Each of these groups of bacteria is subdivided into a number of species

It is worthwhile noting that a bacterial species cannot be defined by the criteria used to define species of higher organisms. Although sexuality exists among bacteria, its occurrence is of no significance in helping to define a species, because true zygotes are never formed, and gene exchange can take place between organisms which are not especially closely related.

Bacterial reproduction is predominantly asexual; genetic variation arises by various types of mutation, by the movement of unstable elements within chromosomes from one site to another, by intra- and interchromosomal recombination, and by the exchange of bacterial plasmids[4] and bacterial viruses[5] (Fig. 7.5).

Species of pathogenic bacteria are often named after the disease they cause. A species frequently contains only a few closely related bacterial strains which have acquired the genetic information required for pathogenic activity. Therefore, for instance, many of the pathogenic strains of *Escherichia coli* can be distinguished from their commensal relatives by their possession of additional chromosomal DNA, containing the genes which encode the virulence determinants. In some cases, some of these virulence genes may be present on extrachromosomal DNA, such as plasmids. **In others, bacteriophages actually introduce the genetic material for exotoxin formation**, and these viruses are therefore entirely responsible for the pathogenicity of the host bacterium (e.g. *Corynebacterium diphtheriae*).

What constitutes a bacterial species remains debatable. Some bacterial genera have been subdivided much more extensively than others, often for historical or practical reasons. Strains of *Salmonella* identified as the cause of epidemics tend to be given species names, but the widely diverse strains of *E. coli* do not. Attempts to rationalize the naming of bacterial species by modern methods based on the comparison of DNA sequences are not yet satisfactory. Bacterial strains are often distinguished by the antigens they carry, by the types of bacteriophage that can infect them, or by the disease syndromes they cause.

In order to explain how a bacterium causes a particular disease, we need to acquire a systematic understanding of the behaviour of the bacterium, outside and inside its host (Fig. 7.6)

In the first instance we need to be sure that we have correctly identified the organism which is causing a particular disease. Then the issues which concern us are: what is the **source** (or **reservoir**) **of infection** for this organism? How does it leave one infected host, and gain access to a new host? **Can it survive in the environment?** If it can, for how long, and in what physical and chemical circumstances? Once inside a new host, what are the key stages in the develop-

4 Plasmids are pieces of genetic material found in the cytoplasm of bacteria. They range widely in size.

5 Viruses that infect bacteria are called **bacteriophages**.

1. Bacterial chromosome: virulence genes may be (a) clustered together, or (b) distributed around the chromosome

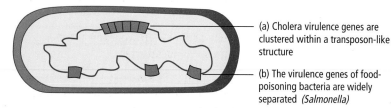

(a) Cholera virulence genes are clustered within a transposon-like structure

(b) The virulence genes of food-poisoning bacteria are widely separated *(Salmonella)*

2. Plasmids: often transferable between bacteria and carry genes which contribute to bacterial disease

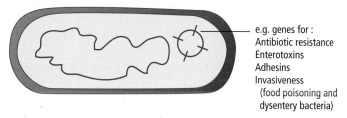

e.g. genes for :
Antibiotic resistance
Enterotoxins
Adhesins
Invasiveness
 (food poisoning and
 dysentery bacteria)

3. Bacteriophages: can introduce DNA which includes a toxin-encoding gene
e.g. diphtheria toxin

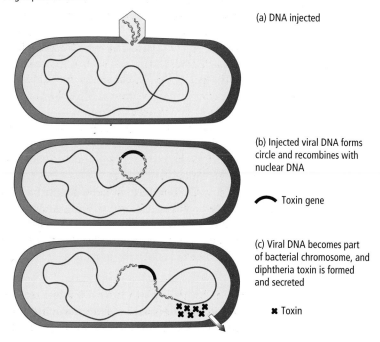

(a) DNA injected

(b) Injected viral DNA forms circle and recombines with nuclear DNA

⌒ Toxin gene

(c) Viral DNA becomes part of bacterial chromosome, and diphtheria toxin is formed and secreted

✖ Toxin

4. Transposons: 'jumping genetic elements' found in plasmids or chromosomes

Transposon DNA   Transposon end: site for recombination

Antibiotic
resistance gene   Bacterial DNA or plasmid DNA

When a transposon jumps, it inserts itself whole into a new site within a plasmid or chromosome, i.e. it remains intact between its ends

Figure 7.5 Location and movement of bacterial virulence genes.

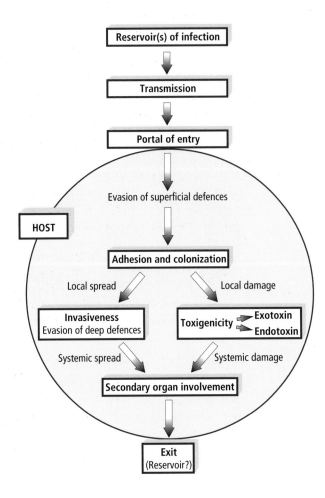

Figure 7.6 Stages of microbial pathogenicity.

ment of the infection, and **how do the bacteria spread within the host**? Which of the stages of association with the host result in the greatest damage, and why? At each step along the way, **which bacterial genes and gene products are crucial to its capacity to cause disease?** Last, but by no means least, we would often like to know why, in molecular and genetic terms, the host is susceptible to infection.

What are the sources from which bacterial pathogens can be acquired?

The source of pathogenic organisms is called the reservoir of infection. Many bacterial diseases originate as a result of contact with infected patients. Active infections in a patient suffering from bacterial disease may result in the bacterial contamination of air, or skin, or faeces, or urine, or the genital tract, depending on the bacterial species and the severity of the infection. If the appropriate exposure to another person takes place, and the means of transmission are available, bacteria from one individual can then be passed on to others. Certain human pathogens are **obligatory human parasites** (for example, the typhoid bacillus, the gonococcus, the meningococcus, the agents of bacterial dysentery, the whooping cough bacillus). In these instances the only possible sources of infection are other humans. These bacterial diseases have evolved so that organisms are shed from infected persons in such a way as to maximize the chances that the bacterium will find a new host. Most of these bacteria can also establish inapparent **carrier states** which provide the organism with a longer period of time in which to be communicated to a fresh host, even after the patient has apparently recovered.

Domestic and wild animals can also serve as reservoirs of human infections. Diseases of animals which are transmissible to humans are known as **zoonoses**. Examples are tuberculosis from cattle, and plague from wild animals, such as rats.

Contaminated air, dusts, soil and water can harbour some bacteria for prolonged periods of time and act as sources of infection. Soil-borne anaerobes—the clostridia—cause a wide variety of diseases in humans and animals, as a result of the profusion of protein toxins produced by different species and strains of these bacteria. **Tetanus** is an example of one such disease.

How are bacterial diseases transmitted?

Respiratory spread is brought about by **the exhalation and inhalation of infected droplets or dusts.** When a person coughs or sneezes an aerosol is formed, and the microscopically small droplets are inhaled by others. Only the smallest droplets reach the alveoli of the lungs.

Outbreaks of food-borne bacterial disease are still extremely common, even in countries in which it ought to be possible to prevent them; hundreds of thousands of such incidents occur each year in the UK alone. Food can become contaminated either as a result of bacteria growing in food animals, or being introduced into food as a result of poor hygiene before, during or after its preparation. The commonest consequences consist of food poisoning, particularly due to *Salmonella* and *Campylobacter* infections and 'traveller's diarrhoea'.[6] Serious systemic infections can be acquired from animals by drinking unpasteurized milk, such as tuberculosis and brucellosis.

Water-borne diseases are commonest in the tropics. This is usually because inadequate sewage disposal and the lack of chlorinated pure water supplies enable pathogenic bacteria to circulate between infected and uninfected individuals via their drinking water. Cholera and typhoid are among the worst of these infections.

Biting arthropods such as fleas, lice and ticks can act as **vectors** of bacterial infection (e.g. plague, by the rat flea). This route of transmission is occasionally mimicked in medical practice, by the inadvertent inoculation of infected blood, or blood products, or intravenous fluids. **Houseflies can transmit infection,** especially if the doses of bacteria needed to establish disease are small (as in bacterial dysentery); in this instance flies can carry bacteria from faeces to food.

6 Traveller's diarrhoea is caused by a wide variety of microorganisms. Pathogenic strains of *Escherichia coli* and intestinal protozoa (see Chapter 13) are especially important.

Exposure to bacterial infection during sexual intercourse can result in the transmission of bacterial agents of sexually transmitted (**venereal**) diseases, such as gonorrhoea, urethritis and syphilis.

Infected inert objects can transmit infection, such as sharp objects contaminated with soil. The use of infected needles for intravenous drug abuse can result in severe local and systemic bacterial infections.

All the methods of transmission considered so far are examples of the **horizontal spread of infection**. **Vertical transmission** is said to occur when the mother is a source of infection for the fetus. **Syphilis** can be acquired congenitally by transfer across the placenta up to the fourth month of pregnancy. **Gonococcal infection** of the eyes of newborn infants by contact with bacteria in the birth canal was once common in the offspring of infected women. **Listeriosis** is usually a mild human and animal infection, due to bacteria (*Listeria*) which are commonly present in the human intestine and in the environment. Infections can be acquired by eating unpasteurized soft cheeses and prepacked salads, because the bacterium is unusually able to grow at low temperatures. *Listeria* can enter a number of different cell types, and can cross the placenta. The consequences in the fetus are variable, but can include stillbirth, premature delivery or severe systemic infection of the newborn infant.

Bacterial infections can also originate as a result of the transfer of organisms from one site to another within the body (endogenous infections)

There are a number of examples of bacterial infections which begin when a bacterium which is living harmlessly as a commensal organism in one site in the body is transferred to another site in which its multiplication results in disease.

The **pneumococcus** is commonly part of the normal flora of the nasopharynx, where it is not known to cause any harm at all. However, if this organism is inhaled into the lungs, **lobar pneumonia** can follow quickly as the pneumococci proliferate.

Staphylococcus aureus is carried inapparently in the nose in most people. From this site it can be transferred by nose-blowing on to the fingers, and thence to minor or major cuts and abrasions elsewhere on the body, where it can establish **purulent wounds**.

The large bowel contains a complex microbial community, made up of literally dozens of bacterial species, some which are **facultative anaerobes**, able to multiply either in the presence or absence of oxygen; most are **obligate anaerobes**, which can only multiply in the absence of oxygen. The individual species of bacteria present in the colon are mostly of low intrinsic pathogenicity. Pure cultures of these gut organisms cannot usually establish infections, except in patients whose immune responsiveness has been destroyed. However, **mixtures of these bacteria can establish severe infections**. The implication is that each individual bacterial species lacks an adequate complement of virulence determinants, but that a functioning set of virulence determinants can be assembled by the mixture of organisms (synergism). Mixed bacterial populations from the gut can gain access to the gut wall after obstruction (e.g. **appendicitis**) or to a skin wound, if the gut is penetrated by trauma or surgery, and faecal contamination occurs. The resulting infections are characterized by their foul smell, due to the production of a range of volatile organic compounds by the anaerobic bacteria present.

Streptococcus viridans are commensal in the human throat. However, after dental treatment or infections in the mouth they may spread in the blood, and form septic foci, or colonize heart valves, especially if these have already been damaged, for example by rheumatic fever.

Different bacterial infections occur with different frequencies in different sections of the population

In this respect it is common to distinguish between community-acquired infections, hospital-acquired infections and occupationally related infections.

Community-acquired infections are by far the commonest and are essentially those which occur in otherwise fit individuals. These infections are generally caused by organisms of high intrinsic pathogenicity, acquired by individuals whose immune system is intact.

Hospital-acquired infections involve a much wider range of bacterial species than community-acquired infections, although the infective agents involved can also overlap. Systemic infections due to Gram-negative bacteria are much commoner in hospitals than in the community. Many different bacterial species are brought into the hospital in and on patients, staff, fruit, flowers and food supplies. Although these bacteria would be unable to establish an infection in healthy individuals, they can sometimes infect patients whose resistance to infection has been lowered by other illnesses, surgery or chemotherapy. Streptococcal pneumonia can be a community-acquired infection—occurring for example following an influenza infection. But it is also much more likely to occur in debilitated, hospitalized individuals, who may inhale their own saliva while lying in bed.

Occupationally related infections occur in veterinarians, farmers, animal attendants, meat inspectors and sewage workers, all of whom may be exposed to zoonotic infections such as brucellosis or tuberculosis.

Overcrowding favours the spread of bacterial infection

Close proximity of infected individuals, coupled with poor hygiene, always favours the transmission of infection, and bacterial disease becomes especially prevalent at times of war or during mass migrations. Tuberculosis became rampant during the early years of the industrial revolution when workers crowded into the cities in search of work.

By contrast, successful containment of infection is often dependent on **isolation**. Infectious disease hospitals used to be known as **isolation hospitals**. Patients with severe infections may still be isolated, or nursed behind barriers within a ward or room of a hospital.

The most extreme form of isolation is **quarantine.** In earlier times ships arriving in port after foreign journeys were obliged to remain isolated for a period so that the authorities could determine whether the sailors were suffering from, or incubating, infectious diseases—of which cholera and smallpox (a virus disease) were the most feared.

Bacterial infections can only become established if an appropriate dose of bacteria is transferred from the source of the infection to a susceptible subject

In thinking about the transmission and onset of bacterial disease it is important to recognize **that different doses of bacteria are needed to initiate different infections**. Only 10–100 *Shigella* bacteria are needed to cause bacterial dysentery. By contrast, cholera or typhoid fever can only begin if millions of bacilli are ingested. The reasons lie in the differing susceptibility of these bacteria to stomach acid. If cholera bacilli are given to volunteers in a concentrated solution of bicarbonate of soda, the infectious dose can be reduced 10 000-fold.

This example indicates that the dose of bacteria needed to establish an infection is not an immutable number; it can vary widely, depending on the level of host resistance. **The influence of host susceptibility on the occurrence of bacterial infections is one of the most important features governing the incidence of bacterial infections.**

Pathogenic bacteria engage in a variety of different relationships with their hosts

Bacterial infections certainly do not follow one single, predictable pattern. Instead we can distinguish between a number of different types of bacterium–host relationships.

Acute infections have a rapid onset and short duration (days to weeks), and are the commonest type of bacterial infection, caused by relatively fast-growing bacteria. Streptococcal and staphylococcal infections of wounds or gastroenteritis due to salmonella food poisoning are good examples of acute infections.

Chronic infections last for weeks or years, and usually arise when the invading bacteria grow slowly, or can hide away in sites which are largely inaccessible to the body's defence mechanisms, or can escape the immune response by varying their surface antigens. Genetic defects in the functions of phagocytes or the immune system or reduced host resistance due to malnutrition can also result in chronic susceptibility to infection, but in some of these instances the episodes of infection more closely resemble repeated acute infections.

Tuberculosis and leprosy are classical examples of chronic bacterial infections. The bacteria which cause these diseases replicate slowly—once every day or so. These bacteria do not produce toxins, but damage their hosts because the combined effect of high bacterial load and the prolonged duration of the infection elicit harmful host responses, particularly sustained or uncontrolled chronic inflammation, and cell-mediated (type IV) reactions.

122

Protected sites within the body, for bacteria that grow in the absence of oxygen, can be found within **necrotic debris**, which is why removal of this debris (debridement) is one of the prime tasks of the surgeon. Protected sites can also be created by medical treatment. Indwelling catheters, for instance, may become colonized by the usually harmless bacterium *Staphylococcus epidermidis*. This bacterium can glue itself to the surface of the catheter by secreting a polysaccharide slime, which also makes it difficult for phagocytic cells to attack the bacteria.

The latent state is a suspension of damaging activity on the part of the bacterium. Tubercle bacilli, for instance (*M. tuberculosis*), can become walled off within fibrosed or calcified lesions, and remain in a latent state for many years, only to be reactivated by a decline in the immune competence of the host. This shows that even in the latent state the body maintains a continuing antibacterial activity, presumably mediated by macrophages.

The carrier state is another important type of host–bacterium relationship; carriers are individuals who can act as a reservoir of infection for others and may not suffer from disease themselves. Individuals most commonly act as carriers when a pathogenic bacterium can either establish a commensal relationship with the host, or give rise to inapparent or chronic, low-grade infections.

Commensal carriage—sometimes transient, sometimes permanent—is common because many human bacterial pathogens are so highly host-adapted. Several species of streptococci and staphylococci, and the meningococci associated with bacterial meningitis, are constantly present in the nose or throat of a proportion of the population. Women who suffer from recurrent cystitis due to specific strains of *E. coli* commonly carry these strains in their colonic microflora; treating the cystitis will not free them of the chance of reinfecting themselves. In an outbreak of diphtheria many more people carry the bacteria in their nasopharynx than suffer from the disease. In the case of commensal carriage and chronic low-grade infections the carrier state is either **asymptomatic or barely apparent.**

Chronic infection can result in the infected person acting as a carrier. This happens in tuberculosis when the infected individual is discharging live bacteria. In the case of tuberculosis the patient will probably be displaying at least mild symptoms of disease, such as a chronic cough. Gonococcal infections in the female urogenital tract may be asymptomatic; nevertheless the carrier is capable of infecting her partner. In fact, communication of gonorrhoea from an asymptomatic woman to her sexual partner can provide a sensitive (and unexpected!) diagnostic test for a low-grade infection which has escaped detection, since gonorrhoea is almost always symptomatic in men. Carriers of salmonella food-poisoning bacteria or of typhoid fever may discharge the bacteria in their faeces for many months after they are free of symptoms. Typhoid carriers commonly have low-grade infections of their gallbladders, and discharge bacilli into the bile (and thence into their faeces) for years after an episode of disease.[7]

7 Typhoid Mary was a cook in New York who infected the families of a series of her employers for some years before being detected.

Epidemics of certain bacterial disease can therefore only be brought fully under control if steps are taken to identify and treat carriers as well as those suffering from disease.

Bacterial infections may be localized or generalized

Some bacterial infections develop at their site of first entry (the **portal of entry**), and rarely if ever invade beyond them. The **cholera bacillus** (*Vibrio cholerae*) attaches itself to the epithelium of the gut, and produces all the symptoms of cholera without either killing the gut epithelial cells or invading the body. The **whooping cough bacillus** (*Bordetella pertussis*) destroys the ciliated epithelium of the bronchial tree, but it does not produce a generalized infection.

In other instances it is common for bacteria to spread away from the initial site of colonization. In the case of some bacteria, such as those which cause bacterial dysentery, the spread may be only local, through adjacent cells of the gut epithelium. In other infections, such as streptococcal infection, bacteria may enter the local lymphatics, or gain access to the blood stream.

Once an epithelial surface has been breached, bacterial spread may occur within a plane of connective tissue, or within the peritoneal, pleural and peri-cardial cavities. However, the details of bacterial behaviour in these sites differ from species to species, and even from strain to strain of bacterium. The presence of the bacteria in the tissues causes acute inflammation, rendering the tissues swollen with exudate. Bacteria can spread through tissues within the inflammatory exudates—the most dramatic example of this is the rapid dissemination of pneumococci within the lungs in **lobar pneumonia**.

Once organisms have gained access to the blood stream, either via the lymphatics, or as a consequence of direct invasion of small blood vessels, a state of **bacteraemia** exists and any organ is open to infection. The activity of sessile macrophages, or antibodies, or acute-phase proteins, or complement may suc-cessfully prevent bacterial multiplication in the blood. But an increase in the numbers of pathogenic organisms in the blood stream (a condition referred to as **septicaemia**, or **sepsis**) is life-threatening. **Meningococcal septicaemia** can be particularly acute, with a patient complaining of flu-like symptoms in the morning and dying a few hours later. Here **sepsis** leads on to infection of the membranes (meninges) surrounding the brain and to **endotoxic shock** in which the bacteria trigger a series of highly damaging events which are difficult to control. These can include vascular endothelial damage, a surge in cytokine output, intravascular coagulation, a dramatic increase in capillary permeability and an uncontrollable fall in blood pressure. These processes are induced by **endotoxins** from Gram-negative bacteria, but shock can also be induced by cell wall components from Gram-positive bacteria, and by certain exotoxins secreted by Gram-positive bacteria.

How do we recognize the presence of bacterial infection?

In its commonest form—that of skin infection—bacterial disease is familiar to anyone who has experienced a cut or scratch which has become infected and turned septic, so that pus is formed.[8] Bacterial infection can also occur inter-nally, for instance when the mucous membranes in the lungs are first damaged by influenza viruses, and the broken membrane is secondarily infected by bacteria. Bacterial infection can occur without prior wounding, if the organism is sufficiently invasive.

8 Pus is a mixture of live and dead bacteria, bacterial products, inflammatory exudate, neutrophils and necrotic debris from cells killed by the bacterial toxins.

124

Intense inflammatory reactions, especially when these are accompanied by the formation of pus, can indicate that bacterial infection is taking place. However, we cannot usually tell from inspecting the wound what kind of bacteria are doing the damage. In order to find out which bacterial species are present we have to **sample the infected site, grow the bacteria in the laboratory and identify the pathogenic bacteria**.

When bacterial infections develop invisibly, deep within the tissues, their presence may be indicated by specific clinical events, as in **tetanus** or **meningitis**. However, the presence of bacterial infection does not always give rise to a diagnostic set of symptoms—the patient may simply complain of feeling unwell, or of having a fever. In this case a search has to be made for possible sites of infection.

Various tests have been developed to aid the diagnosis of specific bacterial infections. For the most part these tests depend on detecting the presence of the bacterium itself, or of antibodies which have been formed in response to it, or of DNA or other products which characterize the bacteria.

Some bacterial pathogens are 'single-disease' organisms; others give rise to a range of disease syndromes

Typhoid fever bacilli (*Salmonella typhi*), tetanus bacilli (*Clostridium tetani*) and cholera vibrios are each essentially associated with a single set of symptoms. Other bacteria crop up in a range of different settings, and may be associated with a number of apparently different diseases.

Many bacterial species cause disease simply because **they cause inflammation and pus formation in whatever tissue they invade**. These are **pyogenic infections**. Staphylococci or streptococci can produce disease in this way anywhere in the body. Pathogenic staphylococci in a hair follicle cause a boil, but in the lungs they can lead to a fatal pneumonia.

Of these more versatile organisms, *E. coli* is a striking example. Most strains of *E. coli* are commensals in the gut. However, others precipitate diseases. Some strains do so in the gut itself. They can produce mild diarrhoea, but some cause dysentery and others, enteric disease with kidney involvement. Different strains commonly lead to urinary infections; others, by contrast, to pneumonia, meningitis and septicaemia. Genetically different forms of *E. coli* give rise to each of these different conditions; they possess disease-forming properties which their commensal relatives lack. In other words, each pathogenic strain of *E. coli* produces a different set of virulence determinants.

Bacterial infection is no longer viewed as a process in which bacteria grow and develop in their hosts in the same mechanical fashion which results in the appearance of a bacterial colony on a plate of nutrient medium

Typhoid bacilli enter the body in contaminated food or water, pass through the stomach into the intestine, attach to specific cells in the epithelium of the gut, and multiply inside them before gaining access to the subepithelial tissue.

They are then ingested by macrophages and transported to the liver and spleen. Obviously these bacteria encounter a rapidly changing set of physical and chemical conditions, and a variety of different protective mechanisms and host cell types along the way. They have to adapt themselves to grow successively: (i) in the gut lumen; (ii) in endocytotic vesicles within epithelial cells; (iii) in the subepithelial tissue fluids; and (iv) within phagocytic vesicles in macrophages. These adaptations are only made possible by swift variations in the expression of genes encoding virulence determinants and metabolic pathways.

Pathogenic bacteria are constantly reorchestrating the expression of their repertoire of virulence genes, in order that the programme of bacterial reproduction within the host can be satisfactorily completed. **It is the possession of a repertoire of virulence genes together with the capacity to coordinate its expression which distinguishes a pathogenic bacterium from a non-pathogenic bacterium.**[9]

The structural components, or soluble products, of a bacterium which are involved in its capacity to cause disease are known as its virulence determinants (Fig. 7.7)

Two major goals of microbiology are to identify the molecules which enable a bacterium to cause disease, and to determine how the genes which encode these molecules are regulated. Considerable progress has been made towards the achievement of these goals.

One way to summarize the properties of pathogenic bacteria is to regard the bacterial cell as a living delivery system for the various macromolecules which eventually result in its capacity to cause disease (Fig. 7.7). These molecules fulfil a number of functions: they may enable the bacteria to fasten themselves to their host, or protect the bacteria from host defence mechanisms, or damage the host's cells, or elicit inflammatory and immune reactions, some of which can be harmful to the host.

Notice that these macromolecules are either derived from structural components of the bacterium, particularly its cell wall, or they are soluble products secreted by the bacteria. In order for infection to occur and disease to result, certain structural components and soluble products are formed in an orderly fashion, so that the bacteria can **adhere to host tissues and establish an initial site of colonization.** Subsequently bacteria may release **toxins and auxiliary factors such as enzymes, invade tissues and multiply within the tissue spaces. Some bacteria also enter host cells** and multiply within them—either transiently, within epithelial or endothelial cells, or for more prolonged periods within macrophages.

The patterns of disease caused by different bacterial species differ, but the above themes continually recur.

In acute infection, the capacity of pathogenic bacteria to multiply much faster than the cells of their hosts becomes overwhelmingly apparent. The host has to gain control over bacterial multiplication rapidly, or the entire host would, within a matter of hours be transformed into bacterial cytoplasm!

9 It is therefore reassuringly unlikely that any single act of gene transfer would convert a commensal bacterium into a pathogen.

126

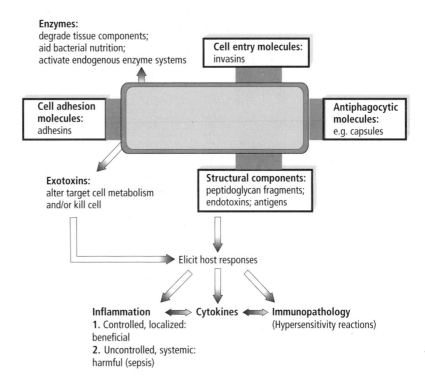

Enzymes:
degrade tissue components;
aid bacterial nutrition;
activate endogenous enzyme systems

Cell entry molecules:
invasins

Cell adhesion
molecules:
adhesins

Antiphagocytic
molecules:
e.g. capsules

Exotoxins:
alter target cell metabolism
and/or kill cell

Structural components:
peptidoglycan fragments;
endotoxins; antigens

Elicit host responses

Inflammation ⟷ Cytokines ⟷ Immunopathology
1. Controlled, localized: (Hypersensitivity reactions)
beneficial
2. Uncontrolled, systemic:
harmful (sepsis)

Figure 7.7 Bacterial virulence
determinants: a diagrammatic
overview.

The mediators of bacterial attachment to their hosts are known as bacterial adhesins

Bacterial adhesins are either sticky prongs, or glues (Fig. 7.8). They enable bacteria to attach themselves to host cells or to tissue matrix proteins, teeth or bone. Attachment is important because it can target bacteria on to the host cell types which they are adapted to enter or damage, and prevent the flow of mucus or tissue fluids washing them away.

Prongs with sticky sides or ends are known as pili. These are formed by Gram-negative bacteria and are filamentous structures whose major function is one of initial longer-range contact with specific carbohydrate or glycolipid receptors on host cell surfaces. The pili bind to their receptors using 'sticky' protein subunits.

Adhesive glues formed by bacteria are usually proteins, slimy glyco-proteins or carbohydrates. In some Gram-negative bacteria, the adhesin proteins do not form a filamentous structure but appear in electron micrographs as amorphous aggregates of surface protein. In other Gram-negative bacteria, proteins found in the outer membrane may act as adhesins, e.g. in the whooping cough bacillus one of the outer membrane proteins may assist binding to ciliated epithelium; similarly, some outer membrane proteins found in salmonella, gonococci and other bacteria act in the same way. The pus-forming streptococci have the outermost surfaces of their thick

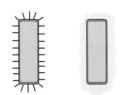

Bacterium with   Bacterium with
pilus adhesins   amorphous adhesins

Figure 7.8 Bacterial mediators
of attachment.

127

cell walls coated with a protein (F protein) which binds strongly to the tissue matrix protein, fibronectin. Tooth-decay bacteria fasten themselves to the surface of teeth by using sugar in the diet to make a slimy carbohydrate glue.

The principal mediators which protect bacteria against host defence mechanisms act against phagocytes and serum-mediated lysis (Table 7.2)

Antibodies and complement can promote the lysis and/or the phagocytosis of bacteria. For this reason **any invasive bacterium has to avoid these mechanisms if it is to survive**. The main ways that bacteria ensure their survival are to coat themselves in capsules which do not activate phagocytosis nor the alternative complement pathway. Alternatively, they may render complement activation ineffective. Bacteria also protect themselves by inhibiting phagocyte migration, by poisoning phagocytes or reducing the effectiveness of antibacterial killing mechanisms, or by degrading serum proteins which promote phagocytosis. Bacteria may also evade the host's immune response by a variety of methods such as switching surface antigens, or coating themselves in host-derived molecules.

Table 7.2 Examples of mechanisms of bacterial evasion of host responses.

Evasion mechanisms	Examples
Forming capsules to prevent phagocytosis	Pneumococci; many other invasive bacteria
Killing phagocytes and/or reducing the efficiency of their killing mechanisms	Exotoxins secreted by many different bacteria have these effects
Antagonizing complement activation (and subsequent bacterial opsonization or lysis). Several mechanisms: e.g. addition of or presence of sialic acid mimics self cell surface, and prevents activation of the alternative complement pathway	Gonococci
Impeding neutrophil chemotaxis and activation by secretion of enzymes which cleave relevant complement component	Streptococcal C5a protease
Ability to resist complement-mediated lysis. Evolution of bacterial strains with more abundant lipopolysaccharide on their outer membrane	More virulent strains of *Salmonella*

Changing surface antigens:
  Switching off pilus adhesin expression to make bacteria less antigenic
  Substituting new surface antigen to 'outwit' immune system
	Meningococci
	Escherichia coli strains which cause meningitis
	Gonococci

The molecular mediators of bacterial entry into cells are known as invasins

A number of different bacteria, particularly those that cause disease in the gut, are able to cross an epithelial cell layer. Some of these bacteria, for instance salmonella, are able to induce cells which are not normally phagocytic to phagocytose them. The molecules in the bacterial outer membrane which mediate these events are known as **invasins**.

The principal mediators of direct host cell damage are the exotoxins

There are many different bacterial exotoxins. In fact, at one time bacterial pathogenicity was thought to consist of little else other than the actions of exotoxins.

Bacterial exotoxins are poisonous proteins. There are two main types of exotoxins: those which act by **damaging cell membranes**, and those which can enter cells and **interfere with some vital aspect of cell metabolism**. The membrane-damaging proteins act either as enzymes which can degrade cell membrane components (e.g. the phospholipases from gas gangrene bacteria) or they form pores in the membranes (e.g. the lysins from staphylococci). The exotoxins which act intracellularly (such as cholera toxin) are enzymes with exquisite substrate specificity.[10] Exotoxins whose modes of action fall outside this neat division are being increasingly recognized. For instance, there are those which can form a bridge between the outside edges of the T-cell antigen receptor, and the antigen-presenting molecule on a macrophage; this fools the T cell into behaving as it would after receiving a specific antigenic stimulus, so that it begins to divide and secrete cytokines. Such toxins are said to behave as **superantigens**.

Other exotoxins are known whose modes of action are not yet understood. For example, some strains of staphylococci release a toxin which attacks the junctions between the superficial and deep layers of the epidermis. Children suffering from such an infection have extensive blistering, as if they have been dropped into scalding hot water.

Enzymes secreted by invasive bacteria may augment toxic tissue damage or enhance invasiveness

The spread of certain bacteria through mucus, connective tissue, pus or necrotic tissue is enhanced by their secretion of degradative enzymes. It is sometimes not clear whether these enzymes are primarily concerned with ensuring bacterial nutrition and growth *in vivo*, or with pathogenicity. The distinction may be artificial: successful bacterial growth *in vivo* is, after all, an essential aspect of bacterial pathogenicity. Bacterial enzymes which activate the host's endogenous enzymes are also known (such as plasminogen activator) and may be important, for example, in promoting bacterial dissolution of blood clots or the penetration of basement membranes underlying epithelial cells.

10 For example, the Shiga toxin, produced by dysentery bacteria, cleaves the *N*-glycosidic bond present in just one out of many thousand adenosine molecules found in ribosomal RNA.

129

Some bacterial components damage the host by triggering one or other of the body's key enzyme cascades to a pathological extent, or by eliciting harmful immune responses

Apart from exotoxins, certain structural components of bacteria also display toxic activity. The toxic constituents of Gram-negative bacteria are known as **endotoxins**. Bacterial endotoxins are **lipopolysaccharides** found in abundance in the outer membrane of Gram-negative bacteria. They are released from dying bacteria, and by the pinching-off of small regions of the outer membrane that can occur during bacterial growth. They become a major cause of host damage when Gram-negative bacteria gain access to the blood stream and multiply there in substantial numbers.

Endotoxins are key initiators of the harmful, elicited host response known as **septic shock**. Their toxicity is due to their capacity to cause the massive release of cytokines from macrophages, to activate the complement and clotting cascades, and to stimulate the formation of other inflammatory mediators such as prostaglandins and leukotrienes. Although small quantities of endotoxin can activate macrophages, the release of substantial quantities of endotoxin into the circulation is very harmful, leading to the formation of thrombi and an uncontrollable, generalized state of inflammation. Eventually the endothelium of small blood vessels in all major organs is so damaged that there is **widespread vasodilatation**; the subsequent fall in blood pressure leads to a failure to oxygenate key organs, and death due to multiple organ failure. In localized infections endotoxins will trigger acute inflammation by activating complement.

Although not endotoxins, certain cleavage products of the cell walls of Gram-positive bacteria can also elicit or enhance shock syndromes in Gram-positive sepsis.

The immunopathological consequences of bacterial infection are most apparent in chronic infections and in certain types of disease due to streptococci. In tuberculosis the sites of bacterial growth become the foci of cell-mediated hypersensitivity reactions. Some streptococcal infections trigger an immune attack on self components in connective tissue, especially in the heart − a condition known as **rheumatic fever**. Other streptococcal infections lead to the accumulation of antigen–antibody complexes in the blood stream. These lodge in kidney glomeruli, and become the sites of highly active and damaging acute inflammatory reactions (poststreptococcal glomerulonephritis).

Summary

In order to cause disease a bacterium needs to be able to attach itself to the host, and begin to multiply. As it does this it must avoid being killed by the defence mechanisms which safeguard the body's epithelial surfaces. As it spreads from its initial site of colonization it must also be able to adapt its metabolism so that it can obtain nutrients to support its growth in different host environments as it encounters them.

If the bacterium gains access to the subepithelial tissues it has to be able to avoid being killed by the mechanisms of innate and acquired resistance which operate within the deep tissues; in particular it needs to resist being lysed by serum complement, or being killed by phagocytic cells. Finally, the bacterium usually needs to be able to replicate in suitable sites within the host which enable it to be transmitted to a new host, or be discharged into the environment in such a way as to favour its chances of survival until it can enter a new host.

The molecular basis for this programme of events is the coordinated expression of genes which encode bacterial virulence determinants.

When bacterial disease occurs, how can we be sure that we have correctly identifed the causative agent of the disease?

The criteria developed for this purpose were first clearly enunciated by the pioneer Robert Koch[11] more than a century ago, in relation to his discovery of the cause of tuberculosis.

A modern statement of these rules would be:

1 the infectious agent should be present in each and every case of the disease, and its distribution in the body (or that of its harmful products) should accord with the pattern of lesions seen;

2 the infectious agent should be recovered from infected individuals, and be established in pure culture in the laboratory;

3 inoculation of samples of the pure cultures into experimental animals (or human volunteers) should cause the same disease;

4 when recultured from the experimental animals or human volunteers, the original bacterium should be recovered.

Koch's postulates cannot always be fulfilled as readily as they were in the case of tuberculosis. There are a number of reasons for this. It may be impossible to grow the infectious agent on the available laboratory nutrient media, or the agent may prove to be a host-specific parasite, in which case it will neither grow in nor reproduce the symptoms of the original disease in laboratory animals. For example, the bacteria which cause gonorrhoea and certain types of meningitis will only grow in humans; these diseases cannot be reproduced in animals exactly as they occur in human beings.

Even today, neither the leprosy bacillus nor the spiral organism which causes syphilis has been grown in nutrient media in the laboratory, although the leprosy bacillus will grow under the skin of the nine-banded armadillo! But it is only because there is a constant association between the presence of certain highly characteristic bacteria and certain equally characteristic lesions that we accept that *Mycobacterium leprae* causes leprosy and that *Treponema pallidum* causes syphilis. Formally, Koch's postulates have never been fulfilled for these diseases.

Another problem which can arise is that the **cultured bacteria may undergo rapid changes in phenotype** and may lose their capacity to initiate human infections when they are subcultured in laboratory media. In this case the lack of host-specific signals results in the bacteria ceasing to express key virulence

11 Robert Koch (1843–1910), German microbiologist; awarded the Nobel prize in 1905.

131

determinants such as adhesins or antiphagocytic capsules. It is no use trying to study which of the macromolecules in such bacteria lead to disease—they have long since disappeared.

Among the many points which can be made concerning the usefulness of Koch's postulates or the difficulties which may be encountered when trying to apply them is the issue of the importance of **factors affecting host suscepti-bility**. Cystic fibrosis patients are uniquely susceptible to damage to their lungs caused by long-term colonization of the thickened mucus present in their lungs by a bacterium called *Pseudomonas aeruginosa*. Koch's postulates cannot be tested simply by inoculating the bacteria into the lungs of a normal animal. Instead, mice belonging to a mutated strain must be used. In these mice the homologue of the gene which is mutated in human cystic fibrosis is also abnormal. In parallel fashion, many hospitalized patients suffer from **oppor-tunistic bacterial infections** which are only ever seen in people whose immune systems are depressed; these are due to bacteria of such low virulence that the infections they cause cannot be meaningfully reproduced in accordance with Koch's postulates.

How are new bacterial diseases recognized?

When a new bacterial disease emerges it is usually recognized by the recurrent observation of a particular pattern of signs and symptoms indicative of the presence of an infectious agent, but differing in some respects from all pre-viously known types of communicable disease. A set of criteria defining the condition are established, and these criteria are given publicity so that phys-icians can be alerted to the existence of the condition. Collaborating physicians and laboratories then report the cases they observe, and provide tissue and serum samples for bacteriological and serological analyses. The major aim is to identify the causative agent as quickly as possible. As far as possible Koch's postulates are used as a guide.

Correctly attributing particular diseases to particular infectious agents can sometimes be difficult. The issues become more complex when disease syn-dromes arise only as a result of mixed infections, or prolonged (chronic) infec-tion. For example, infection of the stomach with a spiral bacterium called *Helicobacter pylori* is associated with the subsequent appearance of stomach disease, including human gastric ulcers, and possibly even gastric cancer, occurring years after the initial infection. When this bacterium was first de-scribed, there was much scepticism that any bacterium could live for long enough in the acid conditions prevailing in the stomach to cause stomach ulcers. Among the crucial experiments was one in which Koch's postulates were put to the test by an Australian scientist who became interested in these stomach-dwelling bacteria. He swallowed a large number of the organisms. When his stomach was monitored by endoscopic examination, and bacterial samples were also taken, it was found that he had developed gastric lesions from which the same bacteria could be isolated.

Another example is the bacterial pneumonia now known as Legionnaire's Disease, first discovered among a number of US war veterans attending a conference in Philadelphia. Some developed severe pneumonia; the reason for this was initially unidentifiable. Only a massive effort coordinated by the Centers for Disease Control in Atlanta, Georgia led, several months later, to the recognition of what was then a previously unidentified bacterium, now called *Legionella pneumophila*, and an established cause of more recent outbreaks of pneumonia in many parts of the world. Large air conditioners and power-station cooling-towers provide reservoirs of this infection unless they are carefully monitored.

Host susceptibility is a crucial factor in determining whether or not bacterial infections occur (Fig. 7.9)

Everyday experience tells us that we seem to be more prone to suffer from infections at some times than at others; also that some individuals are more prone to infection than others. These observations have a sound scientific basis. **The integrity of the body's innate and acquired mechanisms of resistance is overwhelmingly important**; the efficiency of these mechanisms can be enhanced or reduced in ways which materially alter our susceptibility to bacterial infections of any given dose.

Resistance mechanisms operate at two levels in the body: the local defence mechanisms guarding the skin and mucous membranes, and the systemic defence mechanisms guarding the deep tissues and organs

The local defence mechanisms

There is a vast surface area of mucous membrane within the body—estimated at up to 400 m². Much of this area is accessible to pathogenic bacteria. Bacterial binding and survival are antagonized by mucus secretion and flow, aided by

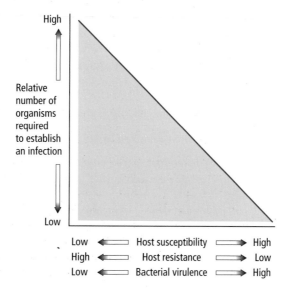

Figure 7.9 Diagrammatic view of the relationship between bacterial virulence and host susceptibility. The slope and shape of the line is different for different bacteria.

133

ciliary action in the upper respiratory tract; the mucus forms a protective layer over the epithelial cells and entangles and removes bacteria. Mucus secretions also contain the bacterial cell wall-degrading enzyme, **lysozyme**, and the iron-binding protein, **lactoferrin**.[12] On the skin, fatty acids in the secretions of sebaceous glands have antibacterial activity. In the gut, bacteria may be killed by stomach acid and by the detergent action of bile salts, which disrupt the bacterial cell membrane. **These innate mechanisms are reinforced by the activity of the local (or mucosal) immune system.** The major function of the mucosal immune system is the formation and secretion of the immuno-globulin A (IgA) isotype of immunoglobulin. More than 70% of the immuno-globulin formed in the body every day is secretory IgA. This form of IgA acts mainly by impeding bacterial binding to epithelial surfaces—agglutinating bacteria within mucus before the individual bacterial cells can bind to receptors on their epithelial cell targets, or binding to bacterial adhesins and blocking their capacity to bind to their receptors.

Bacteria which gain access to the tissues also encounter the activities of the innate and acquired defence systems. The antibacterial activities of the **inflammatory response** come into play, as does the **acute-phase response**, which is essentially a systemic component of acute inflammation. During this response, a number of antibacterial proteins which are made in the liver are released into the circulation. **The alternative complement pathway is activated** by endotoxin, resulting in bacterial opsonization and phagocytosis, or lysis. As in the locally acting mechanisms of bacterial resistance, the presence of **lysozyme and iron-binding proteins is important. Lysozyme** can disrupt the peptide–polysaccharide linkages found in all bacterial cell walls. The enzyme is able to attack Gram-positive bacteria directly, but Gram-negative bacteria are not susceptible because the cell wall is inaccessible to the enzyme unless the outer membrane has been damaged, for example by the complement cascade. Iron-binding activity in plasma increases in infection, because **transferrin** is one of the proteins whose concentration is increased during the acute-phase response.[12]

Acquired immunity

The presence of bacterial antigens in the tissues will lead to an active immune response within a few days of the beginning of an infection, as we have seen.

How can host susceptibility to infection vary?

We can distinguish here between factors which affect the efficiency of the innate resistance mechanisms, and those which affect the development or efficiency of active immunity. Increases in the levels of exposure to bacterial pathogens can overwhelm either of these types of protective mechanism.

Innate resistance

Wounding is probably the single most common cause of enhanced suscepti-

12 Iron is an essential cofactor for key bacterial enzymes. The concentration of free iron in blood and tissue fluids is low, due to the iron-binding proteins such as transferrin and lactoferrin. Pathogenic bacteria possess iron-binding systems of their own, which enable them to grow in the tissues.

bility to infection, especially if the wound is deep or contaminated with dirt. The protective mechanisms safeguarding mucosal surfaces can be disrupted by primary virus infections; in the lungs especially this predisposes to secondary bacterial infection. Excessive exposure to tobacco smoke, alcohol or anaesthesia can paralyse the tracheal and bronchial cilia and counteract the protective action of the cilial escalator. In diabetes, high blood glucose levels tend to depress the function of neutrophils. **Malnourishment results in increased susceptibility to infection.** For example, bacterial dysentery is far more severe, and is more likely to lead to systemic disease, in infants who are malnourished. This may be due to the inability of malnourished individuals to repair or regenerate epithelial cells at a normal rate; they may also be unable to synthesize plasma proteins such as complement components or antibodies quickly enough to prevent the spread of infection.

Acquired immunity is suppressed by inherited or acquired immune deficiencies and enhanced by immunization

Inherited defects can affect the differentiation and function of T cells and B cells, macrophages and other antigen-presenting cells, neutrophils or complement components. Treatment with corticosteroids and other immuno-suppressive drugs enhances the susceptibility of patients (e.g. transplant patients) to infection; the use of cytotoxic drugs or radiation therapy can have similar effects in cancer patients.

Active immunization reduces host susceptibility by priming the immune system to respond so rapidly to the earliest stages of infection that the infectious agent—or its toxins—is effectively neutralized before disease can develop. Immunity to bacterial disease depends principally on inhibiting the binding of bacteria to epithelial surfaces, or enhancing the phagocytosis or complement-mediated lysis of extracellular bacteria, or neutralizing the activity of bacterial toxins. As we have seen, the temporary protection of passive immunization can also sometimes be effective. In the case of intracellular bacteria such as typhoid bacilli, tubercle bacilli or leprosy bacilli, cell-mediated immunity is crucial. This immunity depends mostly on the activation of macrophages by helper T cells.

Control of bacterial infections

The major aims in controlling bacterial infections are to recognize that an outbreak of disease due to a bacterial pathogen is occurring, to identify the bacterium, to eliminate the source of the infection, to interrupt the chain of transmission, and to protect susceptible members of the population from the possibility of becoming infected.

In practice this means that organized systems must exist to monitor the occurrence of bacterial disease in the community, and in hospitals. It is usually the task of public health laboratories to act as centres for diagnosis and surveillance so that outbreaks of disease can be checked quickly. On a broader scale annual and geographical records of infection need to be maintained.

These issues are summarized in Fig. 7.10.

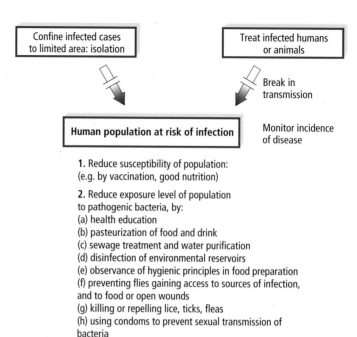

Figure 7.10 Control of bacterial infections: summary.

Summary

Pathogenic bacteria have evolved varied mechanisms of spread between hosts, complex molecular virulence determinants, and ways of evading host responses. Some bacterial diseases can be successfully prevented by immunization or treated by antibiotics, but many, like tuberculosis, typhoid and cholera, remain among the major causes of death; and bacterial evolution continues.

8 Some bacterial diseases

We have looked at the processes underlying bacterial infections, and some of the principles which govern bacterial pathogenicity. Now we will take a closer look at a few well-known bacterial diseases, and see how these principles can be applied in practice.

Tetanus and other clostridial diseases caused by the formation of exotoxins

The possibility that wounding, particularly in warfare, can be followed by severe paralysis and death has been known for centuries. The onset of the symptoms of tetanus is often signalled by the patient displaying an uncontrollable grin, due to spasms of the cheek and jaw muscles. These signs gave tetanus its other name—**lockjaw**. Death is due to muscular spasm (spastic paralysis) extending to involve the muscles of the chest, so that the patient is unable to breathe. A most unpleasant feature of tetanus is that the patient remains fully conscious to touch, pain, sight and sound, is aware of the painful muscular spasms, but completely unable to control them. Even today, with modern intensive care facilities, there is a high mortality.

What has happened to produce the muscle spasm? The story begins with **an anaerobic bacterium that can produce spores**, found in the soil. Spores are small, thick-walled bodies produced by some bacteria in adverse conditions (Fig. 8.1). They are **more resistant than the ordinary vegetative form of the bacterium**, but do not divide. When conditions improve they produce vegetative, dividing cells again. Spores of the Gram-positive bacillus, *Clostridium tetani*, are widely distributed, because the organism is a free-living saprophyte; it is also commonly present in the gut of many animals, so that it is spread with their faeces. Wounding, especially deep penetrating wounds caused by sharp objects contaminated with soil, introduces the spores into the tissues, together with other bacteria. Tetanus is therefore typically **a disease of soldiers, farmers or gardeners.**[1]

At first the spores cannot germinate because the tissue is aerobic, and the bacilli are strict anaerobes. But the wounding can cause local cell death. Other soil bacteria introduced into the wound can grow for a limited period of time, and consume the available oxygen in the microenvironment of the damaged tissue. **As soon as the wound becomes anaerobic, the tetanus spores germinate** to produce vegetative cells, which then multiply. These cells then secrete a potent **neurotoxin**, of which only the tiniest quantities are needed for the disease to develop.

1 This is the potentially fatal disease that can be caused by a rose thorn!

137

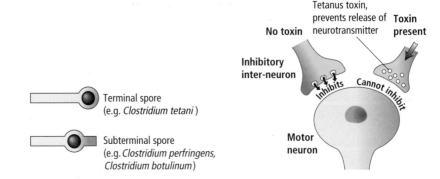

Figure 8.1 Spore-bearers (left).

Figure 8.2 Actions of tetanus toxin (right).

The bacteria producing the exotoxin are completely non-invasive, and lack all other virulence factors except the capacity to produce the toxin.

In some parts of the developing world, mothers smear soil or dung (which will, inevitably, contain tetanus spores) on to the severed umbilical stump of newborn infants to seal it; the result is that a proportion of these infants die of tetanus.

The exotoxin is a protein with several extraordinary properties. It can bind to local nerve endings, travel up the axon to the spinal cord, traverse a synaptic junction, and finally gain entry to the cytoplasm of inhibitory neurons (Fig. 8.2). Within these cells the **toxin exerts a highly specific proteolytic activity on one of the proteins (synaptobrevin)** present in the vesicles which normally deliver neurotransmitter substances to the inhibitory synaptic junction. As a result the inhibitory neuron cannot transmit its impulse, and there is unopposed stimulation of skeletal muscles by the motor neurons.

As in other diseases caused entirely by an exotoxin, **tetanus can be prevented by passive immunization with antitoxin or, better, by vaccination with toxoid**. Antitoxin is also given to patients who have already developed tetanus, but it cannot neutralize any toxin that has already entered neurons.

All clostridia are anaerobic spore-bearing bacilli and produce potent exotoxins that cause different disease. **An even simpler mechanism of pathogenesis than that of tetanus occurs in food poisoning due to a clostridial exotoxin produced by Clostridium botulinum.**[2] This toxin is not usually formed in the body, but is ingested in foodstuffs in which the botulinum toxin has been formed. This happens when food which has been contaminated with *Cl. botulinum* spores has not been cooked at a sufficiently high temperature to kill the spores. If these foodstuffs subsequently become anaerobic, when tinned, for instance, the spores germinate and the bacteria secrete their neurotoxin. This is released in the form of a protein complex; the other proteins present protect the toxin from stomach acid and facilitate its absorption across the stomach wall. Extraordinarily, this toxin too acts to cleave synaptobrevin, but in this instance the toxin targets itself to neuromuscular junctions instead of the spinal cord (Fig. 8.2). Because it blocks the transmission of nerve impulses to voluntary muscles it produces widespread flaccid paralysis.

2 *Botulus* (Latin) = sausage. The name sprang from a German outbreak of botulism from that source in 1793.

Table 8.1 Exotoxins and enzymes of clostridia.

Clostridium tetani	Tetanus toxin (neurotoxin)
Clostridium botulinum	Botulinum toxin (neurotoxin)
Clostridium perfringens	α-Toxin (lecithinase),
	Hyaluronidase,
	Haemolysin,
	Protease and
	Collagenase

Occasionally, infants whose commensal microflora is not yet fully established and who ingest the bacterial spores suffer from a slightly different form of the disease in which *Cl. botulinum* multiplies in the intestine and produces the exotoxin there. Honey is one source; the spores are blown in the wind into plant nectar, and collected inadvertently by honey bees. Although very rare, infant botulism provides an interesting example of what can happen if the protective activities of the intestinal commensal bacteria are inadequate.

Another clostridial disease is known as **gas gangrene**, due mainly to *Cl. perfringens*, although other species are usually also present. Like tetanus, this disease also follows wounding, but in this case the incidence of the condition is highest when someone has suffered really massive wounding and the wound is contaminated with soil. This condition therefore occurs most commonly in warfare. Large wounds can result in extensive tissue necrosis; in gas gangrene the bacteria begin to grow in a necrotic zone and then spread rapidly through the tissue, secreting a whole battery of potent toxins which diffuse into the adjacent tissue and kill the cells here too. The bacteria also secrete a number of enzymes (Table 8.1) which can degrade proteins, fat and connective tissue and cause haemolysis. As a consequence bacterial growth and spread are very rapid; the tissue turns black, and much gas is also produced. Gas gangrene is rapidly fatal unless the affected part is amputated.

Antibiotics are of very little use against anaerobic bacteria like clostridia, because they cannot penetrate the necrotic infected area in sufficient concentration to be effective.

Cholera: disease due to bacterial colonization of an epithelial surface and formation of a toxin with local effects only

Cholera is a bacterial disease, caused by *Vibrio cholerae*, a comma-shaped Gram-negative bacillus, which many people imagine to be a disease of the past. On the contrary, it is very much **a disease of the present day**. In the 19th century there were cholera epidemics in cities such as London and New York, where literally thousands of people would die of the disease each month, especially during the summer. The first example of an epidemic of cholera being stopped was in 1854, when Dr John Snow removed the handle of the pump on the Broad Street well in London, whose water he suspected of being the source of the outbreak. He was right, but the cholera bacillus itself was not identified until several decades later. Efforts to control cholera led to the first systematic study of public health and hygiene, and to the first international agreements on the reporting and control of epidemic disease. Within a few years, **the provision of clean water and the separate disposal of sewage** had eliminated cholera from Europe and North America.

Seven pandemics of cholera have been recorded since 1817. In the late 1980s it appeared that the disease might be within reach of control, as newly developed vaccines began to show improved safety, efficacy and ease of use. Unfortunately, in 1991 a wholly new antigenic subgroup of the organism suddenly emerged within the Indian subcontinent, heralding the evolution of a new form of the cholera bacillus. None of the existing or developing vaccines, nor any immunity acquired previously as a consequence of recovery from infection, is of any value against this bacterium. Meanwhile, also in 1991, a new phase of the previous pandemic resulted in the appearance of epidemic cholera in Peru, possibly due to the discharge of a ship's sewage or ballast water. The disease crossed the continent rapidly, and over 400 000 cases of cholera were reported to the World Health Organization from South America in 1991 (Fig. 8.3).

A patient suffering from full-blown cholera displays some dramatic symptoms, **losing up to 20 litres of liquid each day as a consequence of uncontrollable diarrhoea**. In these circumstances the patient will quickly die unless the body's fluid and electrolyte balances are restored. However, if caught early, the disease can be treated. One of the most significant medical advances of the century, in terms of the number of lives saved, has been the realization that cholera patients and others, especially infants, suffering from any type of acute diarrhoea can be nursed through their acute symptoms if fluids and electrolytes are replaced soon enough. Except in the most severe cases, which require intravenous therapy, **rehydration can be achieved orally**, even if diarrhoea is continuing. This is possible providing that the patient is given water containing glucose as well as electrolytes, because the glucose stimulates the uptake of salts, and hence water, by a mechanism which is unaffected by the simultaneous activity of cholera toxin.

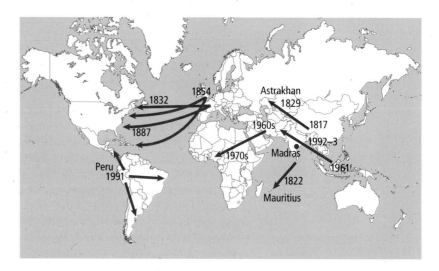

Figure 8.3 Some major cholera outbreaks.

The pathogenesis of cholera is a story of the colonization of the gut epithelium, the secretion and activity of a potent exotoxin, and the formation of a number of other virulence determinants. The activity of the toxin is limited topographically to the epithelial cells most closely adjacent to the colonization sites of the bacterium. Although a good deal is known about cholera and cholera toxin, recent discoveries continue to point to numerous gaps in the details of our understanding of this disease.

Colonization of the epithelium of the small intestine by *V. cholerae* is the essential first step in the development of cholera. This step is known to depend on the presence of pili on the bacterial surface. Pili are particularly valuable for the initial establishment of contact with cell receptors because they can penetrate the mucus which overlies gut epithelial cells. Once colonization begins, cholera vibrios make intimate contact between their outer membranes and the epithelial cells.

The next phase of the development of the infection is the formation and secretion of **cholera enterotoxin**. This exotoxin affects the ion pumps of the epithelial cells and causes reduced sodium chloride uptake and chloride ion secretion, which is accompanied by massive loss of water from the tissues into the gut.

The mechanism by which the cholera toxin leads to this cellular effect has been worked out in some detail. Subunits of the toxin bind to receptors on the epithelial cell surface. Then another subunit penetrates the cell membrane and catalyses an irreversible increase in the intra-cellular messenger, cyclic adenosine monophosphate (cAMP). However, there are some indications that there may be more to the pathogenesis of fluid loss in cholera than has been thought. There are now persistent reports that additional factors, such as the synthesis of prostaglandins and the activity of submucosal nerve plexuses, are required for the ion and water losses to occur. If this is true, it will no longer be possible to confine our explanation of fluid loss in cholera entirely to biochemical events in the epithelial cells.

V. cholerae secretes at least two other toxins which can cause diarrhoea. **Even strains which lack all these toxins will still stimulate minor diarrhoea in some volunteers; this effect appears to be due simply to the adhesion of the bacteria.** The development of cholera vaccines which can be taken by mouth, in order to stimulate local immunity, has proved to be difficult, but has now been successfully achieved. At first it seemed that deletion of a single gene would effectively attenuate the cholera bacilli; then it became apparent that the deletion of the genes encoding the other toxins was also needed.

However, the fact that the most recent pandemic of cholera has begun in a region where cholera has previously been endemic has now pointed vaccine development in a new direction. Since exposure to the pre-existing strains does not confer immunity against the new pandemic strain—all of which produce exactly the same antigenic type of cholera enterotoxin—it has become clear that **the most important element in immunity to cholera is not antitoxin**. Instead it seems that a protective immune response consists predominantly of a mucosal secretory immunoglobulin A (IgA) response directed against polysaccharide components in the bacterial outer membrane. For many years research had been focused on eliciting antitoxic immunity. The realization that this is of little or no significance is due to the experiment performed by nature, revealing the unexpected lack of cross-protection between the old and new pandemic strains of *V. cholerae*.

Why the cholera bacillus should be so well-adapted to causing diarrhoea is surprising when one notes that **the bacterium is not an obligatory parasite**. On the contrary, the organism can survive well in the environment, and its natural habitat appears to be brackish waters and algal blooms. The cholera vibrio can also establish a long-term inapparent carrier state in a significant proportion of individuals in an endemic area. In terms of bacterial survival, the establishment of carrier or disease states provides the bacterium with a means of transport between one area of brackish water and another!

Other enteric diseases: or, beware (especially while travelling)—if one kind of enteric bacterium doesn't get you, another one might

Analysis of the behaviour of bacteria which can cause disease in the gut provides a number of fascinating examples of the intricacies of the interactions between bacteria and their hosts.

We cannot avoid ingesting bacteria which can grow or survive in food and water. Moreover, some bacteria are pathogens of animals whose flesh is eaten by humans. Because of the consistent opportunity presented to them, numerous bacterial species have been able to evolve to exploit our dependence on eating and drinking to gain access to the body. **The enteric route of infection is perhaps the most common mode of acquisition of community-acquired bacterial infections.** The resulting diseases vary greatly in their severity, ranging from mild discomfort, to diarrhoea without any systemic symptoms, to dysentery with ulceration of the intestinal lining, and to even more severe consequences, such as sustained fevers, growth of bacteria in the liver and spleen, and lethal damage to the kidneys.

Diarrhoea, dysentery and fevers which begin with bacterial invasion of the gut (typhoid and paratyphoid fevers) are all caused by Gram-negative bacteria which have evolved differing sets of virulence determinants. As a result, they cause different diseases.

Different cells in the gut provide sites of attachment or entry for different bacteria. The events following attachment also vary in different bacteria.

The simplest examples of enteric disease can be likened to a mild form of cholera. Strains of *Escherichia coli* which colonize the lumen of the small intestine are commensal, and are present in large numbers. Young children and travellers, however, are especially susceptible to infection by pathogenic, gut-adherent strains of *E. coli*, because they **lack mucosal (IgA) antibodies**, which can prevent the bacteria binding to the epithelium. Children have not had time to develop this immunity, and travellers lack it because many antigenically distinct strains of *E. coli* are distributed throughout the world. The basis for these differences in antigenicity lie principally in the surface polysaccharide antigens (known as O antigens) and in the protein subunits of the surface pili.

In the case of bacterial diseases such as diphtheria and whooping cough, there is **essentially only one antigenic form of the infecting organism**, so that vaccines made from one strain of the bacterium will provide worldwide protection against diphtheria and whooping cough. By contrast, **the bacteria which have evolved to cause diarrhoeal diseases exist in numerous forms, all differing antigenically**. For this reason it is possible to suffer repeatedly from diarrhoeal diseasè caused by different strains of E. coli, in different regions of the world.

In the simplest form of illness produced by E. coli, the organisms disrupt the metabolism of gut epithelial cells by proliferating on the surface of cells of the small intestine and releasing **two different kinds of enterotoxin**.

The first toxin appears to have exactly the **same mode of action as cholera toxin**, and its molecular structure is very similar. Curiously, whereas cholera toxin is released from the cell, the E. coli toxin only makes its way as far as the periplasmic space between the bacterial cell wall and the outer membrane. Disruption of the outer membrane by components of the digestive juices, especially bile salts and proteolytic enzymes, is needed to release the toxin.

The second toxin is a much smaller protein and its **mode of action is more like that of a hormone**. It binds to a receptor on the outside of the cell and, without entering the cell, causes a signal to be transmitted across the cell membrane, which exerts a dramatic effect on water balance within the cell. The molecule to which it binds is part of the enzyme guanylate cyclase. This transmembrane protein serves as a receptor for the small toxin. But this is not its normal function. The normal function of this receptor is to bind a peptide hormone known as **guanylin**. Binding of either guanylin or the small E. coli toxin to intestinal guanylate cyclase results in a dramatic rise not in cAMP (as in cholera), but in its close cousin, called cyclic guanosine monophosphate (cGMP). The effect of a dramatic increase in cGMP production is the same, though—the cells secrete chloride ions and water is then lost too.

This is a fascinating example of a bacterium mimicking a hormone in order to exert its effects, but it has led to a further discovery. The normal role of guanylin is probably to maintain sufficient water content in the mucus overlying the epithelial cells. Its activity depends not only on the presence of guanylate cyclase, but also on that of a cell membrane protein which is the same protein that is genetically altered in **cystic fibrosis** sufferers.

The implication of this finding is that an individual who is a carrier of the cystic fibrosis gene may be less prone to suffer from severe diarrhoea due to these bacteria. In other words, just as someone who is a sickle-cell heterozygote is less prone to suffer from severe malaria, so someone who carries the cystic fibrosis gene may be less susceptible to certain types of diarrhoeal disease. Toxigenic strains of E. coli have always been a major cause of death among children in poorer communities. Throughout human evolution there will therefore have been strong selection for any gene diminishing the chances of dying from diarrhoea in infancy. This may perhaps help to explain why cystic fibrosis is now such a common genetic disorder. Clearly, **the genetic structure of human populations has been affected by the selective pressure exerted by pathogenic microorganisms**.

Other kinds of intestinal disease depend on bacteria being more destructive

In some cases, bacterial infection of the gut is followed by blood and mucus being found in the faeces, rather than an excess of fluid. This is indicative of an inflammatory reaction in the gut wall, which does not occur in cholera or traveller's diarrhoea. The appearance of blood and mucus in the faeces is called **dysentery**. The bacteria invade the mucosal cells of the colon, and trigger ulceration and an intense inflammatory response.

Bacterial dysentery, caused by various species of *Shigella*, is highly communicable. Only small numbers (tens or hundreds) of bacteria are needed to start an infection, because the bacteria are resistant to stomach acid. An outbreak of dysentery can therefore be difficult to control. Even **houseflies can spread the bacteria from faeces to food**. Bacterial dysentery used to exert a major influence on the fighting fitness of armies, but nowadays outbreaks tend to occur in nurseries and in refugee camps. The bacteria are obligate human parasites and do not survive for long in the environment.

When an infective dose of the bacteria is swallowed, the bacteria enter and multiply within colonic epithelial cells[3], and then spread laterally from cell to cell. They enter cells by utilizing their specific protein invasins to induce their own **phagocytosis by the epithelial cells**, which are not normally phagocytic. Inside the phagocytic vacuoles, they begin to multiply, then lyse the vacuole and enter the cytoplasm. As the bacteria proliferate, they also induce changes in the cytoskeleton of the epithelial cell, causing the polymerization of actin filaments at one end of the bacterial cell. The actin filaments aggregate in such a way that they act like a sphincter and propel some of the bacteria forward sufficiently vigorously so that they protrude from one cell, and impinge on the next-door cell, entering it within a double membrane, i.e. the membrane of the first host cell, wrapped within that of its neighbour. In no time at all, the bacteria lyse both these membranes, enter the cell cytoplasm and begin to multiply again.

How does this process lead to ulceration of the colonic mucosa? We still do not know all the details. Multiplication of the bacteria kills epithelial cells, either by interfering with the cell's energy metabolism, or by inducing apoptosis. The bacteria produce an exotoxin, called **Shiga toxin**, which can poison protein synthesis; it used to be thought that it was this toxin that killed the cells. This is not the case: bacterial mutants which cannot make the toxin will still invade and kill epithelial cells. Neutrophils and macrophages are attracted to the site of epithelial ulceration and die during the most vigorous phase of bacterial multiplication. The release of lysosomal contents from these cells enhances the damage. Additionally, the Shiga toxin is now known to **damage the endothelial cells of small blood vessels in the wall of the colon**, causing the loss of blood into the faeces. Notice that the end-result of this series of events is that the bacteria can be shed in the faeces, accompanied by a rich brew of nutrients derived from the blood. This helps to ensure that the bacteria are discharged from the infected host in the best possible condition to infect a new host.

3 More accurately, the bacteria first enter specialized phagocytic cells called M cells, distributed among gut epithelial cells.

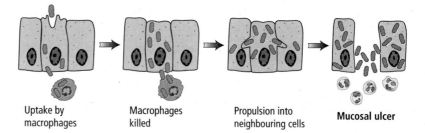

Figure 8.4 *Shigella* in colonic epithelial cells.

Uptake by macrophages

Macrophages killed

Propulsion into neighbouring cells

Mucosal ulcer

Despite the extraordinary gymnastics which enable these bacteria to move from cell to cell within the epithelium (Fig. 8.4), they are unable to invade the body much beyond the basement membrane of the gut epithelium and, within a few days, the immune response leads to healing. Only in malnourished children is it common for these infections to persist, or for systemic symptoms to develop.

Salmonella infections can have more severe consequences than dysentery

These bacteria are among the commonest causes of food poisoning, because so many of them are also pathogens of food animals; chickens are very commonly infected. In poultry the bacteria often infect the ovaries, and hence make their way into eggs. Because salmonella are impossible to eliminate from the food chain, virtually all supermarket chickens contain at least small numbers of these bacteria, and it is important not to eat undercooked poultry or eggs.

The severity of disease caused by these bacteria depends upon the species of salmonella as well as the number of bacteria ingested. **Most salmonella disease consists of gastroenteritis**, in which nausea, vomiting and diarrhoea are experienced within 6–24 h of eating contaminated food. The symptoms can last for a week or more, and some patients may continue to shed bacteria, and hence act as carriers, for weeks or months.

Unlike the shigella, salmonella are able to traverse the brush border of epithelial cells of the small bowel (Fig. 8.5). Their contact with the surface of these cells first induces a characteristic 'ruffling' of the luminal surface. Then bacteria induce the cells to phagocytose them.[4] They use the phagocytic vacuole as a transport device, traverse the cell, and are exocytosed into the subepithelial space, where they multiply, and induce intense local acute inflammation. The diarrhoea which accompanies the disease is thought to be the consequence of either the attraction of neutrophils to the sites of infection, or the release of enterotoxins. Invasion is usually halted by the inflammatory response at the level of the submucosa, unless the bacteria belong to the species which cause **enteric fevers**, including **typhoid** and **paratyphoid fever**.

The characteristic property of *Salmonella typhi*, which causes typhoid fever, is its capacity to spread from the submucosa, multiply in a variety of organs

4 Like shigella, they can also enter via M cells.

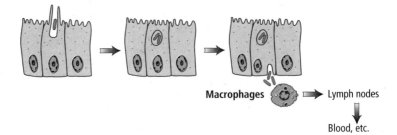

Macrophages ➡ Lymph nodes

Blood, etc.

Figure 8.5 Spread of *Salmonella typhi*.

such as the liver, spleen and bone marrow and, importantly, to survive inside macrophages (Fig. 8.5). Genetic susceptibility to salmonella infection in mice is determined by possession of a gene which determines whether or not the macrophage can kill the bacteria. This gene is of special interest, because it also determines whether macrophages can kill tuberculosis bacteria and leishmania parasites. The gene has now been identified in the human genome, and given the grievously long name: natural resistance-associated macrophage protein gene, or **NRAMP**. It determines whether or not macrophages can be induced to up-regulate their intracellular killing mechanisms very soon after infection.

Studies of different kinds of infective agents have led to the investigation of the genetic basis of macrophage activation. This is important because, if we can learn how to regulate macrophage killing mechanisms, we may be able to augment the activity of antibiotics by boosting the body's natural methods for combating infection!

Lobar pneumonia and meningitis: bacterial diseases which can follow inapparent carriage of bacteria

In the diseases discussed above we saw how disease followed the ingestion of adequate doses of infectious bacteria. A somewhat different circumstance, which can nevertheless lead to life-threatening illness, is where the bacteria are not necessarily newly acquired, but are resident in the nasopharynx as commensals, until a change in the susceptibility of the host, or transport of the bacteria to the lower respiratory tract, initiates disease.

A classic example of this is **lobar pneumonia**, due to *Streptococcus pneumoniae*, which is also known as the pneumococcus. This bacterium is present in the nasopharynx of up to 30% of the population at any one time. If it is transported into the alveoli of the lungs, it begins to multiply, and gives rise to pneumonia, especially if there are predisposing circumstances, such as influenza or heart failure. Once the bacteria gain access to the alveoli they multiply rapidly. They evade phagocytosis by resident alveolar macrophages, because **they possess an antiphagocytic capsule**, polymerized from a number of different sugar residues. There are **84 known different capsular serotypes** of varying virulence. Unfortunately, immunity, when it arises, is specific for one type of capsule. The current pneumococcal vaccines therefore all contain a number of different capsular carbohydrates derived from the commonest strains.

The pneumococcus evokes an intense and rapidly spreading inflammatory response in the lung. This response has the unusual feature that it spreads through a lobe of the lung with astonishing speed, as if the alveolar walls had become porous. Within a few hours the lobe may be entirely clogged with inflammatory exudate, rich in neutrophils. This is in marked contrast to the much commoner pneumonias caused by other bacteria which are much less rapidly spreading, and give rise to the patchy pneumonia known as **bronchopneumonia**.

How do we account for the speed and extent of this inflammation? There is no universal agreement about this yet, but we can make some educated guesses. An important feature of pneumococci is that they are **unusually fragile bacteria**, susceptible to autolysis (digestion from within). Such lysis of the bacteria releases, among other constituents, fragments of peptidoglycan from the cell wall, and a membrane-active cytolysin, or pneumolysin, from within the bacterium. The **peptidoglycan fragments are potent activators of the alternative complement pathway**, and hence proinflammatory. The **pneumolysin attacks a wide variety of cell membranes**, because it has an affinity for cholesterol, a component of all mammalian cell membranes. The damaging action of pneumolysin on capillary endothelial cells may help to account for the characteristic presence of blood in the sputum in lobar pneumonia. Pneumolysin can also activate complement and damage neutrophils sufficiently to suppress their bacterial killing mechanisms. Hence, the cell wall components and the pneumolysin can augment each other's activity.

Lobar pneumonia is brought to a conclusion by the formation of **anticapsule antibodies**, which act as opsonins and tilt the balance in favour of the phagocytes.

Lobar pneumonia can lead to septicaemia and hence sometimes to **meningitis** via the blood stream. Pneumococci can also apparently pass directly from a state of inapparent carriage in the nasopharynx to invasion and multiplication in the blood stream, leading to meningitis. Quite how this happens is uncertain, but it can be rapid and lethal.

Tuberculosis

The last bacterial disease we shall consider here also centres around inflammatory reaction to infection. But whereas pneumococcal pneumonia represents one of the most acute examples of acute infection, tuberculosis represents one of the most chronic of chronic infections!

It may come as a surprise to learn that *Mycobacterium tuberculosis* is as great a killer today as it is. **Each year there are 8 million new cases of tuberculosis and 3 million deaths.** Approximately one-third of the world's population carries the bacterium and is hence at risk of the disease. Recent estimates are that in global terms tuberculosis accounts for 26% of avoidable adult deaths in the developing parts of the world.

Tuberculosis is obviously a highly significant hazard to public health, its incidence is rising, partly because of its association as an opportunistic infection in acquired immunodeficiency syndrome (AIDS), and it is becoming more difficult to treat, as antibiotic-resistant strains are spreading.

Tuberculosis has always been one of the great bacterial plagues. With the coming of the industrial revolution in Europe, and the crowding of the population into cities, the effects of the disease were dreadful; by the mid 19th century it was responsible for a third of all deaths in major cities such as Paris. With the movement of explorers about the world the disease was also introduced into populations which had never before been exposed to it; the South Sea islanders suffered grievously, with the disease at one time affecting more than 80% of all children. Even in the 17th century the poet John Bunyan aptly referred to the disease as 'the Captain of all these Men of Death'. **In all populations, it is particularly the overcrowded, the malnourished and those with other diseases who are most susceptible.**

Despite its past record and current significance we know surprisingly little about the processes by which the bacterium causes disease. This is partly because research into the nature of tuberculosis virtually came to a halt in the 1960s, when it was thought that it might be totally controlled by the combined use of preventive measures and antibiotic treatment, and partly because the bacterium is exceptionally difficult to study. The causative organism, *M. tuberculosis*, grows so slowly in the laboratory that visible bacterial colonies take 3–4 weeks to develop. The cells are heavily armoured with complex lipids and carbohydrates, so that even breaking the cell open to get at its DNA (something every self-respecting microbiologist inevitably wants to do!) is no easy task. In addition, the bacterium is so pathogenic that great care has to be taken to avoid self-infection, or transmission outside the laboratory.

The consequence of this period of neglect in the study of the disease is that **we remain almost completely ignorant about the nature of the bacterial virulence determinants**. What we do know is that the multiplication of the bacteria takes place mostly within macrophages, that this multiplication can only be brought under control by the activation of macrophages by Th1 cells, and that not all humans are equally able to activate their macrophages to the levels of activity required to kill the bacteria.

The outcome of the disease depends crucially on the activity of Th1 cells and a high Th1/Th2 ratio is therefore protective (Fig. 8.6). This is also true of another mycobacterial disease, leprosy, and of the protozoal disease, leishmaniasis, both of which are due to organisms growing inside macrophages.

The commonest form of tuberculosis begins when bacteria (coughed out by infected individuals) are inhaled into the lungs in droplets which are small enough to gain access to the alveoli. These organisms are phagocytosed by alveolar macrophages and in the majority of patients they grow slowly for 1–2 months before cell-mediated immunity develops. This arises because antigens derived from the bacteria are processed by the macrophages and presented to T cells in the local lymph nodes. The T cells circulate, and react by producing cytokines in the lesion (particularly interferon-γ) which activate the killing mechanisms of the macrophages (see Chapter 5). Small focal lesions, or granulomas, develop, and are called tubercles (see Chapter 6). If resistance is high, the lesions are walled off by fibroblasts, and may become calcified. Sometimes not all the bacteria present are killed, and they may remain in a dormant state in these sites for many years.

In less resistant individuals, the lesions may either continue to expand, or a

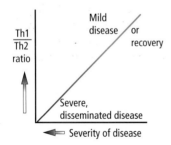

Figure 8.6 Relationship of type of immune response to severity of tuberculosis (or leprosy, or leishmaniasis).

dormant lesion may become reactivated. In progressive disease the bacterial multiplication is not controlled, and the lesions within the lung grow dramatically in size. The death of macrophages results in an **accumulation of necrotic material**. In the worst circumstances the release of hydrolytic enzymes from dying macrophages and other inflammatory cells liquefies this material, and converts it into such a good nutrient medium for growth of the bacteria that huge numbers of bacteria are found—up to 1000 million per millilitre. This liquefaction also creates ideal circumstances for the organisms to **spread to other organs via the blood stream**. Patients with liquefying lesions are highly dangerous to others, because they cough out droplets of the liquid containing large numbers of bacteria.

Patients suffering from progressive tuberculosis become emaciated, and this aspect of the disease is partly due to macrophage activity. Cytokines released from highly activated macrophages switch the balance of metabolic activity in the body from anabolism (building up) to catabolism (a breaking down of the body's reserves of fats and proteins).

In this disease it appears that bacterial virulence is not due to toxins, or other common virulence factors. Instead it appears to arise from the **invasiveness of the bacterium, its capacity to survive within macrophages, to grow to large numbers in liquefied lesions, and to elicit highly active foci of cell-mediated hypersensitivity**.

We are still uncertain as to which of the bacterial constituents represent the antigens which are driving the cell-mediated immune responses. We do know that lipids (called mycolic acids) present in the bacterial cell wall act as potent immune **adjuvants**—substances which are not themselves antigenic, but which enhance immune reactivity to molecules which are. Because of the presence of these adjuvants it is possible that the antigen or antigens responsible for the cell-mediated immune response may only be relatively minor constituents of the bacteria, and therefore difficult to identify.

Summary

We have looked briefly at some examples of the almost infinite variations in bacterial disease. We have seen that rigorous investigations of the mechanisms are necessary in order to attempt to understand the diseases. These investigations are based on the application of molecular and cell biology and genetics. But study of how the diseases occur in human populations reveals how profoundly affected they are by variations in host resistance.

Bacterial diseases, especially their epidemic forms, have truly made history.

9   Viruses

Viruses are obligatory intracellular parasites. They can multiply only inside cells. Different viruses infect plants, animals or the larger microbes such as bacteria. They range in size from 20 nm to about 300 nm in diameter; the largest virus is therefore only about one-tenth the size of *Escherichia coli* (Fig. 9.1). Apart from their small size, viruses are distinguished from other biological entities (i.e. from prokaryotes and eukaryotes) by the **absence of translation machinery or of an adenosine triphosphate (ATP)-generating system**. At their simplest, **viruses are composed of nucleic acids surrounded by a protein coat**, and can be considered as parasitic nucleic acid molecules which code for their own protein coats and for enzymes capable of replicating the viral nucleic acid. The concept of the virus as a parasitic nucleic acid was established from experiments performed half a century ago which showed that the purified nucleic acid extracted from **tobacco mosaic virus**[1] is capable of causing an infection which yields new virus particles. This experiment was one of the foundation stones of modern biology, but the choice of virus was fortunate for, as we shall see, some viruses have nucleic acids which are not infectious.

The virus particle

Different types of nucleic acid comprise the viral genome

Viruses are different from other biological forms in that their genetic material is composed of different sorts of nucleic acid. **The viral genome may consist of either DNA or RNA and may be double-stranded or single-stranded.** Most viruses contain a single piece of nucleic acid but some contain two or more different pieces (segmented genomes). The genome also varies considerably in size. The largest viral nucleic acids are of about 10^8 Da in molecular weight (Mr) (about 100–200 kilobases), the smallest about 2×10^6 Da (about 5 Kb). If an average protein contains about 300 amino acids (Mr about 30000), then 900 bases (300 triplets) are required to code for it. The largest viruses therefore have **coding potential** for 100–200 proteins, while the smallest code for perhaps five proteins.

The protein coat is composed of repeating subunits

The virus nucleic acid (the **genome**) is encased in a protein coat (the **capsid**). Together the genome and the protein coat comprise the **nucleocapsid**, and in many instances the nucleocapsid is the whole virus particle.[2] A nucleic acid can code for about one-tenth its own weight of protein (three nucleotides have a

1 Tobacco mosaic virus is an economically important rod-shaped plant virus that can be grown and purified in large quantities.

2 The virus particle is sometimes called the **virion**.

151

Family	Virion morphology	Species	Disease
Double-stranded DNA genome			
Papovaviridae Icosahedral capsid 45–55 nm. No envelope. 5–8 Kilobase pairs (Kbp)	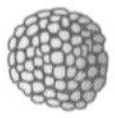	Polyomavirus (mice) Simian virus 40 (SV40) (monkeys)	Tumours in rodents (experimental)
		Papillomavirus	Human warts Cervical carcinoma
Adenoviridae Icosahedral capsid, 80 nm. No envelope. 35 Kbp	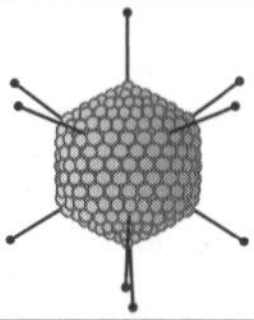	Adenovirus	Acute respiratory disease
Herpesviridae Icosahedral capsid, 120 nm. Envelope. ~150 Kbp	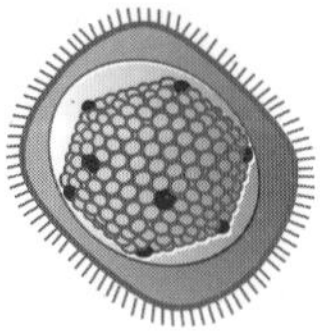	Herpes simplex virus (HSV)	Cold sores (type 1) Genital herpes (type 2)
		Varicella zoster (VZV)	Chickenpox and shingles
		Epstein–Barr virus (EBV)	Glandular fever and Burkitt lymphoma
		Cytomegalovirus (CMV)	Cytomegalic inclusion disease in neonates
		Marek's disease virus	Lymphomas in chickens
Poxviridae Complex capsid (i.e. structure not resolved), 200–300 nm. Envelope, ~200 Kbp. Virion transcriptase	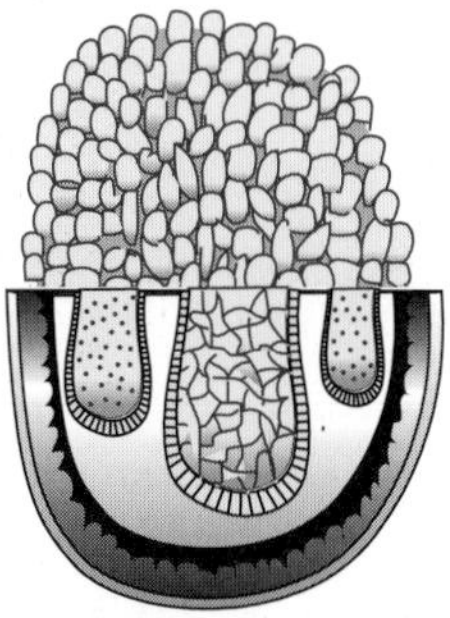	Variola virus	Smallpox
		Vaccinia virus	Vaccine against smallpox
		Myxomavirus	Myxomatosis in rabbits
		Orf virus	Contagious pustular dermatitis in sheep and goats
Single-stranded DNA genome			
Parvovirus Icosahedral virion, 20 nm. No envelope. 5 Kb		Canine parvovirus	
		Feline panleukopenia virus	Cat fever, enteritis
Double-stranded RNA genome			
Reoviridae Icosahedral virion, 60–80 nm. No envelope. Genome has 10–11 fragments. ~20 Kbp. Virion transcriptase	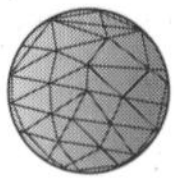	Blue tongue	Catarrhal fever in sheep
		Human rotavirus	Acute infantile gastroenteritis

Figure 9.1 Some examples of virus families and their characteristics.

Family	Virion morphology	Species	Disease
Positive single-stranded RNA genome			
Picornaviridae Icosahedral capsid, 20–30 nm. No envelope. ~7 Kb		Poliovirus	Poliomyelitis
		Rhinovirus	Common cold
		Foot and mouth disease virus (FMDV)	Foot and mouth disease
		Hepatitis A	Acute hepatitis
Togaviridae & Flaviviridae Icosahedral capsid, 40–80 nm. Envelope. 11 Kb	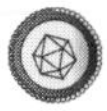	Yellow fever virus	Jungle yellow fever
		Rubella virus	Congenital malformation (German measles)
Negative single-stranded RNA genome			
Orthomyxoviridae Helical capsid and envelope, 80 nm. Genome has 8 fragments. 12 Kb. Virion transcriptase	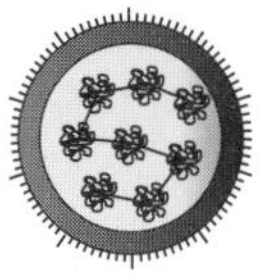	Influenza virus A	Influenza epidemics and pandemics
		Influenza virus B	Influenza epidemics
Arenaviridae Helical capsid and envelope (contains host ribosomes), 50–300 nm. Genome has 2 fragments. 14 Kb. Virion transcriptase	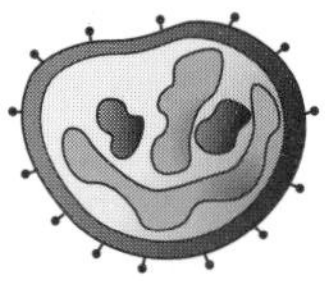	Lymphocytic chorio-meningitis virus of mice	Meningitis
		Lassavirus	Lassa fever
Paramyxoviridae Helical capsid and envelope. Pleomorphic 150 nm. 15 Kb. Virion transcriptase	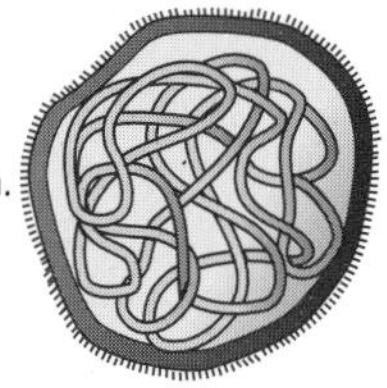	Newcastle disease virus (NDV)	Fowlpest
		Measles virus	Measles
		Distemper virus (CDV)	Canine distemper
Rhabdoviridae Helical capsid and envelope. Bullet-shape 200 x 80 nm. ~10 Kb. Virion transcriptase	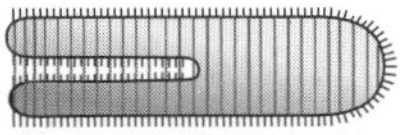	Rabies virus	Rabies
Positive single-stranded RNA genome with DNA intermediate			
Retroviridae Icosahedral capsid, 100 nm, with envelope. 8 Kb. Virion reverse transcriptase	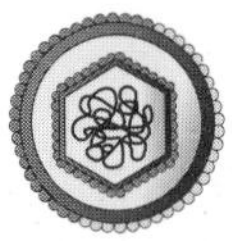	Rous sarcoma virus (RSV)	Sarcomas in fowl
		Feline leukaemia virus	Leukaemia in cats
		Human immuno-deficiency virus (HIV)	Acquired immuno-deficiency syndrome
Double-stranded DNA genome with RNA intermediate			
Hepadnaviridae Icosahedral capsid and envelope, 28 nm. 3 Kbp	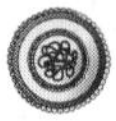	Hepatitis B	Acute and chronic hepatitis. Primary liver cancer

Figure 9.1 *Continued*

153

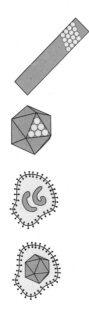

A helical (or rod-shaped) nucleocapsid in which repeating protein subunits wind around the nucleic acid with helical symmetry, e.g. tobacco mosaic virus

An icosahedral nucleocapsid. Protein subunits are arranged in 20 triangular faces with 12 apices, e.g. wart viruses

A helical nucleocapsid surrounded by a lipid bilayer (envelope) in which transmembrane proteins are embedded, e.g. measles

An icosahedral nucleocapsid surrounded by an envelope, e.g. herpes viruses

Figure 9.2 Virus structure.

molecular mass of ~1000: one amino acid has a molecular mass of ~100), and it follows that no nucleic acid could be encased within a single protein molecule for which it codes. All virus capsids are therefore composed of repeating protein subunits. These subunits contact each other to form a symmetrical array (Fig. 9.2) which may exhibit **helical** symmetry (rod-shaped viruses) or **icosahedral** symmetry (spherical particles). Some complex virus particles exhibit both kinds of symmetry: for example the 'head' of bacteriophage T4 is icosahedral while the 'tail' is helical.[3] The simplest virus capsids, e.g. that of the tobacco mosaic virus, are composed of repeating subunits of a single type of polypeptide, but most capsids, including those of all animal viruses, are composed of more than one sort of polypeptide. Indeed, the most complex virus particles have more than 30 different proteins and the details of their structure are as yet uncertain.

Some viruses are surrounded by a lipid bilayer

While many virus particles are composed solely of the nucleocapsid,[4] some are nucleocapsids surrounded by a phospholipid bi-layer. In most instances this **membrane** or **envelope** is acquired from the host cell by the nucleocapsid as it leaves the cell by budding through the plasma membrane. Viruses of this type are said to be **enveloped**. Examples of the various virus particle structures are shown in Fig. 9.2.

3 Bacteriophages (or phages) are viruses that infect bacteria; T4 infects *Escherichia coli*.

4 And are therefore chemically resistant to fat solvents such as ether and mild detergents.

Viruses are classified according to nucleic acid type and particle structure

Although attempts have been made to establish a hierarchical classification of viruses, the resulting schemes are not helpful because they imply evolutionary relationship, and we know nothing of the evolution of different groups of viruses. Indeed, there is no reason to suppose that viruses have arisen from a common ancestor. It is more useful to group viruses according to the type of nucleic acid that they contain because, as we shall see, this determines their multiplication strategy. Within each group we can then identify **families of viruses** that are related by particle structure. Figure 9.1 lists groups of viruses in this way. Each virus family is placed within a group based on nucleic acid type; the size of the genome and structure of the virus particle for each family is described; and within each family examples of individual viruses are given, together with the diseases they cause. This is not a comprehensive list. Note that viruses with single-stranded RNA genomes are divided into two classes—those with **positive**-stranded RNA and those with **negative**-stranded RNA. This is shorthand to illustrate that an RNA molecule can be **coding** or **non-coding**. A positive-strand RNA is a messenger RNA (mRNA) molecule—it can be translated into protein. A **negative**-strand RNA is the complement of the message—a **complementary copy** must be made before the information can be translated into protein.

Multiplication of viruses

Our knowledge of the multiplication cycle of animal viruses derives almost entirely from experiments using animal cells in culture rather than from infection of the host animal. When a culture of animal cells is infected with a large excess of virus particles the subsequent events are described as the **synchronized one-step growth cycle**.[5] The one-step growth cycle is fundamentally similar for all viruses and different from any other infectious agent (Fig. 9.3). The cycle is conveniently divided into three phases: (i) **entry:** virus particles adsorb to the cell surface and penetrate into the cytoplasm; (ii) **eclipse:** immediately after entry the virus particles disappear—no virus particles can be found by electron microscopy and, if we break the cells open, no infectivity can be found. The 'virus' has become a parasitic nucleic acid; and (iii) **assembly and release:** new (progeny) virus particles appear in the host cell and in the surrounding medium, sometimes in huge numbers. The timing of

5 **Synchronized** because, with a large excess of virus, all cells are simultaneously infected; **one-step** because at the end of the cycle there are no uninfected cells remaining to support further virus growth.

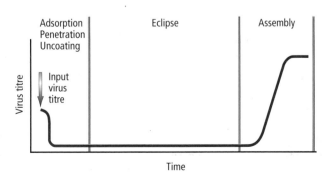

Figure 9.3 The one-step growth cycle.

these events varies from virus to virus and also depends on the condition of the host cell. When T4 phage infects an actively growing *E. coli* the entire process takes about 25 min, whereas the growth cycle of an animal virus takes hours or, in some cases, several days. We will now examine the three phases in more detail.

Entry of virus into the host cell depends on specific attachment to its surface membrane

This is achieved by specific interaction between proteins on the virus and receptors on the cell membrane. The virus proteins involved are present on the capsid surface in the case of **non-enveloped** virus, but in the case of **enveloped** viruses the receptor-binding proteins are glycoproteins embedded in the envelope. For example, the gp160 molecule[6] on the envelope of human immunodeficiency virus (HIV) attaches to the CD4 molecule on the surface of helper T cells, and the haemagglutinin molecule on the influenza virus envelope attaches to sialic acid residues, the terminal sugars on many mammalian cell surface carbohydrates. **The identification of those virus proteins responsible for receptor binding is important, because antibodies directed against these molecules could prevent virus attachment.** Antibodies to HIV gp160 or to influenza haemagglutinin will render the respective virus non-infectious and such antibodies are said to be **neutralizing antibodies**.

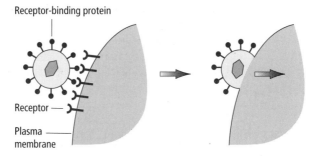

Receptor-binding protein

Receptor —

Plasma membrane

Figure 9.4 Entry of an enveloped virus (human immunodeficiency virus; HIV) by membrane fusion.

The second stage of the entry process is penetration—the transfer of the virion across the plasma membrane. The virus may be taken into the cell by receptor-mediated endocytosis, but this places the virion in a membrane-bound vesicle analogous to a phagosome. To gain entry to the cytoplasm the virus must cross this membrane. Our knowledge of this process is, in most instances, rudimentary. The surfaces of non-enveloped viruses must contain proteins that disrupt the lipid bilayer. The enveloped viruses can gain entry to the cytoplasm by fusion of the envelope with the plasma membrane (Fig. 9.4). This membrane fusion process can take place at the cell surface, as we believe to be true for HIV, or with the vesicle membrane following endocytosis. Thus, for example, influenza virus adsorbs to the cell surface and is then engulfed in an endocytic vesicle. When the pH of the vesicle drops due to lysosomal fusion,

6 Glycoprotein of 160 000 molecular weight.

a change in the conformation of the haemagglutinin molecule takes place. This induces membrane fusion and admits the virus to the cytoplasm.

The eclipse phase is a phase of genetic activity

During this phase of the life cycle, the virus fulfils its function as a **genetic parasite**: the genetic information of the virus programmes the cell to produce new virus particles. The strategy used by different viruses to achieve this varies depending on the type of nucleic acid that comprises the virus genome, but there are some concepts that must be true for all viruses. If new virus particles are to be made, the host cell must make **new virion proteins** for the formation of capsids, and **enzymes which will replicate the virus nucleic acid** to produce progeny genomes. The progeny genome can then be packaged by virion proteins to form new virus particles. The synthesis of new virus-specific proteins requires virus-specific mRNA molecules, and the **strategy** used to subvert the host cell can be thought of as the **route taken to synthesize mRNA**. The different strategies are summarized in Fig. 9.5, and are described briefly below.

Double-stranded DNA viruses (Fig. 9.6; examples: herpesviruses, papillomaviruses)

The use of a double-stranded (ds) DNA genome is familiar to us because this is what **animals** do. The viral ds DNA can be transcribed into mRNA by a host-specific transcriptase (ds DNA-dependent RNA polymerase), and the resulting mRNA is translated into viral proteins in the cytoplasm. These proteins must include new capsid proteins and a virus-specific DNA polymerase to replicate the virus genome. **The virus DNA must be in the cell nucleus** if it is to be transcribed (Fig. 9.6). Replication of viral DNA will also occur in the nucleus and new capsid proteins will therefore contain signals which tell them to go to

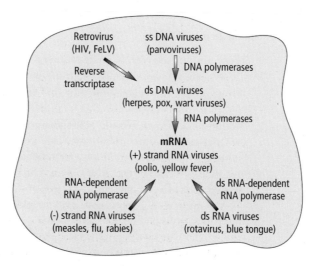

Figure 9.5 Virus gene expression: the routes to messenger RNA.

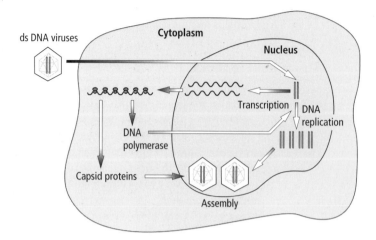

ds DNA viruses

Cytoplasm

Nucleus

Transcription

DNA replication

DNA polymerase

Capsid proteins

Assembly

Figure 9.6 Replication strategies: double-stranded DNA viruses.

the nucleus, where they will package progeny DNA. This is a feature of most DNA viruses–**the viral DNA replicates in the nucleus and new virus particles appear in the nucleus**. Not surprisingly, gross histological changes are frequently seen in the nuclei of cells infected with DNA viruses, and these changes are often of diagnostic value. Note also that, since the first protein involved in this strategy is a **host enzyme** (RNA polymerase), the viral DNA alone is infectious when it is introduced artificially into the host cell.

The strategy of single-stranded DNA viruses, such as parvoviruses, is similar except that the first step is the synthesis of the complementary strand to form a double strand, catalysed by a host enzyme. However, at the end of the process only one strand is packaged.

Positive-stranded RNA viruses (Fig. 9.7; examples: polio, hepatitis A, yellow fever, rubella)

These are viruses with a single-stranded RNA of positive (i.e. coding) sense. Clearly, the cell can do only one thing with such a molecule–translate it: the **virus genome is the message**. The first step then is translation to give virus-specific proteins–both the capsid proteins and an enzyme capable of replicating the RNA molecule. This is a single-strand RNA-dependent RNA polymerase: it makes RNA on an RNA template. The enzyme synthesizes the complementary strand (the minus strand) using the viral RNA as a template and then uses the minus strand as a template to make more plus (positive) strands. The plus strands are packaged and we have new virus. Note that all this can occur in the cytoplasm: there is no requirement for nuclear functions. Indeed, experimentally, many RNA viruses will replicate in cultured cells from which the nuclei have been removed. Note also that the first step is translation by host ribosomes, and we would predict (correctly) that the viral RNA **alone** is infectious if injected artificially into the host cell.

158

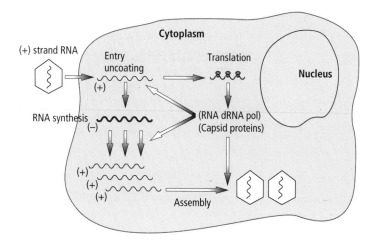

Figure 9.7 Replication strategies: positive-stranded RNA viruses.

Negative-stranded RNA viruses (Fig. 9.8; examples: influenza, measles, rabies)

Unlike the previous group, these viruses contain a single-stranded RNA molecule that is **not** an mRNA; it is the complement of the message. The sequence of events is rather similar, but we have a problem: the cell can neither translate this molecule, nor copy it (cells have no RNA-dependent RNA polymerase). It follows that **negative-strand RNA viruses have to contain an RNA-dependent RNA polymerase within the virus particle**. After the virion enters the cytoplasm, this virion enzyme copies the viral RNA to generate the complementary plus strand (the message), and this is then translated to give new proteins. The plus strand is copied to minus strand, the minus strand (together with the enzyme) is packaged and we have new virus. Note that we have now identified a virus group in which the viral genome alone is **not**

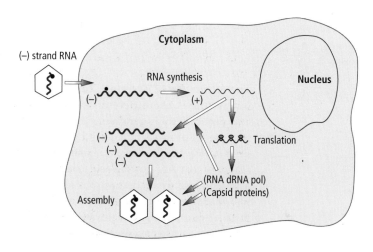

Figure 9.8 Replication strategies: negative-stranded RNA viruses.

infectious, because an enzyme within the virus particle is required to initiate the eclipse phase.

The replication of double-stranded RNA viruses follows a similar strategy: the cell can do nothing with a ds RNA molecule and the first step is to use this molecule as a template for the production of mRNA. This is performed by an enzyme present in the virion—a double-strand RNA-dependent RNA polymerase. The sequence of events is then similar to that of negative-strand RNA viruses except that plus and minus strands are packaged together as double strands (together with the enzyme).

Retroviruses (Fig. 9.9; examples: HIV, feline leukaemia virus)

The members of this important group contain single-stranded RNA but they replicate via a DNA intermediate. The virus particle contains a **reverse transcriptase**, an enzyme that synthesizes DNA from an RNA template. The eclipse phase begins with the synthesis of a DNA copy of the viral genome and this DNA then **integrates** into the chromosomes of the host cell where it is referred to as the **provirus**. Host cell RNA polymerase 'sees' the provirus as a normal set of host genes and uses it as a template to transcribe RNA molecules that can be used as mRNA for the synthesis of viral proteins or as progeny RNA for packaging.

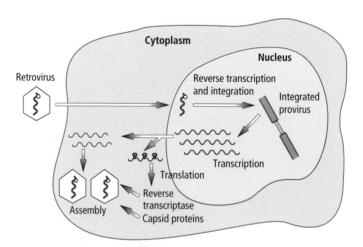

Figure 9.9 Replication strategies: retroviruses.

The eclipse phase, therefore, comprises a variety of processes in which different viruses use different strategies to express their genetic information and replicate their genomes. This variety can seem bewildering, but this is because we are so familiar with just **one** route of information transfer: from DNA to RNA in messenger synthesis and DNA to DNA in replication. The reality is that **any nucleic acid molecule can be copied to any other nucleic acid molecule, given the appropriate enzyme.** Hence there are many routes for information transfer and viruses have evolved that use them all. In considering these eclipse-phase strategies we are led to a number of general conclusions: first, **DNA viruses make use of host transcription machinery**. The viral DNA is therefore found in the nucleus and this is the site of viral DNA replication and virus particle assembly. Since transcription by **host** enzymes is the route to message, the genome alone is infectious. Second, **RNA viruses multiply in the cytoplasm**. **Positive**-strand RNA virus genomes **are** mRNA molecules and the genome alone is therefore infectious. **Negative**-strand and **double**-strand RNA virus genomes are used as templates for mRNA production by virion-associated transcription enzymes. The genome alone is not infectious.

There are two important groups of viruses which do not follow these general rules. We shall come across these viruses in a number of contexts, so we should note their replication strategies.

Poxviruses

These are large double-stranded DNA viruses (the biggest of all) and code for hundreds of proteins. Their replication strategy is the familiar one: mRNA is synthesized using viral DNA as a template and the DNA genome is replicated by DNA-dependent DNA polymerase. However, poxviruses differ from all other DNA viruses in that they do not make use of host cell transcription machinery. The virus particle contains its own DNA-dependent RNA polymerase and the virus is therefore independent of host nuclear functions. Poxviruses set up home in the cytoplasm.

Hepatitis B virus

This is a member of the **hepadnavirus group**. Although these viruses contain double-stranded DNA, the viral genome does not replicate by the familiar DNA→DNA route. The virus DNA enters the nucleus and RNA transcripts are produced by the host RNA polymerase. However these molecules, as well as acting as mRNAs, are used as templates for the synthesis of progeny virus DNA by a virus-specific RNA-dependent DNA polymerase (**reverse transcriptase**). New virus DNA therefore appears in the cytoplasm, where it is packaged into new virus particles. Note that this replication strategy has features in common with those of retroviruses; it involves the synthesis of DNA using an RNA template by reverse transcriptase. For this reason retroviruses and hepadnaviruses are sometimes grouped together as **reversiviruses**. The sequence of events in retrovirus replication is RNA→DNA→RNA, whereas in hepadnavirus replication it is DNA→RNA→DNA. The cycle is similar, but the **packaging** point is different.

New virus particles have to assemble and escape from the cell

Biochemical examination of the virus-infected cell illuminates the mechanisms used by the virus to synthesize new virus proteins and progeny genomes, but tells us little about how these components recognize each other and assemble together to form new virus particles. The process of capsid formation and encapsidation of the viral genome is obviously very specific and must involve the **recognition of particular nucleotide sequences** (packaging signals) because virus particles very rarely contain the wrong piece of nucleic acid. The

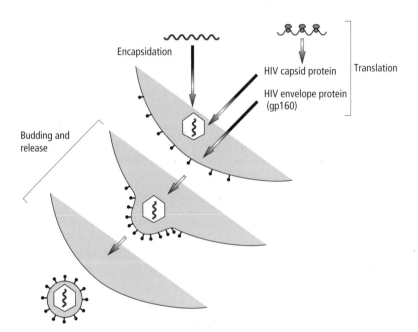

Figure 9.10 Secretion of an enveloped virus (human immunodeficiency virus; HIV).

assembly of helical nucleocapsids seems to be a progressive process in which individual protein subunits or groups of subunits are added sequentially around the nucleic acid from a single growing point. In contrast, icosahedral structures are often formed in the absence of nucleic acid. These empty capsids then eat up a copy of the viral genome to become assembled nucleocapsids.

The simplest mechanism for release of virus particles into the outside world is **host cell death**. The cell lyses and particles are released. Most enveloped viruses, however, acquire their envelope by **budding through the plasma membrane of the host cell**, a process that allows release of virus particles without damaging the cell. Note that, since the envelope of the virus particle must contain proteins responsible for binding and entering the next host cell, the plasma membranes of the infected cell must also contain these proteins, because the plasma membrane will become the viral envelope. Thus, for example, the surface of an HIV-infected cell contains gp160, the glycoprotein present on the surface of the virus particle (Fig. 9.10).

The timing of events in the replication cycle has to be controlled

In this examination of the multiplication of viruses we have considered the virus as a passive intruder; as a group of genes which is translated and replicated. The proteins encoded by the virus genome must include, at a bare minimum, an enzyme capable of replicating the virus nucleic acid, and capsid proteins in which to package the progeny genomes.

It is apparent that some **temporal control** over this process is required. For instance, **replication of the viral nucleic acid should precede synthesis of new capsid proteins**, because there is little point in accumulating capsid proteins

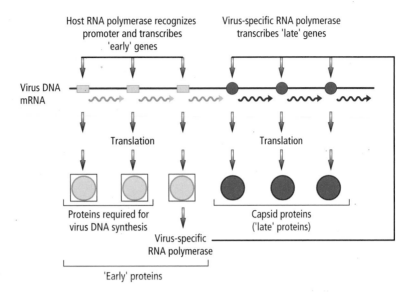

Host RNA polymerase recognizes promoter and transcribes 'early' genes

Virus-specific RNA polymerase transcribes 'late' genes

Virus DNA
mRNA

Translation

Translation

Proteins required for virus DNA synthesis

Virus-specific RNA polymerase

Capsid proteins ('late' proteins)

'Early' proteins

Figure 9.11 Early and late genes: a temporal cascade.

before a pool of replicating nucleic acid is established. Indeed, reference to the different replication strategies shows that, in most instances, newly made viral nucleic acid has two functions: as a template for the synthesis of more nucleic acid and as progeny nucleic acid for encapsidation. It follows that **encapsidation removes viral nucleic acid from the replicating pool and tends to suppress further amplification of the pool**. Efficient viral replication therefore requires regulation of these events. This control is most easily discerned in DNA virus replication, where the expression of different genes occurs during different parts of the eclipse phase. At the beginning of the eclipse, a subset of viral genes is transcribed, including genes which code for enzymes involved in DNA replication. Replication of virus DNA now begins and transcription of a further set of genes now occurs—genes which code for the capsid proteins. This temporal control is found in all DNA viruses and has led to the division of viral genes and viral proteins into **early proteins** (those made early in the cycle) and **late proteins** (those made only after a delay). The means by which temporal control is achieved are many and varied but one simple example is given in Fig. 9.11. This is a transcriptional control system in which the virus genome contains two sets of genes. The first set (the early genes) is recognized by the host cell RNA polymerase and is transcribed immediately after the viral DNA enters the nucleus. The second set is not recognized by the host enzyme (these genes are preceded by different promoter sequences). The early genes code for enzymes involved in DNA synthesis but in addition one of them codes for a new, virus-specific, RNA polymerase. This enzyme recognizes the second set of virus genes, which codes for capsid proteins. The consequence is a positive cascade control system in which expression of one set of genes permits expression of a second set. In the example shown, viral DNA synthesis will precede the accumulation of capsid proteins, ensuring the generation of a pool of replicating virus DNA before the assembly of capsids. This is a simple example. Many DNA viruses, particularly the larger ones, exhibit cascades involving multiple subsets of genes. Furthermore **regulation is not only temporal but also quantitative** because different proteins are required in different amounts.

In this account we have taken a minimalist view of virus replication. We have implied that a virus requires genes that code only for nucleic acid-replicating enzymes and for capsid proteins; and that the only difference between different viruses is the way in which they express and replicate these genes. But some viruses contain hundreds of genes and yet even the most complicated virus particle contains only perhaps 30 different proteins. What do all these genes do? In most cases we do not know, but as we shall see, viruses modify their hosts in a variety of ways. **The virus is not a passive intruder.** It actively modifies its host to create a suitable environment for its multiplication, survival and spread.

Subcellular infectious agents have been discovered that are *not* viruses

During the past 20 years a number of diseases have been identified which are caused by very small infectious agents which are quite different from viruses. Nevertheless, because they are subcellular entities, they are usually considered as falling within the domain of virologists (at least, this is what virologists think) and we will describe these remarkable agents here for want of anywhere better to put them. These agents are of two types.

Viroids are small circular RNA molecules of only a few hundred nucleotides

They have no protein coat and seem not to code for anything—they are not translatable. They survive outside their hosts because the RNA molecule is very heavily base-paired, and base-paired (i.e. double-stranded) RNA is very stable and resistant to enzymic hydrolysis by most RNAases. We do not understand how these molecules multiply but we think they utilize host cell enzymes that process large nuclear RNA molecules to mRNA.

The agents of transmissible spongiform encephalopathies are most mysterious

There are a number of diseases of humans and animals called spongiform encephalopathies because of the spongy appearance of the brain resulting from extensive vacuolation of the cells. These are progressive and invariably fatal diseases, and some, like **kuru in humans, scrapie in sheep** and **bovine spongiform encephalopathy**, are experimentally and naturally transmissible. The nature of the transmissible agents is uncertain but **they are not viruses**: no virus particles have been seen and there is no detectable immune response in these diseases. The agents of these diseases are therefore sometimes called

unconventional agents. There are two opposing views as to the nature of these fascinating entities. One view is that the agent is an aberrant form of a host protein which can catalyse the modification of the normal host protein to the aberrant form (i.e. a positive feedback loop). This view is supported by the fact that highly purified forms of the infectious material are composed of an abnormal form of a protein found in normal neurons. The alternative view is that there must be an infectious nucleic acid associated with infectivity and this view is supported by the fact that different genetic strains of the agent have been isolated from a single species and 'breed true' on passage. Obviously, both of these views cannot be correct. Perhaps neither of them is!

Summary

Viruses are sets of parasitic genes encased in a protein coat, composed of repeating subunits, to allow transmission from host to host. Different viruses contain different types of nucleic acid and this is reflected in the range of strategies that viruses use to subvert the host cell machinery.

10 Viruses and the host cell

When we looked at the nature of viruses and their strategies for multiplication, we reached the conclusion that the virus is **a set of parasitic genes encased in a protein coat**. When these genes are introduced into a cell, the new information is converted into new proteins that are responsible for creating new viruses. Although true, this implies a rather passive process resulting in little change in the cell. In fact, most **viruses cause dramatic changes in cell metabolism and structure**; the virus modifies the cell, subverting it to a vehicle for virus production.

In some instances the changes are so great they can be seen with the light microscope. Virus particles may be so numerous that huge clumps of them produce **inclusion bodies** within the nucleus or the cytoplasm. Multiplication of some viruses, particularly DNA viruses (e.g. herpesviruses), causes **death of the host cells**. Cells infected with certain viruses, such as measles, will fuse with their neighbours and in some instances this can be dramatic, causing the formation of a large multinucleate cytoplasmic mass or **syncytium**, often even larger than the multinucleate cells we have met before. Other viruses induce **cell proliferation**. These gross changes are sometimes of practical medical use because biopsy may allow histological identification of groups of virus-infected cells, which can be used to diagnose the cause of the virus infection. In addition these morphological changes form the basis of simple laboratory assays for virus infectivity, using cells in culture. We will now examine some of these changes that occur in virus-infected cells and try to explain how they occur.

Metabolic changes

The synthesis of hundreds of thousands of new virus particles by an infected cell must place enormous strains on the metabolism of the cell. How does the virus modify the host cell metabolism and harness it for its own ends?

Some viruses shut down host protein synthesis

An animal cell normally makes hundreds of different proteins of its own, and we can observe this simply by feeding cultured cells with radiolabelled amino acids for say 30 min and then examining the various radiolabelled proteins that have been synthesized. If we do the same experiment with poliovirus-infected cells we find, amazingly, that **none of these host cell proteins is made**. Only a few proteins are synthesized and they are all polio-specific. The virus has modified the cell to a factory that makes poliovirus only. This phenomenon is called **host shut-down**. Not surprisingly, the cell produces large numbers of poliovirus particles in a short time and the cell is by then doomed. Host shut-down is seen in many virus infections, though by no means all, and can be achieved by a number of mechanisms. In the case of poliovirus, **the virus synthesizes a protein which modifies ribosomes** so that they no longer recognize host cell messenger RNA (mRNA), but will recognize and translate poliovirus RNA. The distinction is based on the fact that host mRNAs contain a methylated 5′-linked guanosine residue at their 5′ ends. This so-called 5′-cap is absent from poliovirus RNA and the modified ribosomes in polio-infected cells no longer recognize capped RNA (host RNA) but do recognize uncapped RNA (poliovirus RNA).

Some viruses stimulate the cells they infect

Dividing cells are metabolically more active than resting cells. Not surprisingly, therefore, viruses **multiply better in dividing cells than in resting cells**. This is particularly true of DNA viruses, because the synthesis of virus DNA requires deoxyribonucleotides and these are in short supply in non-dividing cells, because the resting cell does not need them. In the animal host, most cells are not dividing and are unsuitable for virus replication.

One group of DNA viruses, the parvoviruses (the smallest viruses of all) are found only in actively dividing cells, but other viruses have found an answer to this problem. **Adenoviruses and papovaviruses stimulate the cells that they infect to enter the cell division cycle**: deoxynucleotides are synthesized and cell DNA synthesis begins. The virus is now in a favourable environment and virus replication can occur. There is an apparent contradiction here: in the last section we saw that many viruses can shut down host cell macromolecular synthesis whereas we are now saying that some viruses stimulate cells. The key is in the **timing** of these events. When a cell is infected by the papovavirus, simian virus 40 (SV40), it first makes a protein called T-antigen which **stimulates** the cell to divide. This is followed by virus DNA replication, capsid protein synthesis, the appearance of new virus particles and host cell death. Host macromolecule synthesis is progressively replaced by virus macromolecule synthesis. **The virus first stimulates the cell to divide, then itself replicates, then kills the cell.** As we noted in the last chapter, viral gene expression is **temporally controlled**. Here we see an example: first T-antigen synthesis (early gene expression), then viral DNA synthesis, then capsid protein synthesis (late gene expression). The ability of some viruses to stimulate host cells into the division cycle is of great interest, and we are beginning to understand the mechanisms involved. For example, the T-antigen of SV40 can form a complex with two cell proteins, called p53 and Rb-105. These host proteins are encoded by **suppressor genes** and their job is to maintain the cell in a non-dividing state. When T-antigen binds to these proteins it inactivates them, and the cell therefore enters the division cycle (see also Chapter 17).

Before leaving this topic we should note that poxviruses also stimulate cell division, but in quite a different way. When a poxvirus infects an epithelial cell it makes an epidermal growth factor which is then secreted by the infected cell, and stimulates growth of surrounding **uninfected** cells. When we examine

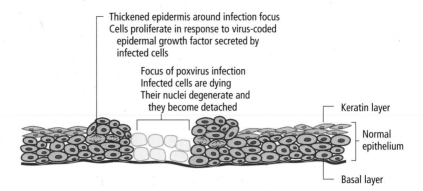

Figure 10.1 Poxvirus infection

a focus of poxvirus infection in epithelium, therefore, we see infected cells that are dying, surrounded by a zone of proliferating uninfected cells (Fig. 10.1). The virus has evolved this mechanism for providing itself with an excellent supply of new host cells.

Large DNA viruses specify enzymes for deoxyribonucleotide synthesis

Stimulating the host cell to enter the division cycle is one way of ensuring a supply of deoxyribonucleotides, but there is another alternative: the virus can itself specify the necessary enzymes for deoxyribonucleotide synthesis. This strategy is adopted by herpesviruses and poxviruses, viruses with a very large coding potential.

These viruses have genes which code for enzymes like **thymidine kinase**, which catalyses the conversion of thymidine to thymidine monophosphate, and **ribonucleotide reductase**, which converts ribonucleotides to deoxyribonucleotides (Fig. 10.2). All cells contain these enzymes, but they are present

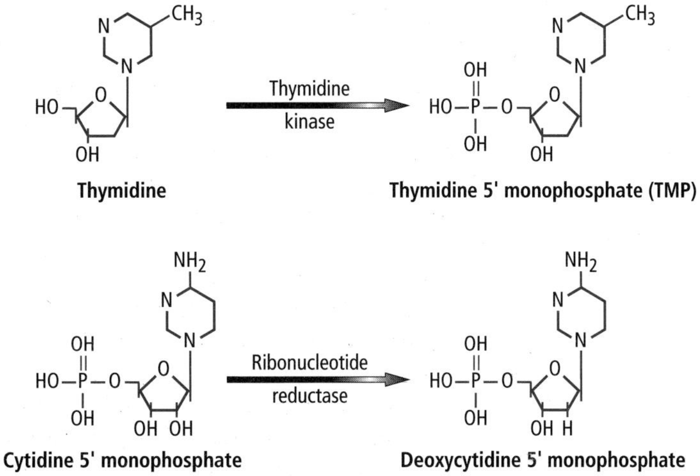

Figure 10.2 Examples of enzymes, encoded by poxviruses and herpesviruses, that increase the deoxyribonucleotide pool in the infected cells.

Thymidine → (Thymidine kinase) → Thymidine 5' monophosphate (TMP)

Cytidine 5' monophosphate → (Ribonucleotide reductase) → Deoxycytidine 5' monophosphate

169

at very low levels in resting cells. If we examine these enzymes in poxvirus- or herpesvirus-infected cells we find that they are abundant. These virus-induced enzymes are **biochemically distinguishable from the host enzymes**: these viruses in fact specify **viral homologues** of host enzymes. An understanding of these enzymes is important: since they are different from the host enzymes, it is possible to find substrate analogues which will react with these virus enzymes but not with the host enzyme. These enzymes are therefore prime targets for antiviral chemotherapy.

Changes at the cell surface

As well as modifying cell metabolism, viruses can make alterations to the cell surface. This is particularly true of **enveloped** viruses. The plasma membrane will become the virus envelope and must therefore have proteins inserted into it that will enable the virus to bind the receptors of other cells. The cell surface contacts and communicates with other cells, the cell surface interacts with soluble factors and the cell surface is recognized by the immune system. We are ignorant about the details of many of these phenomena and of the ways in which viruses interfere with them, but we can consider a few examples.

Some viruses promote cell fusion

An enveloped virus achieves entry into the host cell by binding to the plasma membrane and fusing its envelope with the cell membrane. The nucleocapsid is then released into the cytoplasm. Virus-specific proteins in the virus envelope are responsible for the binding and fusion. These virus-specific proteins must be present in the plasma membrane of the infected cell, because the plasma membrane will become the virus envelope, and it follows that the membrane of the infected cell (like the envelope of the virus) can bind to and fuse with the plasma membrane of an uninfected cell. This is illustrated in Fig. 10.3, which also shows that viruses of this type have two methods of transfer from cell to cell. On the one hand they can bud from the cell and then infect a new cell, while on the other they can pass from cell to cell as a result of

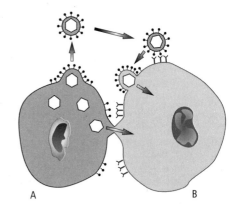

Figure 10.3 Diagram illustrating membrane fusion and transmission of cell-associated virus. The infected cell (A) produces virus nucleocapsids and virus membrane proteins that are inserted in the plasma membrane. Nucleocapsids bud through the plasma membrane to produce the enveloped virus particle which binds to specific receptors on a neighbouring uninfected cell (B) and enters by membrane fusion (see Chapter 11). Alternatively, virus membrane proteins on the surface of the infected cell bind to receptors on the neighbouring cell and fusion is induced. The nucleocapsid may now pass from one cell to the next.

A   B

membrane fusion between neighbouring cells. In the latter case the virus has passed from cell to cell without being outside a cell, and hence without being susceptible to attack by antibody molecules or phagocytes. **Viruses of this type are said to be cell-associated** because infectivity is associated with infected cells rather than with free virus particles. Thus enveloped viruses like measles and mumps (paramyxoviruses) or chickenpox (varicella-zoster—a herpes virus) are circulated around the body primarily in the form of infected cells (i.e. cell-associated), whereas a non-enveloped virus like polio is present as free virions and it cannot get from cell to cell without passing through an extracellular phase.

Viruses can interfere with the immune response

We shall consider the immune response to viruses in more detail later, but since virus-infected cells synthesize foreign antigens we can predict that they will be targets for the humoral and cell-mediated arms of the immune response. Viruses have evolved mechanisms to avoid both. Adenoviruses, which cause acute respiratory disease, make a protein that binds to the major histo-compatibility complex (MHC) Class I antigen and prevents its transfer to the cell surface. Since the Class I MHC antigen is responsible for presenting anti-gens to cytotoxic T cells, adenovirus-infected cells thereby avoid damage from cytotoxic T cells. Some herpesviruses make a cell-surface protein that binds to the Fc portion of immunoglobulin G (IgG); i.e. they make an Fc receptor. If IgG recognizes proteins on the virus-infected cell, it will bind both by its specific binding sites and by its Fc portion. The antibodies react with the infected cell but the cell is spared the consequences, because the Fc portion of the antibody is unavailable for recognition by effector mechanisms such as complement or the Fc receptor on macrophages or neutrophils.

In the last chapter we explored the fundamental principles of virus infec-tion and multiplication. Here we emphasize that the relationship of the virus with the cells is complex. Viruses have evolved many tricks to modify the cell for their own ends—to modify cell metabolism for the purposes of replication, to modify the cell surface to achieve spread of virus by stealth, and to avoid the immune response. These are just a few examples. We should note that many of these modifications are rather subtle ones. They improve the prospects of the virus in its host but they are not absolutely necessary for virus multiplication. We can prove this by attempting artificially to delete individual virus genes from the viral genome. Genes that encode viral capsid proteins or viral polymerases are absolutely essential to the virus and mutants with deletions in these genes cannot replicate. However, if we delete the thymidine kinase gene from a poxvirus or from herpes simplex virus artificially, we obtain mutants which will multiply perfectly well in growing cells in culture, but only poorly in resting cells and very poorly in an animal. Similarly, if we delete the Fc-receptor gene from herpes simplex virus or the epidermal growth factor gene from poxviruses, there is no effect on virus growth in tissue culture, but the mutant viruses survive poorly in an infected animal. **Genes of this type are dispensable in culture, but are important in the multicellular host.**

What is the outcome of infection for the host cell?

The outcome for the cell varies depending on the virus–cell combination. The most common consequence is probably cell death but this is certainly not inevitable and unfortunately there are no simple rules. Here are a few generalizations.

1 Multiplication of DNA viruses usually kills the cell, probably because nuclear function is disrupted.

2 Multiplication of non-enveloped viruses usually kills the cell because the new virus must escape by disrupting the plasma membrane.

3 Multiplication of enveloped RNA viruses and retroviruses is not necessarily lethal for the cell because nuclear function is not disrupted and the virus buds through the plasma membrane, leaving it intact. Some viruses in this group can be used to establish **persistent infection in culture**: cells can be infected and maintained indefinitely while continuing to produce new virus particles. Retroviruses are particularly impressive at establishing persistent infection and are worth exploring in more detail.

Retroviruses can establish latent or persistent infection

We recall that these viruses contain a reverse transcriptase that converts the RNA genome to a DNA molecule, the provirus. The provirus integrates into the host genome and will be transcribed by cellular RNA polymerase. In addition, if the cell divides, both daughter cells will receive a copy of the provirus. The outcome of infection will in turn depend on the efficiency with which the provirus is transcribed into mRNA and this will depend on a number of factors such as site of integration of the provirus, the type of cell infected and the metabolic state of the cell. At one extreme the provirus may not be transcribed at all, no virus-specific mRNA will be made and hence no virus particles. The cell produces no virus but **has the potential to do so because the provirus is present**. The cell is said to be **latently infected**. At the other extreme the cell may transcribe the provirus very actively and very large numbers of virus particles will be produced. This may be incompatible with cell survival and the cell may die (i.e. **lytic infection**). At intermediate levels of virus gene expression, limited numbers of virus particles will be produced and the cells will continue to thrive—the cell is said to be **persistently infected**. The life cycle of retroviruses thus gives the virus a range of options. For example, human immunodeficiency virus (HIV) infection of 'activated' dividing lymphocytes results in extensive virus production and cell death, while infection of resting lymphocytes or resting monocytes results in little or no gene expression, and results in no gross changes in the host cell.

Some viruses can transform cells

Some viruses can induce uncontrolled proliferation of cells in culture. This phenomenon is called **transformation**; but before examining the mechanisms involved we should define what we mean by cell transformation. Normal cells in culture multiply in a controlled way: they stop dividing when they contact each other (contact inhibition) and therefore form an ordered cell sheet or monolayer. A number of physical and chemical agents can cause genetic changes that result in a change in this behaviour. The cells now multiply in a disordered fashion, and no longer show contact inhibition. When a transformed cell arises in a culture of normal cells, it continues to multiply to form a dense multilayered colony, sometimes called a **transformed focus**. Because they exhibit uncontrolled division, transformed cells are reminiscent of cancer cells and indeed these cells will sometimes cause tumours when they are injected into an appropriate animal. The ability of a virus to induce this phenomenon should make us suspicious that the virus might be a factor in causing cancer. This is a possibility we shall return to later, in Chapter 17. Here we are only concerned with the mechanism of virus-induced cell transformation. Two kinds of viruses are involved, DNA viruses and retroviruses, and they cause transformation by quite different mechanisms.

Transformation by DNA viruses results from abortive infection

We have noted earlier that certain DNA viruses, notably adenoviruses and papovaviruses, stimulate the infected cell to divide by causing the synthesis of a protein that binds to host proteins which suppress division. This is normally followed by virus DNA replication, virus capsid protein synthesis and cell death. However, these later stages of the eclipse phase may fail (the infection **aborts**). Thus in SV40 infection, T-antigen synthesis may occur but not viral DNA synthesis or capsid protein synthesis. The cell is stimulated to enter the division cycle but is not subsequently killed by virus replication. The viral DNA will be degraded and, when the cell divides, T-antigen will be diluted out. Occasionally, however, the virus DNA, or perhaps the part of the virus DNA containing the T-antigen gene, fortuitously integrates into the cell chromosome (it turns out that mammalian cells are quite promiscuous in integrating foreign DNA). Now all the daughter cells will receive the T-antigen gene, all will be continuously stimulated and a clone of cells will appear exhibiting uncontrolled growth—a transformed focus. Each of the cells in the focus will contain SV40 T-antigen. We can see now why this protein is called T-antigen. T stands for **t**ransformation or **t**umour (the transformed cells will cause a tumour if injected into an immunocompromised animal). Transformation by SV40 and by some other DNA viruses thus requires two events (Fig. 10.4). The first is **failure of viral DNA synthesis and late gene expression. The second is the integration of the T-antigen gene** (the stimulating gene) **into the chromosome** so that it becomes a stable component of the cell genotype. Not surprisingly, transformation is a rare event, but its frequency can be increased in two ways.

1 Transformation is more efficient in non-permissive cells: infection of primate cells with SV40 normally results in virus replication and cell death (**permissive infection**). Infection of rodent cells results in T-antigen synthesis but the remainder of the virus life cycle fails (these cells are **non-permissive** and abortive infection is the norm). All the cells now fulfil our first requirement for

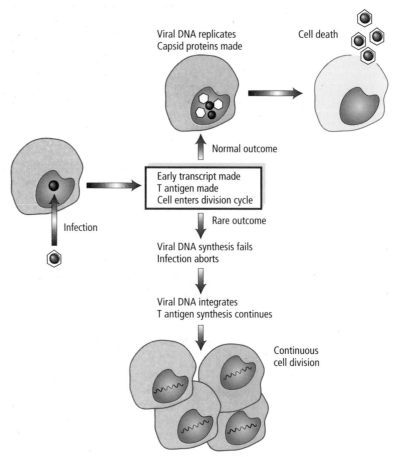

Figure 10.4 Sequence of events in transformation by simian virus 40 (SV40). SV40 contains a circular DNA genome that can be divided into two parts: the 'early region' encodes the T-antigen and can be transcribed from the infecting viral genome by the host polymerase. The 'late region' encodes the capsid proteins and is transcribed only after viral DNA replication. Very rarely, viral DNA replication fails and, again rarely, the viral DNA may integrate into a host chromosome. T-antigen synthesis will continue and the cell will divide. Since the daughter cells receive a copy of the integrated viral DNA, this process of T-antigen synthesis and cell division will continue indefinitely.

transformation (replication failure) and transformation is more readily observed.

2 The T-antigen gene alone transforms cells: genetic engineering allows us to isolate the T-antigen gene from the remainder of the SV40 virus DNA. When the T-antigen gene is introduced into cells, transformation is observed (we have eliminated the problem of virus replication and cell death). This experiment formally proves that T-antigen is the protein responsible for cell transformation. **Genes whose expression causes transformation are called oncogenes.** The SV40 T-antigen gene is therefore a **viral oncogene.**

It is important to recognize that **viruses have not evolved to transform cells**. Unlike the cellular changes described earlier in this chapter, cell transformation offers no advantage to the virus; it is a dead end. Some DNA viruses have evolved to stimulate cells prior to growing in them, but transformation by them is an aberration resulting from failure of the infection cycle.

Transformation by retroviruses is due to acquisition of host genes

Unlike DNA viruses, retroviruses do not code for a stimulating protein as part of their replication strategy and the multiplication of retroviruses does not inevitably result in cell death. Retroviruses therefore transform cells by quite a different mechanism. In fact, **normal retroviruses do not transform cells in culture**, but variants occasionally arise that will transform cells and will cause tumours in a host animal.

The first tumour virus identified was isolated at the beginning of the 20th century by Peyton Rous[1] from a chicken sarcoma (a cancer of muscle cells). Rous showed that an extract of this tumour would cause sarcomas when injected into other chicks. The virus was called Rous sarcoma virus (RSV) and it was not until half a century later, with the advent of cell culture and genetic engineering, that we began to understand why RSV causes tumours and will transform chick fibroblasts. The key is the difference between the genome of RSV and that of most other avian retroviruses. All retroviruses have the same basic genetic content. They are composed of three genes called *gag, pol* and *env*: *gag* stands for group antigen and codes for the capsid, *pol* stands for polymerase (the reverse transcriptase) and *env* stands for envelope (the enve-lope protein). **RSV contains an additional gene** (Fig. 10.5) **which is called *src* (for sarcoma).** We know that the *src* gene is responsible for transformation and tumour formation because mutation or deletion of the *src* gene eliminates these characteristics.

What is the *src* gene and where has it come from? It turns out that the *src* gene in RSV is virtually identical to a gene found in all chicken cells and indeed is closely related to a gene present in all vertebrate cells. **RSV has acquired a host gene** and to distinguish the gene in the virus from the gene in the normal cell we use the terms *v-src* and *c-src*.

What does the *src* gene do and why does *v-src* (the gene in the virus) cause cells to become transformed despite the fact that the gene (in the form of *c-src*) is already present in the uninfected cell? We still do not know precisely what the *src* gene does, but we do know that it codes for a protein that tells the cell to enter the division cycle—*src* is involved in **positive control of the cell cycle**. *v-src* differs from *c-src* in two ways. First, *v-src* is present in the provirus and will therefore be transcribed at high levels, like the other retrovirus genes—it is no longer under the control of cellular transcription signals. Second, during the process of being recombined into the provirus, mutation is likely to occur and as a result *v-src* is not quite identical to *c-src*. Thus *v-src*, a homologue of a normal cellular gene, transforms cells because it is expressed at high levels and because it contains a mutation. In the last section we defined genes whose

1 But Peyton Rous, a New York physician, received a Nobel prize for this discovery only decades later.

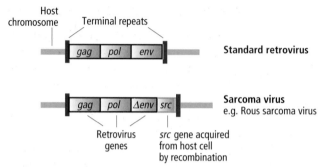

Figure 10.5 Transformation by Rous sarcoma virus (RSV) and the RSV genome. The provirus is a DNA copy of the retrovirus RNA. The mechanism of provirus synthesis and integration is complex and results in the generation of a repeated sequence which includes a strong viral promoter responsible for driving transcription of the viral genes. RSV contains an additional sequence (the *src* gene) which is of host origin. Acquisition of host genes is almost invariably accompanied by loss of some—often most — of the viral genes.

expression results in cell transformation as oncogenes. *v-src* **is therefore an oncogene**. Its cellular homologue, from which it is derived, is sometimes referred to as a **proto-oncogene**.

Many different transforming retroviruses have been isolated from a variety of species. All of these viruses conform to the general description of RSV: they contain **genes of cellular origin which by definition are oncogenes**. Different transforming retroviruses contain different cellular genes and all of these genes are oncogenes. We should not conclude that retroviruses have a particular ability to acquire proto-oncogenes. Retroviruses recombine rather promiscuously and any population of retroviruses will contain virus particles whose genomes include various cellular sequences. In the vast majority of cases this has no consequence: these viruses have no special properties that we can observe. Occasionally, however, the cellular gene acquired will be one that confers upon the virus the ability to transform cells—an oncogene. The significance of the transforming retroviruses to science is that **they have selected oncogenes for us**—they therefore allow us to identify natural host cell genes that play a key role in promoting cell growth and division.

Finally, it would appear at first glance that transforming retroviruses ought to be extremely dangerous entities because they can change normal cells to cancer. In fact, this is not the case because the acquisition of a cellular gene is almost invariably accompanied by the loss of some of the viral genome. As a result, transforming retroviruses grow poorly or not at all–they are **replication-defective**. Thus a virus like RSV may arise in a retrovirus-infected animal and will contribute to the formation of a tumour in that animal, but it will not be efficiently transmitted to other animals. Just as we found in the case of DNA viruses, retroviruses have not evolved to transform. Acquisition of oncogenes is of no value to the virus. It is an accident, but a very interesting one.

The cell can respond to virus infection

We have seen that viruses have evolved different ways of adapting their host cells to their own ends. But of course the host evolves too. The immune response is the most notable defence against virus infection, in the animal host, but individual cells have also evolved defence mechanisms. The best known of these is the production of **interferons**. Interferons are a family of proteins made in response to virus infection. They were discovered about half a century ago by showing that a component in culture medium from infected cells could protect uninfected cells from virus infection. **Interferons are proteins that are secreted by infected cells and act, via interferon receptors, on neighbouring uninfected cells.** These cells respond in a variety of ways, most of which we do not fully understand. One effect of interferon is to 'prime' cells. When primed cells encounter virus (or foreign nucleic acid) they respond by greatly decreasing protein synthesis, thus creating a very hostile environment for virus replication. A second effect of interferon is to increase MHC Class I synthesis, thus making the cell a very good cytotoxic T-cell target (note how this contrasts with the opposite effect of some viruses to **down**-regulate Class I synthesis). The overall effect of interferon is to surround the infected cell with cells which will not support virus multiplication and which will evoke a good immune response—interferon acts at short range and inhibits virus growth and spread in a tissue.

Summary

Viruses cause profound changes in the cells they infect. They can subvert the cell's metabolic machinery to ensure virus replication, change the properties of the cell membrane, persist and hide within the cell, transform the cell, or kill it.

11 Viruses in the multicellular host

In examining the behaviour of viruses in individual cells, we were concerned with the entry of the virus into the cell, its strategy for modifying the cell and multiplying within it, its effects on the cell and its means of exit. In the animal host we are concerned with much more complex questions: **How does the virus enter the host animal? How does it evade non-specific defences and the immune response? What tissues does it infect? How does it gain exit and transmit to new hosts?** Finally, **how does the interaction of virus and host cause disease?** What is the pathogenesis of virus infection?

The study of viruses in individual cells is not easy, but these new questions are an order of magnitude more difficult. Furthermore it is extremely difficult to study human viruses in any detail. How, for example, could we find what tissues are infected in a child with measles? Much of what we think we know comes from indirect evidence and, more importantly, from the **study of human viruses in susceptible animals**, from **studies of veterinary disease** and from the **study of viruses of laboratory animals** (for example, mousepox). We have referred mostly to human viruses simply because we are all more familiar with these viruses and the diseases they cause, but it is important to recognize that much of the good evidence about virus activity comes from studies of veterinary disease.

Virus infections may be superficial or systemic

Superficial infection means that the virus infects skin or a mucosal surface and infection is limited to this tissue. The virus does not penetrate beyond the submucosa and does not spread to other tissues. These diseases are generally of short duration (e.g. respiratory tract infections like the **common cold** or **influenza** and infection of the alimentary canal like **rotavirus diarrhoea**), although **wart viruses** are an obvious exception. These superficial infections seem to be **primarily controlled by non-specific defences** rather than by specific immune responses. This should not be taken to mean that immune responses play no role in recovery, but that they are not crucial. Immunosuppressed people are not at grave risk from superficial virus infection.

Systemic infections are those in which the virus invades the submucosa, is circulated around the body in lymph or blood and infects other organs and tissues. Viruses of this type cause diseases in which there is an incubation period of weeks or months before symptoms occur and recovery from infection is dependent on the immune response, non-specific defences having been evaded. Many systemic infections (e.g. **measles**, **chickenpox**) cause relatively

179

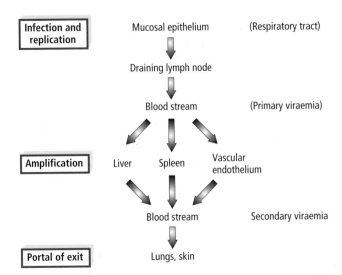

Figure 11.1 Multiplication and spread of ectromelia (mousepox) *in vivo*.

mild diseases of otherwise healthy people but can be severe or fatal in immunosuppressed individuals.

We do not know why some virus infections are superficial while others are systemic but the interaction of viruses with phagocytic cells in the submucosa is likely to be important. Most superficial viruses are destroyed by these cells, just as many bacteria are, while many systemic viruses are resistant to phagocytosis and in some cases (e.g. **smallpox**), will infect phagocytic cells and be spread around the body by them. In a few instances there are simpler explanations. Rhinoviruses (common cold viruses) multiply well at 33 °C but not at 37 °C. It is evident then that these viruses will be limited to the upper respiratory tract and would not survive in the lower respiratory tract or in deep tissues.

Given the number of organs, tissues and cell types within the body it is not surprising that systemic virus infections exhibit great variety, and that in many instances we do not know the details. One of the most thoroughly investigated is ectromelia (**mousepox**), outlined in Fig. 11.1, and this illustrates a number of general features: the virus must have **a portal of entry** (an initial site of infection), **a route of spread** within the body, a **target tissue for amplification** and **a portal of exit** (a tissue which will allow virus release to the outside world). Most viruses use mucosal surfaces as portals of entry, blood and lymph as routes of spread and mucosal surfaces or glandular secretions as routes of exit (Table 11.1), but there are exceptions. **Rabies**, for example, enters through bites or abrasions in the skin, spreads through nerves to the brain and then to the salivary glands where it is excreted in saliva. Some viruses (like **yellow fever virus**) are transmitted from the blood stream of one individual to the blood stream of another by biting insects such as mosquitoes and thus bypass the need to infect entry or exit tissues.

Table 11.1 Some examples of virus infection routes.

Virus	Entry tissue	Exit tissue	Transmission route
Superficial infection			
Rhinoviruses (common cold) } Influenza	Respiratory epithelium	Respiratory epithelium	Respiratory aerosol
Rotavirus (infantile diarrhoea)	Alimentary canal epithelium	Alimentary canal epithelium	Faecal–oral
Systemic infection			
Hepatitis A	Alimentary canal epithelium	Alimentary canal epithelium	Faecal–oral
Poliovirus	Oral epithelium Alimentary canal epithelium	Alimentary canal epithelium	Faecal–oral
Measles } Rubella* } Adenovirus	Respiratory epithelium	Respiratory epithelium	Respiratory aerosol
Herpes simplex (oral) } Epstein–Barr virus	Oral epithelium	Oral epithelium	Oral contact
Herpes simplex (genital)	Genital epithelium	Genital epithelium	Sexual contact
Yellow fever	Blood	Blood	Mosquito-transmitted
Rabies	Submucosa (punctured skin)	Salivary gland	Animal bite
Human immunodeficiency virus (HIV)* } Hepatitis B	Blood Cells of the genital tract epithelium	Blood Genital secretions	Blood contact Blood products Sexual contact
Human cytomegalovirus*	Oral epithelium Genital epithelium	Glandular epithelium and other epithelial surfaces (secreted in breast milk, urine, saliva, semen)	Oral contact Sexual contact Neonatally in breast milk

* Also transmitted transplacentally.

Routes of transmission between hosts are various

Table 11.1 gives some examples of the entry and exit routes of particular viruses and allows us to predict something of the probable epidemiology. If the portals of entry and exit are the respiratory tract, then the virus is usually spread by **respiratory aerosols** (coughing and sneezing)—a very efficient and rapid transmission mechanism. Viruses of this type are therefore highly **contagious**, and cause epidemics in which many susceptible individuals are infected (chickenpox, measles, flu, rubella). Viruses that are secreted into the saliva or from other glands (e.g. sexual secretions, breast milk) are spread much less efficiently and many of these viruses are spread by **contact**, such as genital and oral herpes simplex virus, and Epstein–Barr virus, the cause of glandular fever.[1]

Viruses which are spread by contact are often transmitted particularly efficiently among young children. The behaviour of young children is extremely uninhibited. They explore each other's mouths with their hands and examine the texture of small objects with their mouths, thus achieving a high level of salivary exchange. An equivalent level of contact is achieved by adults only during intimacy or in the front row of a rugby scrum (rugby players can get 'scrumpox', a herpes sore on the side of the face).

Viruses that enter via the gut epithelium (polio, hepatitis A, rotaviruses) are spread by the **faecal–oral** route and usually have to be rather stable viruses because they need to survive in water supplies or on food. We should note that Table 11.1 is somewhat simplified. It is apparent that many systemic viruses must, potentially, be transmissible by **blood contact**. Cytomegalovirus, for example, can be transmitted by blood transfer or organ transplant, but this accounts for only a small proportion of infections. In contrast, blood contact is a major transmission route for human immunodeficiency virus (HIV) and hepatitis B.

Seroepidemiology gives clues to transmission

A knowledge of the entry and exit routes and of the mode of transmission allows an understanding of the **epidemiology** of virus disease but in reality we usually investigate the epidemiology first and then deduce the transmission routes. Epidemiology is detective work. Who gets the virus? When do they get the virus and how can we interpret the data? The simplest way of asking these questions is to search for **serum antibodies** to viruses in the population. When we are infected with a virus we become **antibody-positive** and we are said to have **seroconverted**. By measuring a virus-specific antibody in the population we can ask 'what is the age at which people seroconvert'? That is, 'at what age do they get infected'?

In Fig. 11.2 we illustrate this principle by plotting, for different viruses, the proportion of the population seroconverted against age. We see that most people seroconvert for **flu** early in life, implying a very contagious disease. By contrast, **herpes simplex virus type 2** (genital herpes) antibodies first appear in some of the population in early adulthood, implying sexual transmission. **Epstein–Barr virus** seroconversion occurs in a proportion of the population in early childhood and further seroconversion occurs in early adulthood. This is a **contact disease**, transmitted in saliva, and its seroepidemiology reflects very high contact levels during play in infants, relatively low contact levels during later childhood, followed by contact during intimacy in young adults.[2]

The epidemiological picture in some diseases may be more complex. Table 11.1 shows that human **cytomegalovirus is secreted from many portals of exit**. It can pass transplacentally to the fetus, it is present in breast milk, saliva, urine, blood, and in secretions of the genital tract. It is therefore transmitted by multiple routes and has a complex epidemiology.

1 You can catch flu on the bus but you are unlikely to catch herpes.

2 This is glandular fever, sometimes called the kissing disease.

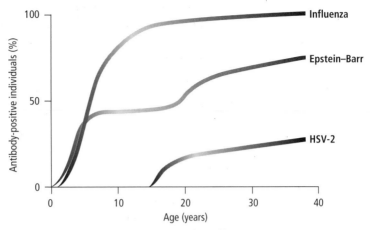

Figure 11.2 Age versus seroconversion for different viruses.

Finally, we should note that the shape of the seroconversion curves depends on factors like **socioeconomic grouping** and **geographical area**. Thus Epstein–Barr virus seroconversion occurs during childhood in developing countries more than in the developed world and, in developed countries, at higher rates in the working class than in higher socioeconomic classes. Working-class children presumably experience a higher level of contact.

The examples quoted above seem straightforward. The pathogenic behaviour of the virus implies mechanisms of transmission which agree well with the observed epidemiology. We seem to know what is going on. But it would be quite wrong to pretend that this is always the case. For example, we know that **hepatitis B virus** is present in the blood and in genital secretions, and in the western world the virus is spread by blood and blood products and by sexual contact. Intravenous drug abusers, recipients of blood products and the sexually promiscuous are therefore the groups most at risk. However, in Africa and parts of Asia, hepatitis B infection is more common and seroconversion in childhood is frequent. Some other mechanism of transmission must be responsible, but we are still not sure what it is.

In this section we have considered, rather briefly, the nature of superficial and systemic infection, the use of entry and exit portals, the transmission mechanism of viruses and the consequent epidemiology of virus infection. Before examining in more detail the interaction of the virus and the animal host we should consider the response of the host to infection.

Virus infection elicits immune responses

At its simplest the response to viruses can be considered as two components: first, the humoral response: production of **antibody** to virus-specific antigens by B cells; and second, **cytotoxic T cells** which recognize virus-specific antigens presented by major histocompatibility complex (MHC) Class I antigens and which kill the presenting cell. B-cell responses **and** cytotoxic T-cell responses both require T-helper cell cooperation. T-helper cells are activated by MHC Class II presentation of exogenous (i.e. phagocytosed) antigens. Antibody production requires only Class II presentation, whereas cytotoxic T-cell responses require presentation of antigen by Class I **and** Class II.

It is apparent that both arms of the immune response (i.e. humoral and cell-mediated) should be of importance in combating virus infection (Fig. 11.3). **Antibodies** will react with free virus particles and inactivate (neutralize) them directly or will **opsonize** the particles such that they are engulfed and destroyed more readily by phagocytes. In addition, virus-infected cells, particularly cells infected by **enveloped** viruses, will bear virus-specific proteins in their plasma membranes and will therefore be recognized by antibody. These cells will then be destroyed by complement-mediated lysis or by effector cells which recognize the Fc portion of antibody molecules. Cytotoxic T cells will recognize and attack virus-infected cells because all cells express Class I antigen and any virus-infected cell will therefore present virus antigen with Class I molecules.

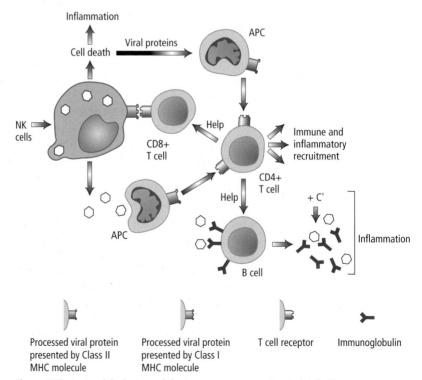

Figure 11.3 A simplified view of the immune response to viral infections.

There is ample evidence to suggest that both arms of the immune response are important in combating virus infections:

1 as we shall see, some viruses mutate to generate variants which evade recognition by antibody made against a previous infection (antigenic variation);

2 some viruses have evolved proteins which bind the Fc portion of antibody;

3 some viruses interfere with Class I antigen presentation in the cells they infect;

4 in experimental infections in inbred mice the outcome of infection with different viruses is profoundly influenced by the Class I genotype, which can influence the **specificity** of Class I presentation.

All these examples provide indirect but compelling evidence that both antibody and Class I-mediated T cells are important.

Nevertheless **the relative importance of these different arms of immunity in individual virus infections is a matter of debate** and is of some consequence because it has **great bearing on vaccine design**: is a vaccine that generates only Class II-mediated responses alone adequate, or must we design a vaccine that will generate Class I-mediated responses as well?

To attempt to assess the relative importance of humoral and cell-mediated responses in virus infections is to tread dangerous ground but we can at least attempt to generalize. **Antibody secreted at mucosal surfaces (immunoglobulin A; IgA) will neutralize incoming virus.** Antibody is therefore likely to be of importance in providing **protective immunity** against incoming virus. **Once infection is established**, recovery and elimination of the virus are likely to require cell-mediated immune responses, and this view is supported by the fact that people with defects in cell-mediated immunity suffer more severe virus infections while those with defects in antibody production recover from most virus infections more or less normally. Cell-mediated responses are of particular importance in eliminating **cell-associated** viruses because these viruses are rarely present as free virus particles—they pass from cell to cell by cell-membrane fusion. In contrast, non-enveloped viruses, like **polio** and other **picornaviruses**, cause rapid cell lysis and are spread as free virus particles. In this case antibody can play a key role in recovery by destroying free virus particles and preventing their spread.

Finally we should note that the immune response is not the sole defence against the virus-infected cell. Natural killer cells, in particular (p. 27), play an important role in killing cells infected by some viruses, though the mechanism by which the targets are recognized is uncertain.

Before leaving this topic we should remind ourselves that the immune response does not act alone. **It acts in concert with the inflammatory response**, the two systems acting together to focus defences on sites of damage or infection. We noted in an earlier chapter that inappropriate immune responses may mediate irrelevant inflammation—**hypersensitivity**. As we shall see, inappropriate responses can also occur during some virus infections and contribute to the virus-induced disease.

How do viruses survive in the population in the face of immunity?

Immunity to virus infection seems very effective. We only catch diseases like measles, mumps and chickenpox once in a lifetime and we are then usually immune for ever. For an obligate parasite this raises a problem: how is the virus to find new susceptible hosts? Take **measles virus**, a member of the para-myxovirus family. Measles is a fragile virus. It survives for only a short time outside the host, it infects only humans and immunity is lifelong. Measles is **very contagious** because it is spread by aerosols and causes short-lived epidemics during which the majority of susceptible individuals in the population are infected (Fig. 11.4). As the epidemic proceeds, the number of non-immune people decreases, producing a high level of **herd immunity**, the epidemic wanes and the next epidemic must await the arrival of new suscep-tible hosts. In some countries, this means the entry into school of non-immune children. During periods **between** epidemics the virus is at risk: it is main-tained only by a small number of susceptible hosts. In small, isolated populations the virus literally runs out of non-immune hosts; **measles is not found in isolated populations of less than 100000 people**. But measles is the exception. Most viruses do survive in small host populations. How do they do it?

Some viruses are stable outside the host

If the virus particle can survive for long periods outside the host, then infecting a new host becomes a matter of less urgency. Viruses of the gut, like polio and rotavirus, have evolved to survive the hostile environment of the alimentary canal and their mechanism of transmission (faecal–oral) requires survival in water and on contaminated foods. These are small non-enveloped viruses and they are unusually stable. Some viruses are even resistant to desiccation. The smallpox virus, for example, would survive for years in dust or bedding.

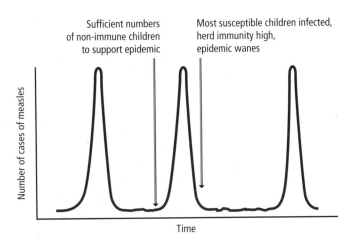

Figure 11.4 Idealized description of measles epidemics prior to vaccination programme.

Infecting multiple species increases the chance of virus survival

Measles infects only humans, so immunity in humans places the virus at risk. But many viruses infect multiple species and if the virus dies out in one species a **reservoir** is present in another. **Yellow fever** is an example. This is a member of a large group of viruses that are spread by insects and can multiply in the insect cells.[3] Yellow fever infects various tropical primates and also proliferates in the mosquito, the transmission vector. The primate–mosquito–primate cycle (the **sylvan cycle**) forms a reservoir from which humans are occasionally infected, and epidemics sometimes occur in which a human–mosquito–human cycle is established (the **urban cycle**). Immunity in the human population is protective to the individual but **the virus cannot be eliminated by human herd immunity because of the persistence of the animal reservoir**.

Antigenic variation in viruses evades host immunity

We catch measles only once but we may be infected by influenza virus many times, despite the fact that we have good immune responses after our first encounter with the influenza virus. The reason is that **influenza virus changes with time**; the influenza virus that circulates this year will be slightly different from the one circulating last year and even more different from the one circulating the year before that. If we examine human antibody samples taken 10 years ago we find that they will react well with influenza viruses that were isolated at the same time, but will react only poorly with more recently isolated influenza strains; the virus has changed. This phenomenon is called **antigenic variation** and the influenza molecule involved is the **haemagglutinin**. This is a molecule on the surface of the virus which is responsible for binding to the host cell via sialic acid residues. Antibody to the haemagglutinin prevents this binding, thus neutralizing the virus, and antihaemagglutinin antibody is the most important component of immunity to influenza. Antigenic variation of the influenza haemagglutinin molecule is due to two phenomena called **antigenic drift** and **antigenic shift**.

Antigenic drift is a slow progressive change in the haemagglutinin which results from **mutations** in the haemagglutinin gene. Influenza viruses in which such mutations have occurred are at a **selective advantage** because we have less immunity to them, and as a result influenza viruses accumulate mutations in their haemagglutinin genes.[4] Antigenic drift is responsible for the recurring epidemics of influenza. The population has only partial immunity to these mutated viruses.

Every decade or so there occurs a dramatic outbreak of influenza which very rapidly sweeps across the world and infects most people. These **influenza pandemics are caused by viruses to which there is virtually no herd immunity**; the antibodies we raised against previous influenza infections do not react at all with the haemagglutinin molecule of the pandemic virus. When we examine the haemagglutinin molecule from pandemic viruses we find that they are so different from those of influenza strains circulating in previous years that it is inconceivable that the differences arose by mutation. This major change is called **antigenic shift**.

3 They are sometimes called **arboviruses** (**ar**thropod-**bo**rne).

4 These result in amino acid substitutions in the haemagglutinin molecule.

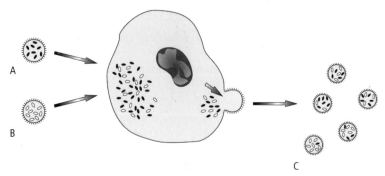

Figure 11.5 Gene reassortment in influenza virus infections. The genome of influenza virus is divided into eight RNA segments. Infection of a cell with two different flu viruses results in progeny with segments from both parents. Progeny virus C has acquired one segment from parent A and seven from parent B. If the segment acquired from parent A is the haemagglutinin gene, then progeny C will inherit all the characteristics of virus B but will make a new haemagglutinin.

The precise source of these pandemic viruses is unknown, but it seems certain that they arise not by **mutation** but by **recombination**. In Table 11.1 we saw that, unlike most viruses, the genome of influenza virus is composed not of one piece of ribonucleic acid but of several; the genome is **segmented** and each segment corresponds to a gene. When two different viruses infect a cell, **segment reassortment** can occur (i.e. genetic recombination) so that progeny viruses can contain RNA segments from both parent viruses (Fig. 11.5). Pandemic viruses are recombinant viruses that contain a new haemagglutinin gene, probably derived by recombination of a human influenza virus with an influenza virus of a domestic animal (swine or avian flu). Influenza does not have an animal reservoir as such, but it **does** have a **genetic** reservoir in animals—a source of new haemagglutinin genes with which to evade human immunity.

The consequence of antigenic shift is that influenza is the last great pandemic disease (or was, before the advent of acquired immunodeficiency syndrome, or AIDS). Because of their selective advantage in evading the immune response, pandemic viruses entirely replace the viruses that were circulating in previous years. After a pandemic the new virus again **drifts** (i.e. accumulates mutations) and causes occasional epidemics. Pandemics have occurred in 1918, 1957 and 1968. The virus which caused the last pandemic[5] has been drifting ever since and we have no idea when the next pandemic will occur. Nor, since we cannot predict what the next pandemic virus will be like, can we do much about it. It's a bit like living in an earthquake zone!

Measles, polio, yellow fever and influenza are **acute** infections. They are eliminated from the host by immune and non-specific defence mechanisms and their survival is dependent upon survival outside the host or on rapid transmission to new non-immune hosts. As we have seen, measles fails in small populations. Many viruses however have evolved strategies which require neither survival outside the host nor efficient transmission to new hosts; **they persist within the host**.

5 Called influenza H3—i.e. haemagglutinin 3.

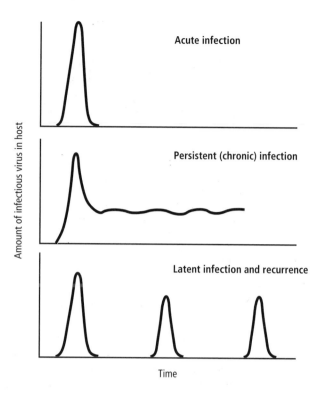

Figure 11.6 Acute, persistent and latent infections.

Persistent and latent infections

Virus infections may be broadly placed in one of three categories (Fig. 11.6): (i) **acute** infections are those which are eliminated by the host response; (ii) **persistent** infections (or **chronic** infections) are those in which the virus is not eliminated and can be consistently isolated from the host over a long period, perhaps for the lifetime of the host; and (iii) **latent** infections are those in which the virus is apparently eliminated but reappears, perhaps many years later.

Persistent infections

Persistent infection implies continuous growth of the virus in the face of the immune response.

It would be foolish to believe that we understand how this immune evasion occurs, but we can give some examples where we have an inkling. Persistent infection also implies that the virus involved cannot be highly cytotoxic. If virus multiplication caused rapid cell death then continuous virus production would inevitably result in tissue destruction and would be incompatible with host survival: there would be no point in evolving to evade the host response, only to kill the goose that lays the golden egg.

Hepatitis B virus (sometimes called serum hepatitis) is a relatively infrequent infection in Europe and North America but is very common in the underdeveloped world. In parts of Africa and Asia the majority of the population becomes infected and many people are persistently infected. Infectious virus can be continuously isolated from the blood of a patient for decades. It is estimated that, **worldwide, there are several hundred million such carriers**. Hepatitis B virus (HBV) grows, as far as we know, only in liver cells and is secreted into the blood. The virus is non-cytolytic and, although liver injury occurs during the acute phase of disease and chronic damage occurs in persistent infection, most of this damage seems to result from the immune response directed against virus-infected liver cells.

We do not know why the virus persists in so many people but two possible reasons are proposed. First, liver cells normally express very little MHC class I antigen and, when infected with HBV, are not very efficient at presenting peptides and inciting cytotoxic T cells. Second, HBV seems to have evolved a mechanism for overwhelming the humoral responses. The surface protein of HBV is called the hepatitis B surface antigen (Hbs antigen) and antibodies against this protein (Hbs antibodies) neutralize the virus. Chronically infected individuals have very high concentrations of Hbs antigen in their blood stream. The antigen is in the form of spherical or rod-shaped aggregates which look like virus particles but contain no viral nucleic acid—they are composed solely of Hbs antigen. Real virus particles are also present, of course, but for each virus particle there are about 100 Hbs antigen particles. This great excess of Hbs antigen seems to swamp the antibody response.

Individuals who become infected with HBV fall into two categories: those who eliminate the virus are **Hbs antigen-negative** and **Hbs antibody-positive** and are immune to reinfection; those who become chronically infected are Hbs antigen-positive. The probability of chronic infection varies with age. Infection in early life frequently leads to chronic infection—a feature of infection by many of the persistent viruses. Infection of adults more commonly results in acute disease and clearance of the virus.

Retroviruses are persistent viruses *par excellence.* We noted, in the previous chapter, that the replication strategy of retroviruses offers the virus a number of options. The key points are that the genome of a retrovirus is converted to an integrated provirus and that virus replication is non-cytolytic. We can see that **an infected animal will contain different types of infected cells**. Some cells will be producing large amounts of virus and these will be good targets for the immune response. Other cells will contain the integrated provirus but may be producing little or no virus. These cells will not be recognized by the immune response and, provided that they are long-lived cells, will maintain the infection in the host. At some point the quiescent cell may become an active virus-producer in response to some stimulus such as a differentiation signal. We see that this is a dynamic situation in which, at any one time, some infected cells are producing virus, and are immune targets, while others are not. In consequence retroviruses are difficult to eliminate and frequently persist. One example is **feline leukaemia virus**, a retrovirus of cats that infects many circulating cell types. It causes a wide range of diseases including leukaemia. This virus often establishes a persistent infection in cats and, just as we noted for HBV, infection of young animals is more likely to lead to persistent infection than is infection of adults. It appears that **an immature immune system improves the chances of the virus establishing itself**.

One group of retroviruses is spectacularly successful at establishing persistent infection. These are the **lentiviruses** and they include HIV, simian immunodeficiency virus, visna (a disease of sheep) and equine infectious anaemia virus. As far as we can tell, **infection by these viruses always results in persistent infection and the virus is never eliminated**. We are not sure why this is, but all of these viruses share the notable characteristic of antigenic variation. The surface glycoprotein (gp160), against which neutralizing antibody is directed, accumulates mutations during the course of infection and antigenic variants are selected by the humoral response. There is also evidence that mutations cause changes in virus T-cell epitopes, creating variants that can escape the attentions of cytotoxic T cells. This **antigenic drift** is very reminiscent of the phenomenon observed with influenza virus, but here we observe this drift in a single infected individual and this doubtless contributes to the ability of the virus to persist.

Latent infection implies the disappearance of the virus after the acute phase of disease and its reappearance at some later time

The phenomenon is exemplified by herpesviruses, and perhaps the most dramatic example is varicella-zoster virus, the virus which causes chickenpox. After catching chickenpox in childhood, the virus remains with us for the rest of our lives. But we are entirely unaware of it until it reappears, often many decades later, to cause **shingles**[6] (**herpes zoster**). The pathogenesis of the disease is illustrated in Fig. 11.7. The inhaled virus first infects respiratory epithelium, invades the submucosa and is transmitted around the blood stream in a cell-associated form. After an incubation period of a few weeks it enters the epidermis and causes the characteristic vesicles we associate with chickenpox. **The virus then passes from the skin along sensory axons to neurons of the sensory ganglia, and in these nerve cells the virus establishes a latent infection.** We do not understand the nature of latent infection but it appears that during latency no virus proteins are synthesized. The virus genome is present in the sensory neurons, but the virus is entirely quiescent and is not a target for immune attack. Under some conditions the virus will **reactivate in the sensory neuron, pass back down the sensory axons and infect the skin to cause the syndrome known as shingles or herpes zoster**. The distribution of a shingles rash corresponds to a **dermatome**, the area of skin served by a particular sensory nerve branch.

Herpes simplex virus is genetically similar to varicella-zoster virus and its pathogenesis is also related. The virus usually infects the lip, often as a result of a mother's kiss, but does not penetrate the submucosa, its growth being first limited to the epithelium around the site of infection. The virus then enters sensory nerve endings and passes axonally to the neurons of the trigeminal ganglia, where latent infection is established. Reactivation results in transmission of the virus from the trigeminal ganglion to the skin where it grows to cause a recurrent **cold sore**.[7]

6 **Shingles** is from *cingulum* (Latin), a belt, referring to the band-like distribution of the rash.

7 Genital herpes behaves similarly but the portal of entry is genital epithelium.

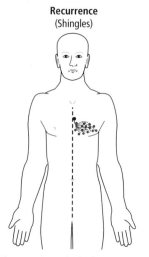

Primary infection
(Chickenpox)

Recurrence
(Shingles)

1. Infection by respiratory route
2. Systemic spread and amplification
3. Skin infected from capillaries. Chickenpox vesicles
4. Virus enters sensory nerve endings and travels to sensory ganglia. Latent infection established

1. Virus reactivates in single sensory ganglion and travels to skin along sensory nerves
2. Virus multiplies in skin to give vesicles in single dermatome

Figure 11.7 Primary and recurrent infection by varicella-zoster virus.

In the case of herpes simplex virus we can formally demonstrate latent infection because the human infection can be mimicked in the laboratory mouse. Infection of the mouse skin with herpes simplex virus results in a cold sore-like lesion, which disappears after a few days. If we now examine the sensory ganglion which innervates the infection site, we find that it contains no virus particles and no detectable infectivity. However, if we cultivate the ganglion with epithelial cells, infectious virus will appear and grow in these cells. The ganglion harbours virus in a latent form and does so for the mouse's whole life-time.

The key to latency exhibited by herpes simplex virus and varicella-zoster virus is that these viruses behave differently in different cells: in epithelial cells they cause productive, lytic infection, while in sensory neurons they establish quiescent latent infection. The choice of the neurons as a site of latent infection is an excellent one—neurons are non-replaceable cells and live for the whole life-time of the host. We do not know what induces the virus to reactivate from the latently infected neuron, but we have a problem here in that we cannot observe **reactivation**. What we observe is the clinical consequence—infection of the epithelium (**recrudescence**). It is probable that reactivation from the neuron occurs quite frequently, but that only under certain conditions does this result in visible infection of epithelium. Thus a recurrent lesion probably requires two independent events: the **reactivation trigger** in the neuron and an immune state that allows virus multiplication in the epithelium.

We think that all herpesviruses are capable of establishing latent infection, but different viruses use different cell types. **Epstein–Barr virus** grows productively in oral epithelium and **establishes latent infection in B lymphocytes**. In B lymphocytes the virus synthesizes a protein which **immortalizes the cell** (i.e. interrupts the terminal differentiation programme), thus ensuring the long-term survival of the latently infected cell. In other instances we do not know the cell type involved. We know, for example, that cytomegalovirus productively infects glandular epithelium but we are not sure which cell type becomes latently infected. Indeed our knowledge of latent infection is rather rudimentary. What is the molecular basis of latent infection? How is the virus maintained in a latent state, what factors trigger reactivation and what is the outcome of reactivation for the latently infected cell? Whatever the mechanisms involved, the ability to establish latent infection is of great survival value to the virus. Measles can be maintained only in large populations, but varicella-zoster virus has been found in closed communities of fewer than 50 people.

Here, and in Fig. 11.6, we have implied that there are clear distinctions between acute, persistent and latent infections, and the examples chosen highlight these distinctions. Nevertheless, there are cloudy areas. Some viruses do not persist for the life-time of the host but do take a very long time to disappear. A good example is **papillomavirus**; skin warts take months or years to eliminate. Mouse cytomegalovirus (an animal model for studying human cytomegalovirus) is secreted from glandular epithelium for long periods. It has been proposed that **epithelial cells may represent a privileged site**, under rather poor surveillance by the immune and inflammatory responses.

The central nervous system is also regarded as an immunologically privileged site—Class I antigens are present at very low concentration in neurons, and there is evidence that some viruses can establish an unusual form of persistence at this site. We used measles as a classic example of an acute infection but there is a rare chronic demyelinating disease of the brain called (would you believe) subacute sclerosing panencephalitis (SSPE) that is a sequel to measles infection. This disease occurs several years after a measles infection and measles virus proteins and nucleic acid can be found in the brain of patients who have died of the disease, though infectious virus is very difficult to isolate. It is clear, from this evidence, that measles virus **can** persist for years within the infected person and that this may have fatal results.[8] Nevertheless the epidemiology of measles virus infections points to measles being an acute rather than a persistent infection and there is no evidence that SSPE patients, or any other people, can transmit measles except during the acute phase of measles infection. Thus this persistence is of no value to the virus. For herpesviruses and retroviruses persistence is a way of life, but measles persistence appears to be a rare accident.

Pathological consequences of infection

8 We know that measles virus is the causative agent of SSPE because the disease has disappeared from populations vaccinated against measles.

The outcome of infection for the multicellular host is the most difficult of the questions that we have tried to address, because to answer it we need to know which cells the virus infects, the effects of infection on these cells and the response of the host to the infection.

Virus-infected cells may be destroyed

We noted in the last chapter that many viruses destroy the cells that they infect, and in some instances this will have inevitable pathological consequences. The most obvious example is the destruction of intestinal epithelium by rotaviruses and consequent diarrhoea because of the inability of the mucosa to maintain water and solute gradients. Similarly, rhinoviruses, the common cold viruses, destroy ciliated epithelial cells of the upper respiratory tract. We are left with a raw, inflamed mucosal surface which is no longer cleansed by beating cilia and which is susceptible to bacterial infection. Poliovirus infection occasionally leads to the severe or fatal disease poliomyelitis, in which motor neurons are infected. The disease is characterized by the rapid destruction of these neurons by the virus and a resulting paralysis.

Rotaviruses and rhinoviruses are picornaviruses, which are lytic *in vitro* and *in vivo*, and there are many other examples. But many viruses are not cytolytic and we must look to other mechanisms for induction of disease.

Virus interference with cell function can cause disease

Virus infection may interfere with the specialized function of a cell without destroying the cell. **Rabies**, for example, is not a cytolytic virus, and neurons infected with rabies virus show few obvious signs of virus damage—a situation very different from that observed with polio. Nervertheless, rabies infection of neurons has dire consequences due to the loss of function of the infected cells. We know of few examples of functional impairment by human viruses, but we can be confident that this is a widespread phenomenon because it has been demonstrated very clearly in infections of laboratory mice. Lactate dehydrogenase virus (an arenavirus) infects macrophages of mice and impairs their phagocytic competence without affecting their viability or morphology. Lymphocytic choriomeningitis virus (LCMV—also an arenavirus) establishes a persistent infection in young mice and infects many cell types including the cells of the anterior pituitary gland. The gland then secretes reduced levels of growth hormone, though the cells appear normal, and this probably accounts for the reduced growth of infected animals.

Disease often results from immune and inflammatory responses to viruses

In many—perhaps most—instances **the diseases caused by viruses cannot be accounted for by the direct effect of the virus on individual cells.** Histological examination of lung tissue from fatal cases of cytomegalovirus pneumonia suggests that few cells are infected and that the disease results from the extensive inflammatory infiltrate which fills the alveolar spaces. Disease of this kind, which results from response to infection, is particularly noticeable in persistent or chronic infections. The destruction of liver cells in chronic hepatitis B infection is thought to result not from direct cell killing by the virus but from immune attack on infected liver cells by cytotoxic T cells and by antibody-mediated cytotoxicity (i.e. type II and type IV hypersensitivity reactions). Animals persistently infected with feline leu-kaemia virus or equine infectious anaemia (retroviruses) suffer disease due to the deposition of immune complexes (type III hypersensitivity). Epstein–Barr virus infects B lymphocytes, but the number of infected cells is rather small and the disease symptoms of glandular fever result from the massive T-cell activation and proliferation which occur in response to infection.

Although disease can result from activity of the immune and inflammatory responses, we should not take this to mean that in the absence of this response there would be no disease. Epstein–Barr virus infection in the absence of T-cell responses does not result in glandular fever—instead the virus causes a B-cell proliferation that may be fatal. **Immunopathology is the price to be paid for eliminating or controlling the virus.** Nevertheless, in some instances the re-sponse to infection appears inappropriate. Infection with an insect-borne virus called **dengue** (a flavivirus) results in the production of antibody which confers protection against reinfection with the same virus strain. However, infection with other dengue strains can still occur and these infections are much more serious when there is pre-existing immunity. Infection with strain B is more severe if the patient has already encountered strain A. It appears that antibody against strain A will react with dengue strain B, but this is a low-affinity reaction and neutralization does not occur. However, the bound antibody allows opsonization and efficient uptake of the virus by phagocytic cells, within which the virus grows, and one explanation of these severe infections is that the **low-affinity antibody**, raised against a different strain, **enhances the infectivity of the virus**.

A dramatic example of an inappropriate response is **seen in infections by LCMV**. We have noted that infection of young mice is persistent and many cell types are infected. The animal suffers some defects in growth but there is no gross disease. Infection of the mouse as an adult, however, results in a fatal meningitis, the outcome of a vigorous cell-mediated immune response to infec-tion and consequent inflammation. No such dramatic examples are found in human disease, but a number of virus diseases of adults (flu, mumps, Epstein–Barr virus) can occasionally result in inflammatory disturbance of multiple nerves.[9] This neuritis may take months or years to resolve. We do not under-stand the mechanism of this disease, but it is associated with response to virus infection; the response persists after the infection has cleared and is clearly inappropriate.

We have tried to offer plausible explanations of disease induction by viruses, but we should recognize that this is an area where there are more theories than facts. Our ignorance is exemplified by **HIV, the cause of AIDS**. We know that the most notable feature of the disease is immune dysfunction and that this is accompanied by loss of T-helper cells. We also know that the virus infects T-helper cells. Logically, then, the virus infects and destroys or disables these cells and immune deficiency is the result. However, the proportion of the cells infected at any one time appears to be too small to account for the observed reduction in numbers. Recent evidence suggests that large numbers of T-helper cells become infected, but that the cells are very rapidly killed by cytotoxic T cells. Thus, while the observed number of infected T-helper cells is small,

9. Acute demyelinating polyneuropathy or Guillain–Barré syndrome.

infection and immune response do contribute to the rate of turnover of these cells.

Nevertheless, it is difficult to see why this imbalance often takes more than a decade to become catastrophic. Most of our observations on HIV pathogenesis are made by examining cells in the circulation (because these can be sampled easily), but it is likely that **events in the lymphoid organs** are of great importance; the combined effects of infection and the response to it may cause long-term destruction of organ architecture and consequent loss of function. Of course, HIV infects, in addition to T-helper cells, other CD4+ cell types—monocytes, macrophages and dendritic cells—and it may be that infection of these antigen-presenting cells is a key factor in AIDS. There is no shortage of theories, but despite intensive study we do not know how HIV causes immune deficiency.

Finally, we should note that the pathogenesis of persistent infections confronts us with a particular problem. We have noted that HIV exhibits antigenic variation in the infected individual, but this may be the tip of the iceberg: the virus may be varying in other ways. **If we become infected with a virus which continues to multiply within us for 10 years, it is reasonable to suppose that we will now be infected with a considerable mixture of mutant viruses.** This is certainly the case for feline leukaemia virus. Chronically infected cats have been shown, by genetic engineering techniques, to contain a wide variety of integrated feline leukaemia virus proviruses. When we isolate viruses in cell culture from an infected cat we obtain only part of this variety—in fact only those viruses which grow best in culture. The key question, and a very difficult one, is which of the variants is responsible for the observed disease?

The outcome of infection depends on the state of the host

Like other parasites, **most viruses are well adapted to their hosts**. Our viruses have in most cases evolved with us for millenia and we have achieved an uneasy balance with them to the extent that we are unaware of most virus infections. No such balance exists when we are infected with a new virus such as pandemic flu, or HIV or with a virus for which humans are not the primary host, for example yellow fever. The balance is also lost when the condition of the host is abnormal with respect to age or immune status. **Rubella** is a mild infection of children or adults but severely disrupts the development of the fetus. Herpes simplex is frequently a trivial and at worst a distressing recurrent disease, but it is hardly ever life-threatening. However if the virus is acquired in the birth canal from an infected mother it can cause a fatal generalized disease, destroying the cells of many organs and tissues. Most of the population is asymptomatically infected with human cytomegalovirus but, like rubella, transplacental transmission leads to fetal abnormality, and infection of the immune-suppressed individual can be extremely severe. Cytomegalovirus pneumonia is one of the most common causes of death in transplant patients receiving immune-suppressant drugs, and AIDS patients may lose their sight from cytomegalovirus retinitis. The weak pathogen may become a severe pathogen in the abnormal host.

Viruses can cause cancer

In the previous chapter we noted that certain groups of viruses are capable of inducing cell proliferation in culture and that this should make us suspicious that some viruses might be able to induce similar events *in vivo*; that is, viruses may play a role in the induction of cancer. In fact, there is excellent epidemiological and experimental evidence that **infection with certain viruses does increase the risk of cancer**, as we shall see.

Summary

The ways that viruses spread from their reservoirs to the susceptible host are affected not only by virus behaviour but also by host factors just as varied as those for bacterial disease. The complexities of the host tissues and of the inflammatory and immune responses have resulted in variations in the patterns of virus disease. These include persistence and latency, cell killing and transformation, and immunopathology.

12

Intervention against viruses

The battles against virus diseases include notable victories. **Smallpox has been eradicated**. Paralytic **poliomyelitis**, a disease which terrified parents before 1960, is now little more than a memory in rich countries. **Measles, mumps** and **congenital rubella** appear to be under control. We should note, however, that some of these battles have yet to be won in the developing world, where **measles, polio and hepatitis B, for example, remain major killers**. Controlling these infections is, in part, a matter of political will, though as we shall see, there are specific problems associated with control programmes in the developing world.

In the developed world, too, we have no grounds for complacency. The appearance of **human immunodeficiency virus** (HIV) has exposed dramatically our vulnerability to new viruses in particular, but there are many older viruses that continue to threaten us. We have no adequate defence against **influenza pandemics**, and we have no idea when the next one will arrive. We think of **chickenpox** as a relatively mild disease of childhood, but reactivation of the latent virus (**shingles**) is a lengthy and painful disease in the elderly. Perhaps one in five of us can expect to suffer from shingles in our old age.

Genital infections are underestimated; people don't talk about them. But genital **herpes simplex** and **genital warts** are common infections which, in addition to being physically painful, destroy sexual relationships and therefore can have profound psychological effects. Furthermore, we believe that some genital wart viruses are important factors in the development of **genital cancers**. At the other extreme, diseases like the **common cold** are little more than a nuisance, but we could certainly do without them.

In the veterinary world, viruses like **foot and mouth disease** in cattle and **Marek's disease** in poultry remain a constant economic threat and changing practices in animal husbandry may encourage the emergence of new diseases.

In this chapter we will examine the strategies available for combating viruses and virus diseases and consider the prospects for the future. The strategies for intervention can be summarized as: (i) **interrupting transmission**; (ii) **vaccination**; and (iii) **therapy**. Many of the underlying principles apply to other infectious agents as well as viruses.

Diagnosis and surveillance are crucial in combating virus disease

It is obvious that if we wish to intervene against a particular virus and to assess the success of that intervention, then we must first be able to **measure the infection rates in the community and to detect and record outbreaks and**

epidemics. It is frequently assumed that the elimination of smallpox was achieved by mass vaccination but it is difficult to achieve vaccination of whole populations, particularly in underdeveloped countries and, in any case, some vaccinated individuals may be capable of harbouring a mild smallpox infection. An important part of the smallpox eradication programme mounted by the World Health Organization was a **thorough surveillance operation**, the **isolation of suspected cases** and **intensive vaccination** in those localities where cases were diagnosed (**ring vaccination**).

Diagnosis of a virus infection can sometimes be made confidently on clinical grounds alone but the **laboratory isolation**, cultivation and characterization of the virus are more certain. **Virus culture** is labour-intensive and often difficult. Other methods are available, such as observation of the virus in a clinical specimen using the **electron microscope** (particularly useful for detection of rotavirus in infant diarrhoea), and recently methods have been developed that allow the **specific detection of minute amounts of virus nucleic acid in clinical specimens**.

It is not, however, essential to detect a virus in order to prove that infection has occurred. Virus infection is accompanied by **seroconversion** (the appearance of antibodies to the virus) and good evidence for recent infection by a particular virus can be obtained by demonstrating a rapidly **rising antibody titre** in the patient. In principle, then, virus diagnosis is straightforward, though in practice there are many pitfalls. The important point is that surveillance of the community for virus infection requires an expensive organized network of physicians and authorized laboratories, efficient reporting to central authorities and effective collation of the data.

Before leaving this subject we should note that **some viruses present us with particular surveillance problems**. Infection with HIV may result in symptoms only after several years, so it is likely that the majority of infected people have no symptoms, and are unidentified. Yet we need to know how rapidly the virus is spreading in different groups in the community and we need to know whether intervention strategies are having any effect (e.g. public education, clean needles to intravenous drug abusers). How should this be done? Is it reasonable to screen the population for HIV on a compulsory basis? Is it ethical to screen anonymously, and hence not to inform people of the fact that they are infected? These are difficult issues and ones which the AIDS epidemic has highlighted.

Interrupting virus transmission requires a thorough knowledge of the epidemiology and transmission routes. There are many routes of transmission, but the major ones are via **vectors, faecal–oral spread, sexual transmission, blood contact** and **respiratory routes**.

The vector can be controlled

Insect vector populations can be controlled, at least in urban areas. Urban **yellow fever** (human-to-human transmission by mosquito) can be controlled by the simple expedient of storing water in covered vessels and by treating open pools of water with insecticides. In rural areas, mosquito control is much more difficult.

Rabies is transmitted to humans from wild animal reservoirs by domestic animals, mainly by the dog. In areas where rabies is endemic the vector should be controlled by strict dog licensing and leash laws, by destroying strays and by vaccinating dogs against rabies. It is sometimes possible to reduce the virus load in the reservoir. In Europe, foxes are the major source of rabies: fox numbers are controlled and attempts are being made to vaccinate foxes against rabies using vaccine-loaded bait. In the USA many wild mammals harbour the virus and control by this method will be more difficult.

Faecal–oral spread can be reduced by public health measures

Picornaviruses (e.g. polio and hepatitis A) and rotaviruses are spread by the faecal–oral route and their transmission can be reduced by effective sewage treatment, chlorination of water supplies and screening water supplies for the presence of virus. Other measures include thorough cooking of food and the use of different working areas and equipment for cooked and uncooked food in the catering industry.

Blood and blood products can be screened

Blood transfusions and therapy involving blood products (e.g. clotting factors) carry a significant risk of transmission of virus from donor to recipient. Blood can be screened for the presence of high-risk viruses (e.g. HIV, hepatitis B) and blood products can be treated to inactivate viruses that may be present. None the less, thousands of haemophiliacs were infected with HIV via contaminated doses of clotting factor VIII and this tragedy was an important piece of evidence in determining the cause of AIDS. Transmission of HIV by this route is now eliminated by heat treatment of clotting factors.

Other viruses remain a problem in blood transfusion of certain patients. Some 100 000 organ transplants are now performed each year and recipients are given immunosuppressive therapy to reduce graft rejection. Graft recipients frequently require blood transfusion and these individuals are at risk from blood-borne viruses that, in normal people, would be no great problem. For example, we noted in an earlier chapter that human cytomegalovirus causes severe disease in immunosuppressed people and, since many healthy blood donors carry the virus, immunosuppressed blood recipients are at significant risk.

The remaining major transmission routes are sexual and respiratory. Our ability to intervene here is very limited. We can attempt to reduce sexual transmission through programmes of education and barrier contraception but the level of success is very uncertain. If we wish to interrupt respiratory transmission completely, we must resort to patient isolation, but in the richer countries respiratory transmission has already gradually decreased as a result of less overcrowded living conditions.

Inducing a protective immune response: vaccination

The concept of vaccination is a very simple one: since infection with a virus usually results in an immune response that protects the individual from further attack by the virus, it follows that if we can induce a similar response with **a related virus, a modified virus or with some component of the virus**, then the recipient will be similarly protected. Before examining the types of vaccines that can be used we should consider the **aims of vaccination**, the inherent risks and the strategies.

Vaccination strategy

Smallpox was controlled and ultimately eradicated by a combination of mass vaccination and surveillance. In the developed world a similar strategy is used for measles vaccination: all infants are offered measles vaccine. Such mass vaccination aims not only to provide **protection to the individual** but also to establish high levels of **herd immunity**. Herd immunity reduces the epidemic spread of the virus, reduces the virus load in the population and, provided that there is no animal reservoir, has the potential to eliminate the virus.

A similar strategy would be inappropriate for **rabies** vaccination. The virus load in the human population is irrelevant. The source of infection is the reservoir in wild animals and human herd immunity can have no effect on virus prevalence. The only purpose of vaccination is to protect the individual. We therefore vaccinate 'at-risk' people such as laboratory workers and people who may contact rabid animals and, of course, we vaccinate the vector (the dog).

We can now consider one rather less obvious example. **Rubella** is a mild infection in children but, if acquired in the early months of pregnancy, the virus crosses the placenta and causes grave damage to the fetus (**congenital rubella syndrome**). The main reason for rubella vaccination is to prevent this congenital infection. What is the best vaccination strategy? If we vaccinate young girls than we protect the individuals at risk, because they cannot be infected later in life during pregnancy. However, we achieve no significant **herd immunity** and the frequency of rubella epidemics will remain more or less unchanged. Any girls who for one reason or another did not receive a successful vaccination would face the same risk of congenital rubella as they did before the vaccination programme began. The second option is to vaccinate all children in infancy, a policy which would create herd immunity in children, interrupt epidemic spread and reduce or eliminate the virus load in the community. Note that this policy requires the vaccination of boys against a virus that presents them with no risk. They receive vaccine for the communal good–to establish herd immunity. This is perceived by some as an ethical dilemma. In the UK, rubella vaccination used to be given only to young girls, but the second option is the current policy.

Types of vaccines

The purpose of vaccination is to induce a protective immune response. This can, potentially, be achieved in a variety of ways. The vaccine may be an infectious but non-pathogenic strain of the virus (**a live attenuated vaccine**); it may be composed of inactivated virus particles (**a killed vaccine**) or it may be a component of the virus (**a subunit vaccine**). Table 12.1 gives examples of

Table 12.1 Examples of vaccines.

Virus	Vaccine type
Polio	Live attenuated (Sabin oral)
	Killed (Salk)
Measles	Live attenuated
Mumps	Live attenuated
Rubella	Live attenuated
Yellow fever	Live attenuated
Canine distemper	Live attenuated
Smallpox	Antigenically related virus (vaccinia)
Marek's disease (chicken herpesvirus)	Antigenically related virus (turkey herpesvirus)
Foot and mouth disease	Killed virus
Rabies	Killed virus
Influenza	Killed virus
Hepatitis B	Subunit (hepatitis B surface antigen expressed in yeast)
Pseudorabies (pig herpesvirus)	Rationally attenuated (engineered deletion mutant)

vaccines in current use. We can now consider the nature and properties of these vaccines.

Most vaccines in current use are live attenuated vaccines

Attenuated means that the virus has been **mutated to a non-pathogenic form**, and this is most commonly achieved in the laboratory by growing the virus in tissue culture cells for many generations. This places new selection pressure on the virus so that mutations accumulate that favour rapid virus growth in the particular cell type used and, it sometimes turns out, simultaneously reduce the ability of the virus to grow *in vivo*. Note that this approach is entirely empirical. It requires no knowledge of the underlying mechanisms of viral pathogenesis or of the nature of the immune response to the virus.[1] The production of an attenuated vaccine is based on two observations: first, **that infection with the 'normal' virus protects against reinfection;** and second, **that growth of the virus in tissue culture reduces its pathogenicity**.

The overwhelming virtue of a live attenuated vaccine is that it will induce a 'natural' immunity: it will induce the same range of immune responses as the virus infection itself. In addition, attenuated vaccines are cheap because a very small dose is required—sufficient to initiate an infection. Attenuated vaccines do, however, have a number of disadvantages. First, since they are 'live' infections, they may cause disease in some individuals, particularly in immune-suppressed people. Second, the vaccine may not always take—the recipient may fail to become infected with the vaccine. Note that the vaccine dose is, itself, too small to be immunogenic; an immune response requires multiplication of the vaccine in the recipient. This has been a problem with the live oral polio vaccine, because other enteric pathogens can interfere with infection by

1 It would be nice to imagine that knowledge of the immune response resulted in the development of vaccines. The truth is different. Remember Jenner and his milkmaids!

polio—a particular problem in the developing world, where there is a heavy enteric pathogen load. Third, because the vaccine is live it must be maintained in a viable state. Many viruses are fragile, and attenuated vaccines must be kept in cold storage—a significant problem in remote parts of the world. The final, and perhaps most unsatisfactory aspect of attenuated vaccines, is that in most instances we do not understand the significance of the individual mutations that accumulate during the attenuation process, and we cannot assume that the attenuated virus is **genetically stable**—it may revert (back-mutate) to a pathogenic form. In making the vaccine we achieve loss of virulence by passaging the virus in tissue culture, but when the virus is introduced into the multicellular host this selection process is reversed and we now favour back-mutation to the original virus.

Killed vaccines do not cause infection

Killed vaccines are preparations of purified or partially purified virus particles that have been inactivated by chemical or physical treatment (e.g. formalin or heat). The objective is to introduce enough antigen to raise a response. As a result **a large dose is necessary**, and this is expensive. Killed vaccines have the virtues that they do not require cold storage, because they are already inactivated, and they present no infectious risk. Their major disadvantage is that, because they are not infectious, they do not induce a natural immunity. Like other antigens, they will be taken up by phagocytic cells and presented to the immune system by Class II major histocompatibility complex (MHC) molecules but, unlike a live virus, they will not be efficiently presented by Class I MHC molecules. They therefore induce **good humoral responses but relatively poor cell-mediated responses**. They will not, for example, induce the production of cytotoxic T cells. Killed vaccines are therefore not applicable to all virus infections. In addition, killed antigens, unlike live infections, induce relatively short-lived responses and booster vaccinations are required to maintain immunity.

We do not know why live infections induce long-lasting immune memory, while dead antigen fails to do so. One popular theory is that live antigens become sequestered at some unknown site, rather than being completely eliminated from the body, and that small amounts of antigen therefore continue to be present to jog the immune memory.

Subunit vaccines are difficult to produce

Gene cloning and gene expression techniques allow us to produce individual proteins in very large amounts. We can identify a particular protein (or subunit) of a virus particle, identify the virus gene that encodes it and then express the gene product in *Escherichia coli* or in yeast or in mammalian cells. In theory, this technology should, by now, have revolutionized vaccine production. In practice these techniques have had little impact because of the level of immunological knowledge that is required to exploit them. We noted that the development of live attenuated vaccines preceded immunological knowledge. By contrast, the development of a subunit vaccine requires us to know the relative importance of different components of the virus in inducing a protective response. Furthermore, subunit antigens, like killed vaccines, induce poor cell-mediated immunity. To date, only one genetically engineered subunit vaccine is used in humans. The hepatitis B vaccine is a preparation of the hepatitis B surface antigen synthesized in a yeast expression system. Antibodies against this protein in the vaccine recipient will neutralize hepatitis B virus.

Recent developments in vaccines

Rationally attenuated vaccines

Attenuated vaccines have the great virtue that they induce a natural immunity, but to date the attenuating mutations have been introduced empirically and, since the mutations are base-pair substitutions, they are reversible. Given adequate knowledge of pathogenic mechanisms it should be possible to **engineer attenuated viruses in a rational way**. Some large viruses have many genes that are not absolutely essential for virus growth, but which help the virus in the multicellular host by, for example, increasing the nucleotide pool size (e.g. the thymidine kinase gene of herpesviruses) or are involved in immune evasion. If we remove these genes, the virus will still grow in tissue culture but will perform poorly *in vivo*—it will be rationally attenuated. This has been done for an economically important herpesvirus of pigs (called pseudorabies virus or Aujesky's disease). The thymidine kinase gene has been removed from the virus and the resulting vaccine strain has been used throughout Europe. Note that **because a segment of DNA has been removed, reversion to virulence** (i.e. back-mutation) **is not possible**.

Live subunit delivery

We noted that viral subunits (i.e. individual viral proteins) can be manufactured by genetic engineering techniques but that these antigen preparations induce poor cell-mediated responses. One way round this problem is to deliver the subunit inside a live vector. Vaccinia virus (the virus used to vaccinate against smallpox) is a large virus that can accommodate additional genes. If we introduce a gene from another virus (say rabies) into vaccinia then the **recombinant vaccinia virus vector** will now make, in addition to vaccinia proteins, a rabiesvirus protein, and because the vector is live, we will achieve a full range of humoral and cell-mediated responses against this protein The principle is outlined in Fig. 12.1. The rabies vaccine that is being used in bait for foxes in Europe is in fact a recombinant vaccinia virus of this type.

Will vaccines work against all virus infections?

Most human vaccines currently in use are directed against acute virus infection, caused by viruses that are usually cleared by the immune system. We are on solid ground here. Since we know that the immune system usually eliminates the virus (e.g. smallpox, measles, mumps, rubella, polio) we can confi-

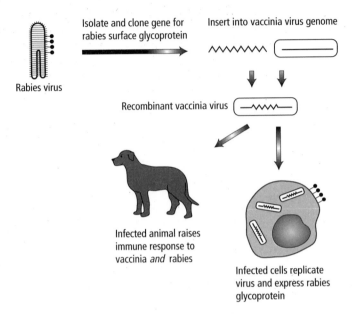

Isolate and clone gene for rabies surface glycoprotein

Insert into vaccinia virus genome

Rabies virus

Recombinant vaccinia virus

Infected animal raises immune response to vaccinia *and* rabies

Infected cells replicate virus and express rabies glycoprotein

Figure 12.1 Strategy for production of vaccinia virus delivery vector (e.g. for delivery of rabies vaccine).

dently predict that a pre-existing response will clear these infections very quickly—the vaccine will work. When we consider viruses that usually persist in the host we are faced with a conundrum. If the virus is capable of persisting in the face of the immune response and can evade acquired immunity, how can we be confident that a pre-existing response will be effective against a challenge infection? This question is particularly pertinent to our efforts to produce a vaccine against HIV, a virus that is apparently never eliminated by the immune system. Will an HIV vaccine work? The answer is that we don't know, but what is obvious is that the rather simple principles which underlie the development of measles and polio vaccines are not adequate for developing an AIDS vaccine. Success, if it is possible, will require a detailed understanding of the processes of HIV infection and of the immune response to HIV.

Therapy of virus infection

While antibiotic therapy of bacterial infection has been standard practice for half a century, antiviral therapy is in its infancy. Before considering recent progress in this field we should note that even if effective antiviral agents were available, their widespread therapeutic use might be difficult, because **the symptoms of virus disease frequently occur after the main phase of virus replication**. Thus by the time we suffer the symptoms of respiratory infection by a **rhinovirus (the common cold)** the virus has done its damage; by the time we diagnose **glandular fever, Epstein–Barr virus** (the causative agent) has probably completed its major replication phase and the patient is suffering the debilitating effects of mounting a massive cell-mediated response. Interfering with virus replication through the use of antiviral agents would not, in these instances, appear to be very useful. We cannot be dogmatic on this subject because our experience and knowledge are very limited. Nevertheless the major use of antiviral therapy is likely to be in particular circumstances, such as: (i) the treatment of infections that persist for long periods (e.g. HIV, wart viruses, hepatitis B); (ii) the treatment of patients who fail to combat virus disease (e.g. varicella-zoster in the newborn, cytomegalovirus in the immunocompromised); and (iii) prophylactic treatment of at-risk patients.

Therapeutic approaches can be divided broadly into two categories, immune therapy and chemotherapy.

Passive immune therapy

Active immunization is the induction of an immune response by administration of antigen (e.g. vaccination). **Passive immunization** is the direct administration of the products of the response—antibodies, cytokines or immune effector cells. The current explosion in our knowledge of immune mechanisms and of immune and inflammatory mediators offers great potential for future immune therapy of virus infections. **At present only passive antibody and interferon therapy have been used.** Passive administration of antibody has proved useful in combating some infections. Newborn babies (particularly premature babies) are defenceless against varicella-zoster virus (chickenpox) and benefit from doses of human immunoglobulin containing high-titre varicella-zoster antibodies. Immunosuppressed transplant recipients have been given human immunoglobulin containing cytomegalovirus antibodies and some success has been achieved. People suspected of being bitten by a rabid animal can be given serum containing anti-rabies antibodies. The use of passive antibody therapy should be much more widely applicable with the production of human (or humanized) monoclonal antibodies against a wide variety of viruses.

The discovery of **interferons** as antiviral agents was originally expected to herald a major breakthrough in the therapy of virus infections. In fact, interferon therapy has proved of little value in combating virus diseases, probably because this cytokine acts at short range to limit virus spread during the initial phase of infection. Systemic therapy of established infection seems not to be beneficial. One success of interferon, however, has been in the treatment of chronic hepatitis B infection. Elimination of the virus has been achieved with an extended course of systemic therapy, but it is not clear that this is achieved through the direct antiviral action of interferon. Some believe that the success of this treatment is due to the up-regulation of MHC Class I molecules on hepatocytes and the subsequent killing of virus-infected cells by cytotoxic T cells.[2]

2 This view is supported by the fact that clearance of the virus is accompanied by a period of severe clinical hepatitis due to attack by cytotoxic lymphocytes.

Chemotherapy

It is an axiom of viral infection that viruses replicate using host cell machinery: most drugs that interfere with virus replication will therefore also affect the metabolism of normal host cells and will have toxic side-effects. But there are some aspects of the viral life cycle that are unique, for example, the binding and entry of the virus into the host cell, specific protein–protein interactions required for the assembly of the virus capsid, specific nucleic acid–protein interactions involved in packaging the virus genome and specific enzyme reactions involved in replication of the viral nucleic acid. A detailed understanding of these processes should allow the design of **specific antagonists of parts of the virus life cycle**. To date the only clinically useful antiviral compounds available are those which **interfere with viral nucleic acid replication**. These are exemplified by two compounds, **acyclovir** (which acts against herpesviruses) and **azidothymidine** (AZT), which acts against HIV. The mechanism of action of these drugs is outlined below.

Acyclovir

This is a nucleoside analogue with an incomplete ribose ring which, importantly, lacks carbon 3 and hence the 3′ hydroxyl group (Fig. 12.2). In mammalian cells this compound is inactive because it cannot be phosphorylated to give the nucleotide. We may recall however, that herpes simplex virus (and some other herpesviruses) synthesize a thymidine kinase in order to increase nucleotide pool size in the infected cell, and this virus-specific enzyme has broader substrate specificity than the related cellular enzymes. **The viral enzyme will phosphorylate acyclovir** and the drug is therefore converted into the **nucleotide analogue**, but only in infected cells. Once phosphorylated, the analogue is incorporated into the viral DNA by the herpes DNA polymerase, but since it lacks a 3′ hydroxyl group, further nucleotides cannot be added and the nucleotide analogue therefore acts as a **chain terminator**, a molecule which interrupts a growing DNA chain. The antiviral specificity of acyclovir is thus based on recognition by two herpesvirus enzymes. The drug is **activated by the thymidine kinase** and is then **incorporated into DNA** by the DNA polymerase.

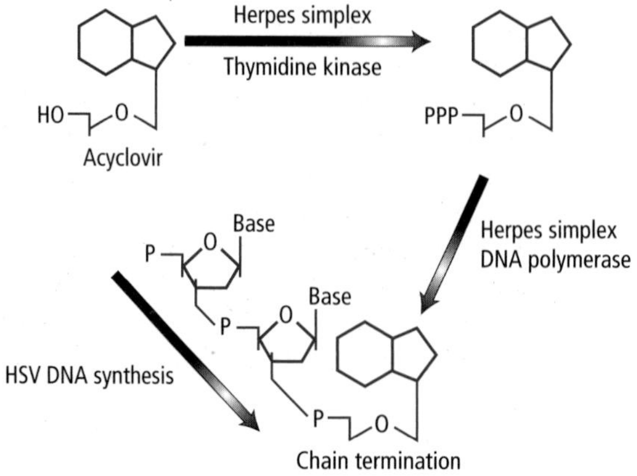

Figure 12.2 Action of acyclovir.

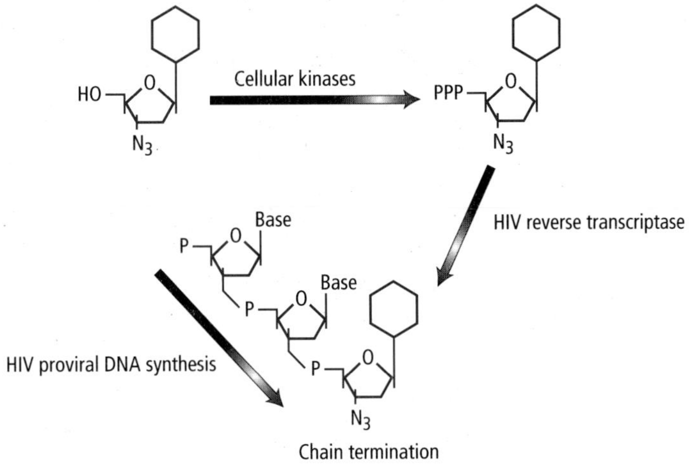

Figure 12.3 Action of azidothymidine (AZT).

Azidothymidine

Like acyclovir, AZT is a nucleoside (thymidine) analogue which lacks a 3′ hydroxyl group (Fig. 12.3). In this case the ribose ring is complete, but the 3′ hydroxyl is substituted by a nitrogen atom. This molecule **is phosphorylated to the nucleotide analogue by cellular kinases**, but the nucleotide analogue is not recognized by DNA polymerases. It is, however, recognized by the reverse transcriptase of HIV and is incorporated into the proviral DNA during reverse transcription of the RNA template (p. 160). Like acyclovir, AZT acts as a chain terminator because it lacks a 3′ hydroxyl so that addition of the next nucleotide cannot occur. Resistance to AZT is a real problem. HIV has a high mutation rate, probably because of the error rate of reverse transcriptase, and base-pair substitutions arise very rapidly in the HIV genome. Within a year of AZT treatment, resistant HIV mutants can be isolated from patients. These mutants have changes in the reverse transcriptase such that the enzyme no longer recognizes AZT as a substrate.

To date the development of antiviral compounds has been largely fortuitous. Both acyclovir and AZT were originally synthesized as potential anticancer drugs and were subsequently found to be effective against herpesviruses and HIV respectively during random screening of large numbers of compounds. The development of new antiviral drugs is becoming increasingly rational as our understanding of the mechanisms of drug activation and action improve, and as more is learned of the pharmacological characteristics of different classes of nucleotide analogues. A major aim is the determination of the detailed three-dimensional structure of virus-specific enzymes by X-ray crystallography (this has been achieved recently with HIV reverse transcriptase) in the hope that this information will allow the design of molecules that will interfere in a specific way with the enzymes in question.

The battle against virus diseases is truly an uphill struggle.

13 Parasites and disease

Parasites are organisms which depend on their hosts to supply their nutrients

The term 'parasite' comes from the Greek word *parasitos*, which was used in antiquity to express disapproval of a person who ate habitually at someone else's expense. In contrast to commensal relationships, which are generally either harmless or of mutual benefit to both the host and the commensal organism, parasitism amounts to the selfish **exploitation of one creature by another, to the sole benefit of the parasite**. Parasites are predators, and many of them actively seek out their prey as effectively as a hunting lion, if less conspicuously. You may not be able to see the schistosome larvae swimming with you in a tropical river, but they can sense your presence, swim towards you, attach themselves to your skin, and penetrate through it—all within a few minutes.

Pathogenic bacteria and viruses also live as parasites in their hosts, but virology and bacteriology have developed as separate fields of inquiry. So **parasitology** is confined, rather arbitrarily, to **the study of protozoan and metazoan parasites**. These are **eukaryotic organisms**,[1] which have evolved to live in other creatures (**endoparasites**) or on their surface (**ectoparasites**). Parasites are to be found in almost every type of living being.[2]

Ectoparasites are not just an irritation

Anyone who has been bitten by ticks, lice, fleas or mites will be well aware of their nuisance value. Some are more adventurous; the mite that causes **scabies**, for instance, burrows beneath the skin and elicits hypersensitivity reactions which can be unsightly and intensely itchy.

Ectoparasites may also spread pathogenic microorganisms from host to host. Lice transmit typhus, fleas carry plague and ticks spread Lyme disease.[3]

Although ectoparasites are therefore of considerable importance, **we shall concentrate on endoparasites, because their impact on human health is of a higher order of magnitude**.

Endoparasites have evolved among various groups of organisms

There is no distinct evolutionary lineage which is composed solely of parasites —many different kinds of organisms have adapted to a parasitic mode of life. Nevertheless, certain groups within the animal kingdom contain a large number of parasitic forms (Table 13.1). Usually parasites occupy characteristic

1 Cells whose chromosomes are contained within a nuclear membrane are referred to as eukaryotes; those whose chromosomes lie within the cytoplasm are known as prokaryotes.

2 There is even a bacterium, bdellovibrio, which is a parasite of other bacteria!

3 Named after Lyme, in Connecticut, where an outbreak was investigated in 1975; this disease is due to a spirochaete.

Table 13.1 Endoparasites: a simple classification and some of the diseases they cause.

Multicellular (macroparasites; metazoa)
Roundworms (e.g. intestinal ascariasis; filariasis)
Cestodes, or tapeworms (e.g. hydatid disease)
Trematodes, or flukes (e.g. schistosomiasis)

Single-celled (microparasites; protozoa)
Amoeba (amoebic dysentery)
Kinetoplastid flagellates (e.g. African sleeping sickness; leishmaniasis)
Apicomplexa (e.g. malaria, toxoplasmosis)

sites or **ecological niches** in their hosts, where their nutritional needs can be satisfied with the minimum of metabolic effort on the part of the parasite.

The biochemical pathways present in many parasites are commonly simpler than those of their hosts, because the parasite can rely on its host to provide it with many of its nutrients ready-made.

The metazoan parasites are often referred to as macroparasites, whilst the protozoa (together with viruses and bacteria) are known as microparasites. In mammals, different parasites have found ways of living within virtually any of the tissues of the body. Indeed, one protozoan parasite, *Toxoplasma gondii*, is sometimes referred to as the **most successful parasite**, since it appears to be able to parasitize many cell types in a variety of mammals.

The life history of parasites is often complex

A **life cycle** describes the parasite's host or hosts, the various forms of the parasite which develop in the host or hosts and how the parasite is transmitted. **Life cycles may be direct or indirect.** Parasites with direct life cycles need only a single host species. They may be transmitted from person to person, as in the case of the venereal transmission of a ciliated protozoan called *Trichomonas vaginalis* (Fig. 13.1). Alternatively, free-living, non-replicating forms of a parasite may be shed into the environment, and transmitted by the faecal–oral route—as in the case of the common human intestinal **roundworms** (Fig. 13.2). Here eggs which are shed in faeces can survive desiccation in dusts for months or years. Children are especially likely to pick up the eggs, and swallow them inadvertently after touching their fingers to their lips.

Direct life cycles are less common than indirect life cycles, which involve at least two different host species. Malaria, leishmaniasis and schistosomiasis are examples of parasitic diseases with indirect life cycles involving definitive and intermediate hosts. A **definitive host** is the host in which parasite sexual maturation and mating occur. An **intermediate host** is the host in which immature forms are found, and within which the parasite may replicate asexually. A **vector** is an insect or other invertebrate which transmits a parasite from one host to another. Some vectors act as purely mechanical agents of transmission (flying syringes!); in other cases, e.g. malaria parasites, the mosquito vector is also the definitive host.

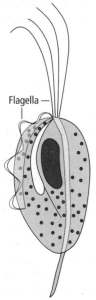

Flagella —

Figure 13.1 *Trichomonas vaginalis* (10–30 μm long).

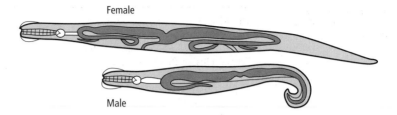

Female

Male

Figure 13.2 *Enterobius vermicularis* (female 8–13 mm, male 3 mm). (Pinworm, a variety of roundworm.)

An important feature of **macroparasites** is that (unlike microparasites) they **do not replicate directly** in their definitive hosts. One roundworm cannot simply divide itself into many more roundworms. It reproduces by laying eggs which usually have to be shed into the environment, where they hatch as larvae. These larvae moult several times before they become infective to new hosts, and commonly undergo part or all of this process of growth and maturation in their intermediate host. Some, such as the larvae of the hookworm, are free-living.

The inability of macroparasites to replicate themselves directly means that their number, and hence the severity of the disease, depends upon how many larval forms enter the definitive host and of those, how many survive and mature. This parasite load is described as the **intensity of infection**.

Diseases caused by microparasites are driven towards increasing severity by their multiplication in the host, so a small infective dose of a virus, bacterium or protozoan can often still lead to disease. In contrast, exposure to small numbers of macroparasites does not necessarily result in disease, since there is usually a **threshold level of intensity of infection below which clinical effects are not noticeable**.

The different stages of a parasite's life cycle usually have different morphological forms

Parasitologists often give complicated names to different stages in the life cycle, but the way to simplify matters is to **focus on the disease**. It is more important to learn about the tissues or cells in which the particular parasite develops.

For example, **when malaria parasites[4] are inoculated into their hosts by infected mosquitoes, the infective forms quickly pass to the liver** via the blood stream, and enter liver cells. There they divide, rupture the liver cell and break free into the circulation, where they **enter red blood cells**. Once inside a red cell the parasite's development can follow one of two courses. In the majority of red cells, the parasite grows and divides; eventually the divided forms disrupt the cell and are released into the blood stream. These released parasites can only infect other red cells but, in a minority of red cells, the parasites **develop into a different form**, which is **only infective to mosquitoes** (Fig. 13.3).

4 Malaria parasites all belong to the genus *Plasmodium*.

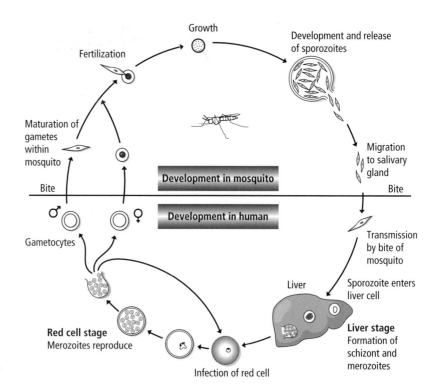

Figure 13.3 Life cycle of malaria parasites.

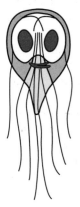

Figure 13.4 *Giardia lamblia* (10–20 μm). Note eight flagella.

It is perfectly permissible to think of the various stages of development of the malaria parasite as **human infective forms** when they are present in the salivary glands of the mosquito, **liver-cell forms** when they are present in liver cells, **red blood-cell forms** and **mosquito-infective** forms. When you've mastered the sequence of events, and understand the differences between the stages, you can give them their proper names.

In developed nations in temperate zones, parasitic diseases make only a small impact on human health and welfare

Human parasitic diseases certainly occur in temperate climates, but are much less common than in the tropics. Examples include intestinal roundworms and some protozoal diseases, such as genital infections with *Trichomonas*, intestinal infection by *Giardia* (Fig. 13.4), and toxoplasmosis, caused by *Toxoplasma gondii*, mentioned above (Fig. 13.5). It is not easy to assess the incidence of infections, which are often too mild to be noticed, such as toxoplasmosis. However, to judge from the numbers of people who are found to have antitoxoplasma antibodies, up to 20% of the UK population have been infected, most without realizing it. One source of *Toxoplasma* is raw meat; those who like to eat it are much more likely to have antibodies (up to 85%). Although usually mild, toxoplasmosis can be life-threatening in special circumstances, such as transplacental spread to the fetus, and in the immunosuppressed.

214

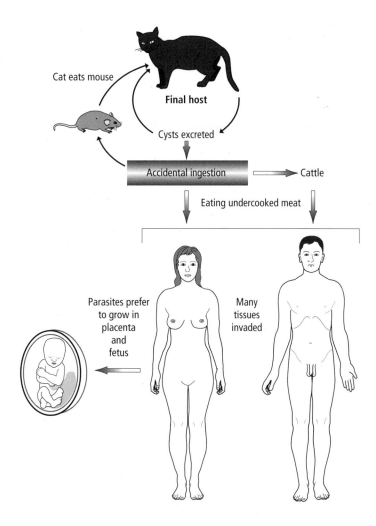

Figure 13.5 Spread of *Toxoplasma gondii* to humans.

5 The commonest parasitic diseases in travellers coming back from the tropics are diarrhoea and dysentery. These can be caused by *Giardia lamblia* or by pathogenic amoebae, which ulcerate the gut.

6 Malaria may at first be mistaken for influenza or other acute viral illness, but it can develop into life-threatening cerebral malaria within a few hours if untreated.

On the whole, these parasitic diseases of temperate climates do not present a major health problem. So why are parasitic diseases important? Here are some facts to consider.

1 First, and most importantly, parasitic diseases are a major cause of ill health in human populations in poor countries in the tropics. Table 13.2 reveals the scale of the impact of a selected group of parasitic diseases on human health in the tropics and subtropics.

2 Owing to their higher prevalence in the tropics, **parasitic diseases also occur among returning travellers.**[5] Physicians in temperate countries see so few parasitic infections that they may be difficult for them to recognize.[6]

3 Armed forces are often sent in large numbers to tropical regions and need to be accompanied by expert medical personnel if their health is to be safeguarded.

4 Acquired immunodeficiency syndrome (AIDS)-related parasitic disorders are increasing in incidence as the human immunodeficiency virus (HIV) pan-

Table 13.2 Impact of some parasitic diseases on world health in the 1980s.

Disease	No. of people infected	Deaths per year	Disease: cases per year	Relative disability caused*
Malaria	800 million	1.5 million	150 million	1–2
Leishmaniasis	12 million	1000	1 million	3
South American trypanosomiasis	12 million	60 000	1.2 million	2
African trypanosomiasis	1 million	5000	10 000	1
Amoebiasis	400 million	30 000	1.5 million	3
Ascariasis	1 billion	20 000	1 million	3
Hookworms	800 million	60 000	1.5 million	2–4
River blindness	30 million	35 000	350 000	1–2
Schistosomiasis	200 million	750 000	20 million	2–4

Adapted from Warren K.S. (1989); based on estimates from the World Health Organization and its special programme for research and training in tropical diseases.
*1, Bed-ridden; 2, able to function on one's own to some extent; 3, ambulatory; 4, minor.

demic continues, and opportunist infections due to pathogenic protozoa, such as *Toxoplasma gondii* and *Pneumocystis carinii*, are becoming more frequent.

5 Parasitic organisms are major causes of disease in domestic livestock and in household pets; some of these animal parasites are transmissible to humans.

Let us look at the first of these points in more detail.

Why should parasitic diseases be commoner in the tropics and subtropics?

Parasites are most often acquired by swallowing **contaminated food or water**, or by exposure to **infected biting insects**, both more likely in these climates. A few parasites can be acquired by sexual contact, and some can be vertically transmitted from mother to fetus. The respiratory route of infection, so important for the spread of bacteria and viruses, is not used by eukaryotic parasites. Throughout much of the tropics it is inevitable that the prevalence of diseases which are associated with poor hygiene should remain high; clean water is often unavailable, human and animal excreta frequently contaminate food and water supplies, and populations of insects are abundant and difficult to control. Although the incidence of most parasitic diseases could be greatly reduced by applying simple public health measures on a broad scale, lack of knowledge, poor administration and, above all, poverty may prevent people from being able to protect themselves against infection.

For example, villagers bathing in rivers and streams in many tropical countries will inevitably expose themselves to the risk of **schistosome infection** unless all members of the local population understand that urinating or defecating in or near water will spread the parasite if the intermediate host—a snail—is present. This means that school teachers need to devise attractively presented lessons about the local risk of parasite infection, so that children grow up understanding the measures they need to take to protect themselves. Even so, many villagers will still be unable to avoid infection—it will be carried down to them in the water from the villages upstream. Therefore, health education tends to carry more weight if it is offered alongside programmes of diagnosis and treatment.

Other factors complicate the prevention of parasitic diseases, and make them more difficult to control than, say, measles or diphtheria

Whereas the control of measles and diphtheria is a relatively straightforward matter, which depends chiefly on combining surveillance of a population for the presence of these agents with the vaccination of an adequate proportion of that population, parasitic diseases are usually much more difficult to control.

There are many reasons for this. The first is that the life cycles of most human parasites are indirect and cannot be completed without **transmission between a definitive host and an intermediate host**. To devise strategies to control a parasitic disease we need to understand the biology of both the parasite and its hosts. This involves finding the answers to a large array of questions: What proportion of the human population is infected, and what determines this? How is the overall burden of the parasite distributed among people who are infected? Does everyone who becomes infected suffer equally badly, as seems to occur with African sleeping sickness, or is there, as more commonly happens, much variability in the clinical response? Is there evidence that immunity can be acquired as a consequence of natural exposure? How long does it take to develop this immunity? When immunity develops, is it partial or complete? If the parasite is vector-borne, what are the key factors which affect the abundance of the vector? Where and when does contact occur between the vector and the host? What proportion of the vectors are infected, and what determines this? Is the parasite only found in humans, or does it also occur in domestic or wild animals? If it is found in these animals, how is it transmitted to humans?

Answering these questions accurately can call for years of painstaking field research. **Understanding the ecology of parasitic disease is a vital aspect of its study.** When mathematical models based on field observations can accurately predict the course of outbreaks of parasitic disease, then we can begin to feel confident that we have correctly identified the factors which regulate the occurrence and the extent of these outbreaks.

Human ecology has a profound effect on the prevalence of parasitic disease

The settlement of new areas of land can bring people into contact with the insect vectors of animal parasites, to which humans may sometimes also be susceptible. When people migrate from rural areas into the towns they may carry their parasites with them. These may then spread more rapidly in densely populated urban areas or the parasites may fail to find their secondary hosts, and die out. **Domestic animals** kept as pets can act as reservoirs of parasite infection both in towns and in rural areas. In the countryside especially, these pets may range more widely, and come into contact with both domestic and wild animals and with insect vectors. **Vector abundance** and the **degree of human exposure to insect vectors** can be affected by such factors as seasonal changes in the weather, the distribution of vegetation around dwellings, or the proximity of human dwellings to farm animal houses.[7] In Brazil, the sandflies which transmit **leishmaniasis** bite dogs and humans equally readily, yet dogs are more commonly infected with these protozoan parasites than are humans. The reason is that the sandflies bite at night, when most people have retreated indoors.

Adequate knowledge of parasite ecology can be crucial in devising control strategies. The success of any control programme depends on a commitment to continue the programme until its goals have been achieved. Schistosomiasis was brought under control in China during the era of Mao Tse-Tung by a simultaneous programme of diagnosis and treatment of infected individuals, and by an immense effort to eliminate the snails which act as intermediate hosts. Villagers were mobilized to pick the snails by hand out of the local streams and ditches! Few countries are able to motivate their people to accomplish such a task. Hence, **political factors can make the difference between the success and failure of disease control programmes**, since only the politicians may be able to ensure that adequate financial resources are made available, that people are adequately educated, and that their cooperation is secured on a sufficiently large scale.

The impact of parasitic disease in the tropics

For people who live in temperate countries it can be hard to appreciate that the prevalence of parasitic disease in many tropical countries can reach levels which would challenge the capacity of the health authorities in any country, let alone those that are impoverished. The difficulties of controlling any one parasitic disease may be compounded by the number of different parasites present in a particular area. **Villagers in much of rural Africa are quite likely to be exposed to the possibility of infection with schistosomes, hookworms, roundworms, malaria and, in some areas, sleeping sickness!** Which physician elsewhere would want to be confronted with a situation in which many patients were suffering from even one such disease?

As a consequence, it is not surprising that people in developing countries often suffer from chronic and untreated parasitic disease. It has been aptly remarked that in these countries people are **poor because they are sick, and sick because they are poor**. And, because the symptoms caused by macroparasites can be slow in onset, and subtle in appearance, the effects of parasitic disease are much less visible than those of acute illnesses. **Most macroparasitic diseases cause relatively few deaths. The toll that such parasites take is principally experienced as a steadily diminishing quality of health.** Except for those individuals suffering from acute infections with protozoan parasites, and those whose burden of macroparasites is so large and so long-lasting that they are seriously ill, the predominant effect that parasitic

7 Even the types of roofing materials used in simple huts can make a difference—many more insects can hide in thatched roofs than under corrugated iron.

disease has on a community is to make people feel generally unwell. Infected individuals are less productive than those who remain uninfected: they are therefore even more likely to remain poor.

The effects of parasitism on livestock can be significant

Although all diseases have direct and indirect effects on the people and populations affected, the insidious nature of the effects of parasitic disease on the economy of nations needs to be emphasized. For example, Table 13.2 refers to **African trypanosomiasis** (sleeping sickness) as a human infection. In fact, **trypanosomiasis is not a single disease, but a group of diseases** which has a far greater impact on human health and welfare than is apparent from counting the number of cases of sleeping sickness Trypanosomes (Fig. 13.6) also infect and kill domestic livestock, and because of the broad geographic spread of the various species of **tsetse fly**, which act as vectors, these organisms interfere with the rearing of domestic animals over much of Africa, from just south of the Sahara to the north of South Africa—an area which is much larger than that of the USA. Trypanosomiasis has a dramatic effect on the rural economy: a peasant family able to keep a draught ox is three to five times more productive than a family that uses hand cultivation alone. So not being able to keep livestock does not just reduce the quantities of available milk and meat; it also has a significant effect on the production of other staple foodstuffs.

The parasite may evade the immune response

Although a parasite finds dependable nourishment and constancy of environment within its host, the host also normally reacts against its presence, and attempts to expel or kill the parasite. Any parasite has to survive in its host for a sufficient length of time (on average) to ensure that infectious forms are successfully transmitted to a new host. The process of transmission is often precarious, with the majority of infectious forms dying before they find a new host. For this reason, many parasites secure their survival by using ingenious methods to avoid being damaged or expelled prematurely from their hosts.

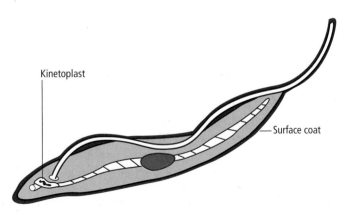

Figure 13.6 *Trypanosoma brucei.*

Indeed, **some parasitic organisms devote a substantial proportion of their genetic and metabolic resources to combating vigorous host responses**. The pathogenic African trypanosomes evade their hosts' immune responses by substituting one surface coat protein for another, for months or years on end. As many as 1000 genes are involved in this process. Successive immune responses, which take place at intervals of just a few days, are able to eliminate all the parasites with one type of surface coat. But, because the parasite can switch its coat faster than the host can respond, the host never manages to eliminate the infection. Malaria parasites also exploit antigenic variability.

Many protozoan parasites, such as leishmaniae and plasmodia, live inside host cells, like some bacteria, and thus evade antibodies. Other parasites, such as adult schistosomes, have developed surfaces that are resistant to even the most active immune effector mechanisms.

So parasites can hide by wearing coats, or cloak themselves in host cells, and try to blend into the background.

A parasite may injure its host directly and by consuming host components

Simple mechanical effects can lead to damage. For example, parasite cysts may press against, and hence obstruct, blood vessels, the gut or the ureter. A profusion of roundworms can sometimes obstruct the intestine.[8] Parasites can also interfere directly with the health of their hosts by **depriving them of nutrients**. Some do this sparingly, and some are positively gluttonous. Hookworms attach to the gut lining and feed so wastefully on host blood that they take in many times the volume of blood that they can absorb, and excrete the rest. **Iron-deficiency anaemia** is a common consequence. There is also evidence that some roundworms and tapeworms can interfere with the absorption, transport and metabolism of key nutrients.

Malaria parasites feed on the contents of red blood cells and destroy them directly from within. Extracellular parasites, such as the pathogenic amoebae, cause extensive ulceration of the intestinal epithelium, which is then followed by dysentery.[9] Both these parasites possess highly active proteolytic enzymes to enable them to digest host proteins rapidly.

Parasites elicit a wider range of immune reactions than is common in other infectious diseases

8 Pinworms are a common cause of appendicitis, due to their blocking the lumen of the appendix.

9 Dysentery is diarrhoea with blood and mucus in the faeces.

10 For this reason it has proved difficult to identify protective antigens which might be used as vaccine components.

The varied nature of the immune reactions mounted against parasites is due to a number of factors. The chronicity of parasitic disease activates a broad range of host responses. Immune reactions form a key component of these responses, owing to the persistent presence of numerous parasite antigens. Eukaryotic parasites have large genomes, with the potential to encode thousands of antigens. These antigens are introduced into the host by the different stages of a parasite's life cycle, and each stage has different antigens. Very few of these activate effector mechanisms that protect the host[10] and, even when they do, different mechanisms are needed to kill the different stages in the life cycle. For example, cell-mediated immunity is needed to kill the liver stages of the malaria parasite, whilst antibodies can block the binding of these parasites to red blood cells.

Some parasites stimulate the overproduction of antibodies by the immune system: increases in the amounts of circulating immunoglobulin M (IgM) and IgG are seen in sleeping sickness and malaria respectively. But these antibodies do not seem to be protective. They are formed because certain parasite components are able to trigger sustained polyclonal B-cell multiplication.

Parasites can cause immunosuppression

In parts of Africa where malaria is endemic, children need to be given higher doses of vaccines against tetanus, diphtheria and whooping cough than do children elsewhere, because their immune systems are working overtime to cope with the challenges of restraining the growth of malaria parasites. **Immunosuppression is common in many different types of parasitic disease**. For example, the pathogenic African trypanosomes immunosuppress their hosts by stimulating macrophages to secrete substances which inhibit the multiplication of helper T cells.

Parasites elicit characteristic immune reactions

Type I, or immediate-type reactions

Helminth (worm) infections are potent stimulators of **high IgE levels**, and increased numbers of eosinophils and mast cells are commonly seen in the tissues of patients infected with worms. A significant increase in the amount of IgE and the number of eosinophils in the blood should always alert the clinician to hunt for the presence of helminth parasites.

It is thought that certain worm components selectively trigger the activity of helper T-cell subsets (Th2) which secrete cytokines able to increase the rate of immunoglobulin class switching to IgE in B cells, and stimulate the **production of increased numbers of eosinophils and mast cells by the bone marrow**. The mast cells act in concert with the eosinophils, since mediators released from mast cells attract eosinophils, and also improve the capacity of eosinophils to kill parasite larvae. Eosinophils migrate into tissues in which helminth parasites are present, and attack the parasite by **exocytosis**, as previously described.

Another result of mast cell degranulation is that **smooth muscle of the bowel wall contracts**, tending to expel parasites. Meanwhile, within the gut epithelium, the mucus-forming cells are stimulated,[11] the excess mucus covers the parasites, and this makes it more difficult for them to bind to the wall of the gut. Mast cells can even deprive worms of the cells to which they are trying to attach themselves by releasing a proteolytic enzyme which strips away localized areas of the gut epithelium.[12]

Type I reactions essentially act as fast-acting amplifiers of acute inflammatory reactions; **these reactions are protective when they expel gut parasites or recruit cells and serum factors which can kill tissue-dwelling parasites**. Harmful reactions involving IgE, mast cells and eosinophils include tropical

11 Just like the excess mucus secreted by the bronchial epithelium, in asthma.

12 Do not worry: this is very quickly regenerated from local stem cells in the crypts!

pulmonary eosinophilia, which accompanies infection with filarial worms[13] in some patients, and the generalized anaphylactic shock which can accompany the rupture of hydatid cysts.[14]

Type II, or antibody-dependent cytotoxic reactions

These can be activated during parasite infections. **Trypanosomes, and malaria parasites following their release from red blood cells, are susceptible to lysis mediated by antibodies and complement.** Some parasites, such as leishmania, can shield themselves against complement because they have molecules on their surface which render the cell membrane resistant to complement-mediated attack.

Antibody and C3b binding will opsonize microparasites for phagocytosis by macrophages. Antibody can also initiate cell-dependent cytotoxic reactions. These cytotoxic reactions are predominantly directed against macroparasite larvae in the tissues.

Type III, or immune complex-mediated reactions

In view of the long life-span of many worms, and the prolonged presence of the parasites of, for example, malaria or sleeping sickness in infected hosts, substantial quantities of antiparasite antibodies are produced. Ageing and death of parasites, or immune attack, may release antigen, which will then initiate the formation of immune complexes. Chemotherapeutic treatment therefore often has to be used cautiously. It may work wonders in terms of its effects on the parasites, but the patient may suffer from severe immune complex reactions if a large population of parasites is killed within a short space of time.

Antigen–antibody complexes may give rise to lesions locally in the tissues adjacent to the parasites, or they may become lodged in capillary beds in other organs. Kidney function can be badly affected if circulating complexes are deposited within the glomeruli. Immune complex reactions have been associated with kidney disease in malaria and lesions in the connective tissues in animal trypanosomiasis. They may also be an important element of lymphatic filariasis.

Type IV, or T-cell-mediated immune reactions

These reactions will have protective effects if they are directed against intracellular parasites which live within the macrophages, such as leishmania, because macrophage activation may result in the death of intracellular parasites. But when macrophage activation occurs in response to T-cell reactions against some extracellular parasites, chronic granulomas may arise, which can be harmful, for example in schistosomiasis.

Cytotoxic T cells are less frequently involved in immune responses to parasites than in virus infections, but cytotoxic T cells can kill some host cells presenting parasite antigens via Class I major histocompatibility complex

13 Filarial worms are tissue-dwelling nematodes (roundworms).

14 A stage in the life cycle of a tapeworm spread from dogs to sheep and humans.

(MHC) proteins. The liver stage of the malaria parasite is attacked by this mechanism.

Summary

Both macroparasitic and microparasitic infections can result in the release of antigens into the tissues, which trigger a variety of immune responses. These responses are important mediators of the cellular pathology of the lesions seen in parasitic disease. Some of the issues which arise in trying to gain an adequate understanding of the pathogenesis of parasitic disease may become clearer if we now consider a few individual parasitic diseases. The aim is to see how these diseases differ from those caused by bacteria and viruses. The parasites concerned continue to affect millions of people and represent major challenges to pathology. If you are looking for problems to solve, read on!

Malaria: a disease whose impact on human health is unmatched by any other parasite

Probably about 150 million people are infected annually with malaria in the tropics and subtropics; and 1–2 million, mostly children, die

The disease was once common in temperate countries too.[15] Although malaria has been eradicated from most of Europe and North America, the mosquito vectors able to carry the parasite remain prevalent in the USA and southern Europe, and the potential for at least seasonal outbreaks of the disease still exists in these regions (Fig. 13.7).

In the 1940s and 1950s it was thought that **the use of insecticides** would quickly lead to the conquest of malaria. With the introduction of DDT at the time of the Second World War, the recorded number of malaria infections in the Indian subcontinent fell from many millions each year to a few tens of thousands. However, the widespread application of DDT and other agents resulted in the **selection of insecticide-resistant mosquitoes**. Also, many developing countries found themselves unable to implement adequate measures of mosquito control. Subsequently, concern arose about the environmental impact of the near-indiscriminate use of insecticides. This combination of factors has resulted in a continuing increase in the incidence of malaria in the tropics.

Virtually all tropical land-dwelling mammals, birds and reptiles harbour their own malaria parasites, but these are not transmissible to humans. **Four species of human malaria parasites are known,** of which three give rise to relatively benign infections. All of these infections are characterized by **bouts of high fever,** separated by periods of normal or subnormal temperature. The fever comes on when a freshly divided batch of parasites breaks out of the remains of the red cell in which it has grown. Just one of the four species, *Plasmodium falciparum*, **is the great killer** because, in a small proportion of

15 Shakespeare wrote of the 'ague'.

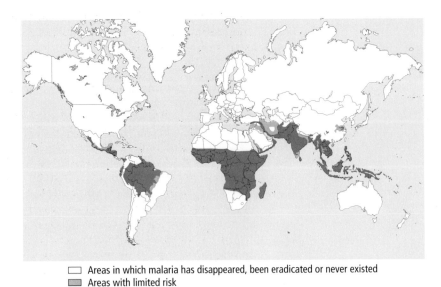

☐ Areas in which malaria has disappeared, been eradicated or never existed
▨ Areas with limited risk
■ Areas where malaria transmission occurs

Figure 13.7 World map of malaria.

cases, untreated infections with this parasite can rapidly lead to multiorgan failure. This parasite is also unique in its evolutionary origins; it is more closely related to the malaria parasites of birds than it is to the monkey malarias, which the other human malaria parasites resemble. The more benign species of human malaria parasite can still prove dangerous, however, leading to anaemia, kidney failure and enlarged spleens which occasionally can even rupture spontaneously.

Plasmodia are protozoan parasites of red blood cells

The parasites all undergo a cycle of sexual development in their definitive host (the mosquito) and cycles of asexual development in their intermediate host (humans; see Fig. 13.3). Female anopheline mosquitoes need a blood meal before they can breed. The males feed harmlessly on plant sap![16] Mosquitoes that have ingested blood from a malarial patient subsequently inoculate parasites, which have meanwhile multiplied in their salivary glands, into new hosts. **These parasites quickly invade liver cells, multiply and release forms that invade red cells. Repeated cycles of multiplication occur within red cells**, each concluding with parasite release, followed by reinvasion of fresh red cells. The parasites digest the contents of the red cell as they grow, ultimately destroying it.

The most significant differences between the development of the various species of human malaria parasite in their hosts are: (i) the propensity of the less pathogenic species to remain dormant in the liver for varying periods of time before releasing parasites which will infect red blood cells; (ii) the ability of *P. falciparum* to develop in red cells of all ages; the other, less pathogenic species are limited to growing in subpopulations of red cells—either very young or very mature cells. *P. falciparum* can therefore reach higher levels

16 We thought that we'd mention this, because it's almost the only good news in this chapter.

of parasitaemia, and hence cause more severe degrees of anaemia; and (iii) the distinctive behaviour of *P. falciparum*-infected red cells, which become adhesive, as described later.

Malaria infections are highly variable in severity

Although 99% of people who become infected with *P. falciparum* develop fever, only about 1% suffer from cerebral malaria or severe anaemia. Why is this? It is clear that in malarial areas people display **a range of innate resistance to malaria infection**, and can also develop some degree of active, acquired immunity. The best-known source of natural resistance is inheritance of the haemoglobin variant known as **sickle-cell haemoglobin** (HbS). The possession of HbS reduces the severity of the disease and an individual with HbS is much less likely to fall among the 1% of severely affected individuals. However, it offers no protection at all against mild malaria. The underlying mechanism of protection appears to be that the parasite is less able to grow in cells which contain HbS, in the low oxygen tensions of the capillaries in which the parasitized cells pool, because these cells have lower than normal levels of intracellular potassium. Other individuals are protected from infection with *P. vivax* because they lack the receptor on their red cells to which the parasites can bind.

Recently, it has been shown that **parasite-driven natural selection** has also operated within the immune system. The MHC Class I antigen human leukocyte antigen (HLA)-Bw53 is associated with protection against severe malaria. The frequency of this allele is only about 1% in European populations, but it reaches 14–40% in West African peoples. This difference is believed to be a direct consequence of natural selection due to malarial infection in Africa. Whereas 25% of all Gambians carry this allele, it is found among only 14% of those patients presenting with severe malaria in the Gambia. It is thought that possession of the allele permits early presentation of a parasite epitope eliciting cytotoxic T cells, and thereby conferring protection.

Acquired immunity also develops in endemic areas

People living in such areas become less susceptible to severe malaria as they grow older, which is why the highest mortality from severe malaria is seen in children. Tourists, who lack any previous exposure to the parasite, are especially prone to suffer severely if they become infected with *P. falciparum*. Both these observations are compatible with the idea that **living in an endemic area results in the gradual acquisition of immunity**. What is more surprising is the finding that children in the most susceptible age groups in endemic areas may quite often be found to be heavily parasitized, and yet not display any clinical symptoms. However, they have not lost their susceptibility to malaria, because they may subsequently become ill with it. We cannot yet explain these findings. **Are some parasite strains quite innocuous, and others harmful?** Eventually, people in endemic areas show a much diminished incidence of parasitaemic episodes, which argues that, in the later stages of the development of naturally acquired immunity, the immunity is directed against the parasite itself.

Clearly, **we still know all too little about the basis for immunity to malaria**, yet we need to understand how naturally acquired immunity develops, in order to try to produce an effective antimalarial vaccine. Which are the most important protective antigens, and what are the most important protective effector responses? Can the immune effector mechanisms operate against one or more stages of the parasite?

The infecting form inoculated by the mosquito, the liver-cell forms and the red blood-cell forms all possess characteristic and different antigens. The liver stages are attacked by cytotoxic T cells, which recognize the presence of malaria epitopes within the Class I MHC molecules on the surface of the liver cells. Additionally, certain T cells produce interferon-γ, which can prevent the intracellular replication of the parasites. The antigens associated with the surface of the infected red blood cell represent targets for immune attack, but these are so numerous that it is difficult to identify any single antigen which can serve as a vaccine constituent. Additionally, the structures of several of the surface proteins which have been identified on the parasitized red blood cells appear to have evolved so that they can assist the parasite to evade the host's immune response. These antigens all contain a large number of repeat sequences, which are strongly immunodominant. However, they induce T-independent antibody responses, which generate only low-affinity antibodies. Such antibodies are unable to trigger effector mechanisms which can eliminate the parasites.

One awkward question which has to be faced during the development of a malaria vaccine is whether its use will increase antigenic diversity within the population of malaria parasites. The existence of an obligatory sexual stage during the parasite's development in the mosquito vector means that each transmission event is preceded by a meiosis. This allows the generation of recombinant parasites, antigenically distinct from their progenitors; the use of a vaccine which does not provide protection against a diverse range of antigenic variants among the malaria parasites will simply result in novel antigenic types quickly replacing those in current circulation, and the vaccine becoming ineffective.

How do malignant malaria parasites cause severe disease?

Most malaria fatalities arise from the 1% or so of *P. falciparum* infections in endemic areas which progress beyond intermittent fever and moderate degrees of anaemia via a cascade of events to a multisystem disease, which involves metabolic disturbances and cerebral malaria with or without severe anaemia. The percentage of severe infections is much higher among travellers who contract malaria, owing to their lack of any acquired immunity.

An important feature of *P. falciparum* infections is that **growth of *P. falciparum* within a red cell results in that cell acquiring a new and dangerous property, that of stickiness to the endothelium of blood vessels.** This dramatic change coincides with the appearance of electron-dense 'knobs', which represent parasite-derived antigens, associated with the red cell surface. Some of these antigens have been identified, as have the molecules on endothelial cells to which they bind. The small venules in many tissues may be obstructed by this adherence of parasitized red blood cells. The tissues are therefore forced into an anaerobic mode of metabolism, and lactic acid formation can be sufficient to exceed the buffering capacity of the blood. The consequent metabolic acidosis can lead to fatal cardiac impairment; at sublethal concentrations the acidosis further enhances the red cell adherence. The acid–base status of children suffering from *P. falciparum* malaria is a good indicator of whether recovery is likely.

Cerebral malaria is due to microvascular obstruction by the adherent red cells. Not all small vessels are affected, and ischaemia is not total. The patients become comatose. Although the symptoms are severe, most patients recover completely if they are treated promptly with antimalarial drugs.

A fall in blood glucose (**hypoglycaemia**) may also occur, and this may be the consequence of the insulin-like activity of a glycolipid toxin released from ruptured red cells as the parasites complete a round of asexual multiplication. But it is also known that quinine—still one of the most effective antimalarials—causes an increased insulin output, and use of quinine therefore worsens the hypoglycaemia. Intravenous glucose has been found to be life-saving.

An area of major interest is the **role of cytokines** derived from macrophages and endothelium in this series of events. The release of cytokines, including interleukin-1, and tumour necrosis factor (TNF-α) from macrophages accounts for the very high fevers which are characteristic of malaria, and the same cytokines are known to activate endothelial cells.[17] Recent evidence suggests that some people are genetically predisposed to release large quantities of TNF-α in response to malaria infection and that these patients are much more likely to die of cerebral malaria than individuals whose output of TNF-α is more restrained.[18]

One of the most important long-term consequences of chronic malarial infection is the increased risk that it brings of suffering from a form of cancer known as **Burkitt's lymphoma**, associated with co-infection with the virus which causes glandular fever (Epstein–Barr virus). The mechanism is unknown, but the correlation presumably represents another indication of the profound changes in the immune system which take place in malaria infections.

Leishmaniasis: a disease with a bewildering variety of clinical forms

Leishmaniasis is the name given to a whole group of diseases, caused by protozoa characterized by their possession of a unique cellular organelle—the **kinetoplast**. This lies immediately adjacent to the point of origin of the flagellum and consists largely of DNA, which provides a genome for the single, big mitochondrion in these organisms.

About 12 million people are infected with leishmania at present, and up to 350 million people live in areas which place them at some risk of infection. **Leishmaniasis is a vector-borne disease, transmitted by female sandflies** (Fig. 13.8). It is difficult to control because the various species of the parasite are also

17 This will enhance the adhesion of parasitized red blood cells.

18 See also cutaneous leishmaniasis, where moderate tumour necrosis factor-α responses are protective, but high levels are associated with one form of disseminated disease.

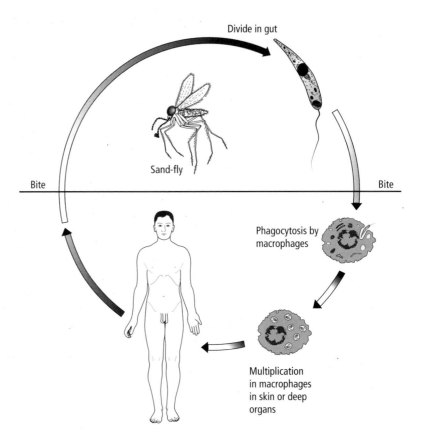

Figure 13.8 Life cycle of *Leishmania*.

found in animals which function as reservoir hosts. About **13 different species of leishmania** in the Americas can infect humans, which can be transmitted by several species of sandfly and are found at times in literally **dozens of species of mammalian hosts**. It is often difficult to tell how much danger the parasites in a particular animal host pose to humans, because finding the parasite in a reservoir host does not yet enable us to tell whether that strain of the parasite will be able to cause disease in humans or how severe that disease is likely to be. **Dogs are particularly important domestic reservoirs** for the severest (visceral) form of the disease.

The protozoa multiply in the gut of the fly, and infective forms are inoculated when the flies feed on host blood. The organisms are taken into macrophages, where they are able to thrive, even within phagocytic vacuoles which have fused with lysosomes, and are acidic. The multiplication of the organisms, coupled with the subsequent death of macrophages and reinfection of new macrophages, results either in large skin sores, or in disseminated lesions in mucous membranes.[19] Certain species of leishmania cause **visceral leishmaniasis**, in which the infected macrophages move to deep organs. Most of the skin lesions heal spontaneously within a few months. Some, however, may spread locally, resulting in the erosion of skin, mucous membranes

19 The disfiguring skin lesions are variously known as oriental sore, Baghdad boil or Chiclero's ulcer.

and cartilage from the face and nose, and causing terrible discomfort and disfigurement.

Leishmaniasis has been called a spectrum disease

This spectrum of severity ranges from rapid control and resolution of the infection on the one hand to progressive cutaneous or visceral disease on the other. How do we account for the spectrum?

There appear to be several strands to the answer.

1 The species and strain of the parasite exert an important effect, since some species are only associated with cutaneous leishmaniasis, or only with visceral leishmaniasis, whilst others can be associated with a broader spectrum of lesions, ranging from cutaneous to visceral.

2 Some individuals may be genetically less susceptible to the disease than others because they possess the appropriate allele of a gene we met earlier, called natural resistance-associated macrophage protein (NRAMP),[20] which enables macrophages to kill any leishmania which enter them.[21]

3 The form taken by the immune response appears to be critical. In order to clear an infection it is vitally important that the right subset of T-helper cells should be activated in the early stages of the disease. The correct subset is the one that is associated with activation of macrophages, namely the T-helper 1 subset, enhancing cell-mediated responses, just as we saw earlier, in tuberculosis (see Fig. 8.6). T-helper 2 responses result in susceptibility to progressive disease.

We are still not sure exactly how leishmania cause disease

In the commonest form of the disease, that of localized cutaneous leishmaniasis, the skin ulcerates over an underlying granuloma, in which many lymphocytes are present, as well as macrophages containing relatively few parasites. In this form of the disease the infection is effectively controlled. CD4+ T-helper 1 cells in the lesions can activate macrophages, so that the replication of the parasites is restrained. During the time that it takes for the cell-mediated immunity to become established, the lysis of infected macrophages, with the inevitable release of tissue-damaging components, is presumed to contribute to the death of the overlying epidermis. However, the important point is that the responding T-cell populations are characteristically those which are required for a good cell-mediated response.

In addition to localized cutaneous leishmaniasis, there are two other cutaneous forms of the disease in which the parasite is more widely disseminated through the skin and adjacent mucous membranes. In one form (**diffuse cutaneous**) it appears that tissue destruction is associated with a **lack of cell-mediated immunity**; here the macrophages contain large numbers of parasites, and there are few lymphocytes in the lesions. In this form there is preferential multiplication of T-helper 2 cells, and the host makes antibodies—uselessly, since these cannot limit the multiplication of an intracellular parasite.

In the second form (**mucocutaneous**) it appears that **the cell-mediated reac-**

20 The equivalent gene also confers early protection against salmonella and tuberculosis infections in mice.

21 At present this is only an inference, based on observations in mice.

tion to the parasites runs out of control, since the macrophages in the lesions contain few parasites, but the granulomas themselves spread and destroy the oral and nasal cavities. This severe form of the disease is associated with relative overproduction of TNF-α. In this respect the effects of TNF-α in leishmaniasis may parallel those observed in malaria. People who are genetically predisposed to respond to infection by making moderate levels of TNF-α are protected against severe disease; those who make too much TNF-α suffer unusually severe symptoms—destructive granulomatous lesions in leishmaniasis, and cerebral involvement in malaria.

Schistosomiasis, or how much damage can be done by an egg?

The characteristic presence of blood in the urine which indicates urinary schistosomiasis is referred to repeatedly in Egyptian medical papyri, and the calcified eggs of the parasite have been identified in mummified human remains from about 1200 BC. But it was not until the 19th century that Bilharz,[22] working in Egypt, showed that parasitic worms which live in the blood vessels adjacent to the intestine or urinary bladder were associated with the occurrence of the disease which was first named after him (**bilharzia**), but which is now more usually called **schistosomiasis**.

Three major species of schistosome parasite can infect humans and, except in people who acquire massive acute infection later in life, such as tourists inadvertently bathing in heavily infected streams, the disease arises slowly over one to two decades. Granulomatous reactions occur due to the deposition of parasite eggs in the wall of the intestine, and in the liver, or in the bladder and urinary tract. The affected sites differ, depending on the species of schistosome.

More than 200 million people are infected with schistosomes

The disease exists in over 70 countries in Africa, the Middle East, South America, China and parts of South-East Asia.

In any community in which the parasite is found, the majority of affected individuals are found to carry only light infections, while a few—often less than 5% of the total—are heavily infected, and suffer clinical symptoms. **This aggregation of most of the parasites present in a human population within a relatively small number of people is characteristic of many helminth infections** in humans and other animals.

There are several possible reasons why this uneven distribution of parasites occurs, and probably no single explanation covers all the circumstances. **Variations in exposure to infection** may occur as a consequence of differences in human behaviour. Some individuals may regularly undertake tasks which expose them to higher numbers of infective forms, such as entering water while tending domestic livestock, washing clothes, fishing, cleaning irrigation canals or working flooded rice fields. **Some people may inherit genes which make them unusually susceptible** to infection, while less susceptible individ-

22 Theodor Bilharz (1825–1862), a German helminthologist.

uals presumably inherit more protective alleles of these genes. **Genetically different strains of the parasite may exist**.

As with most disease due to helminth parasites in the definitive host, **the severity of clinical disease is related to the intensity and duration of infection**. The severest form of the disease usually develops among heavily infected older children and young adults.

Human infections develop following exposure to water contaminated with larval forms of the worms, which are released from freshwater snails (Fig. 13.9)

Each larva is capable of developing into a single adult worm, and is either male or female. **The larvae enter moist skin** after attaching themselves to it using a pair of suckers. Then they release proteolytic enzymes, and penetrate the skin within a few minutes. Once through the epidermis they pause for a couple of days. During this pause remarkable changes take place in the larvae, which have to adapt from living in a freshwater environment to the saline environment of the body. Whether as a reaction to this change, or to enable them to resist the onslaught of the host's immune system, they add an additional layer to their outer membrane. Many larvae fail to complete this process of adaptation without accident. Up to 60% die, even in non-immune hosts, at this stage.

Subsequently **the larvae migrate through the blood stream to the liver**, where they mature into adult worms. At this stage the males and females also

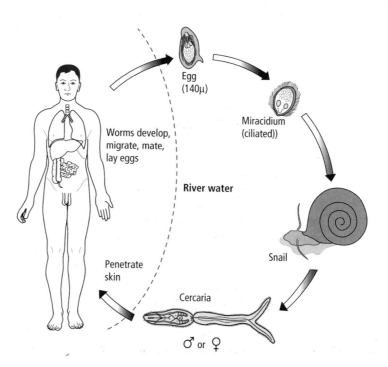

Figure 13.9 Life cycle of *Schistosoma mansoni*.

find each other. In the blood vessels adjacent to the intestine or urinary bladder, the worms mate and settle down to years of active egg-laying.

The eggs contain larvae which can only develop further if they are released into fresh water, where the appropriate species of snails can act as intermediate hosts. However, in order to get back into fresh water the eggs have first to find their way into the faeces or urine. They achieve this by eroding their way through the wall of the venule in which they were laid, into the tissues of the wall of the gut or bladder. In one species, the eggs are armed with a hooked spine, so that they tend to move in one direction only as smooth-muscle contractions occur around them. In addition digestive enzymes are secreted by the larva from within the egg. The eggs finally emerge into the lumen of the gut or the urinary bladder and are discharged. If they reach fresh water the eggs hatch, and the free-swimming larvae search out the snails to begin the cycle again. One infected snail can subsequently release up to 200 000 free-living infective forms.

The development of disease is a consequence of the immune response to the schistosome eggs

The eggs are highly antigenic, and elicit granulomas at their sites of deposition. The schistosome granulomas consist of an accumulation of lymphocytes, macrophages and eosinophils, surrounded by fibroblasts. In the early stages of the disease the granulomas can occupy up to 100 times the volume of the egg itself. Therefore relatively few eggs can disrupt the function of a disproportionately large volume of tissue. Later in the disease, the granulomas diminish in size. Lodging of an egg in the liver is followed by the gradual onset of severe fibrosis. This can have grave consequences if the extent of the fibrosis interferes with the normal flow of blood through the liver.

In urinary schistosomiasis, the egg granulomas form in the wall of the bladder, and the fibrosis involves both the bladder wall, which loses its elasticity, and the urethra, which can eventually become obstructed.

Schistosome granulomas represent delayed-type hypersensitivity reactions to egg antigens

Previously infected experimental animals show enhanced and accelerated cell-mediated reactions to the intravenous inoculation of schistosome eggs. Such reactions are specific to egg antigens, and can be transferred to naïve animals by T lymphocytes. Granuloma formation is classically a sign of the activity of Th1 helper T cells. However, schistosome infections are also characterized by raised levels of IgE and eosinophilia.

There is also a case for regarding the granulomas as fulfilling a protective function

Mice which are depleted of T cells and then infected with schistosomes are only capable of forming very small granulomas, and more of these mice die of the infection. Schistosome eggs are known to release factors which are directly toxic to liver cells. The formation of a granuloma around an egg probably shields the liver from these factors.

At least three of the types of hypersensitivity reactions occur in this disease

The repeated exposure of individuals in endemic areas to free-swimming, skin-penetrating larvae released from infected snails can result in the development of immediate (type I) hypersensitivity skin reactions to the larvae, called **swimmer's itch**.[23] At different stages of parasite maturation, immune responses can result in severe systemic reactions, including high fever. When these occur, 1–2 weeks after infection, they probably represent reactions precipitated by the release of antigens from worms which die before they mature. In this case it is the formation and systemic deposition of immune complexes which are thought to be responsible for the clinical signs (type III).

When similarly acute fever is seen 1–2 months after infection, it coincides with the onset of egg-laying and the formation of granulomas around the first eggs to be deposited in the tissues (type IV). Here the clinical signs may be due to the systemic effects of cytokines released from macrophages.

Immunity to schistosomiasis is slow to develop

In endemic areas, people who have been infected in childhood gradually acquire increasing resistance to reinfection. This immunity depends on the presence of adult worms but, curiously enough, the immune response leaves these adult worms unharmed. Instead, the acquired resistance is directed against incoming larvae. **A prominent feature of this immunity is that it takes 7–8 years to develop.** During the intervening years, schistosome-infected children are certainly mounting antibody responses to antigens found on schistosome larvae. These early antibody responses, however, **do not confer any protection against infection**. How can this be the case? The answer is that during the early years of exposure to infection the major stimulus to antibody formation comes from egg-derived antigens, because of the very large quantities of eggs deposited in the tissues. These antigens are mostly polysaccharides. They elicit T-cell-independent IgM antibody responses which fail to trigger eosinophil binding and degranulation, and actually get in the way of antibodies of other isotypes which can bind eosinophils and thereby kill the larvae.

With the passage of time, older children develop IgE antibody responses against antigens present in adult worms and later, as adults, they develop similarly directed IgA antibody responses. **These responses are both highly protective**, and are thought to mediate antibody- and eosinophil-dependent attack against larvae as they migrate through the tissues. Why these protective responses should take so long to develop is unclear. If the epitopes which elicit these responses are only present on the incoming larvae, the doses of immunogenic material may be very small. Even allowing for this possibility, antibody responses which take a decade or more to mount represent yet another fascinating and curious aspect of parasite immunology.

23 In other instances, skin reactions can also occur in unsensitized individuals, due to the trauma caused by the invading larvae.

Control of parasite diseases

Since parasitic diseases are caused by communicable agents, many of the principles which we encountered in relation to the control of bacterial and viral diseases also recur here (see Fig. 7.10). The main differences lie in the fact that so many parasitic diseases have indirect life cycles involving secondary hosts, or vectors. Also, animals can act as reservoirs of infection for leishmania, trypanosomes, *Toxoplasma* and some species of schistosome. The control of parasitic diseases currently centres around the treatment (chemotherapy) of infected individuals, coupled with programmes of vector control (e.g. the use of insecticide-impregnated bed nets against malaria mosquitos) or the control of intermediate hosts (e.g. the use of molluscicides to kill snails carrying schistosomes, in streams or irrigation canals). Vaccines are in their infancy; the occurrence of antigenic variation and of other mechanisms for evasion of the immune response greatly complicates parasite vaccine development. Nevertheless, the first antimalarial vaccine has been tested in South America and in Africa, and shown to have a significant effect in combating the incidence of the disease. However, the levels of protection observed are lower than we would expect when using bacterial or viral vaccines.

Summary

These few examples of parasitic disease illustrate the complexities of the interactions between parasite and host, which are much greater than those in bacterial and viral diseases. They also illustrate, better than most diseases, how the incidence and the severity of human disease can be influenced by myriad factors, from genes to social behaviour.

The logistic difficulties and expense of improving public hygiene to interrupt the parasites' life cycle are immense. Notable successes have included the development of new antinematode and antischistosome drugs. But mutations to drug resistance in malaria are posing new and daunting difficulties. Antiparasite vaccines are proving difficult to develop; it is hard to identify the best antigens to use and difficult to obtain protective immune responses using single, purified antigens.

14 Cardiovascular disease

It may seem unusual, in a general account of disease, to single out one organ system for special attention. The reason is not just that cardiovascular diseases are the commonest cause of death in the industrialized world. It is that these diseases clearly show how abnormalities of one part of the body can affect other parts. They also illustrate, better than most, certain pathological principles which are important.

1 Disease may occur as a result of quantitative changes in physiological variables, rather than by novel exogenous injury.

2 Many different forms of injury may produce the same disease.

3 Innate reactions to injury may themselves do harm.

We shall return to these principles at the end of the chapter, but first we must look at the most important forms of cardiovascular disease, beginning with anaemia.

Anaemia

Anaemia is insufficient oxygen-carrying capacity of the blood

The oxygen-carrying capacity depends on the quantity of haemoglobin present in the red blood cells in a given volume of the blood and, as shown in Table 14.1, there is a range of haemoglobin concentrations commonly accepted as normal, which vary with both sex and age. The total red cell count is also variable.

Anaemia is usually defined as a reduction in the blood haemoglobin concentration below these normal ranges and is usually accompanied by a reduction in the number of circulating red blood cells. The difference from normal is therefore essentially quantitative. Usually, however, there are also recognizable changes in the appearance of the red cells, which are different in different types of anaemia.

Table 14.1 Normal ranges of haemoglobin concentrations.

	Women		Men	
	Mean	95% range	Mean	95% range
Adults				
Red cell count, $\times 10^6/\mu l$ (or $\times 10^{12}/l$)	4.6	4.1–5.1	5.1	4.5–5.9
Haemoglobin (g/dl)	13.9	12.2–15.0	15.3	14.2–16.9

Children (6–14 years) are normally within the same range as adult women. Under 6 years, 11 g/dl is the acceptable lower limit of normal

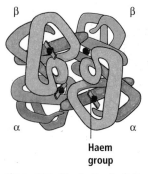

Figure 14.1 The bulk of adult haemoglobin consists of four haem groups and four globin chains.

Haemoglobin is a large, complex molecule

The elements of the molecule are folded around the oxygen which is transported in its centre. Haemoglobin has properties which, in combination with other molecules present in red cells, allows the oxygen to be taken up by it, when in the pulmonary capillary circulation, and yet released within the tissues, where it is required.

Haemoglobin consists of **four haem molecules and four globin chains**. Each flat haem molecule contains a single ferrous ion in its centre and is set cross-wise into a globin chain, which then allows the chain to fold into the correct configuration (Fig. 14.1). Normal haemoglobins contain two pairs of globin chains which are different from each other, but their structure allows them to self-assemble to form a stable, large molecule. Most of the normal haemoglobin in adults has two α and two β chains; the haemoglobin of the fetus is different and consists of two α and two δ chains. This is because its function is different, picking up oxygen from the placenta, not the lungs.

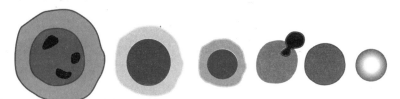

Figure 14.2 During development, the erythroblasts and their nuclei decrease in size. The nucleus is finally extruded to give the reticulocyte, which matures with further size reduction to a circulating red cell.

Haemoglobin is packaged within red blood cells or erythrocytes

Although red cell precursors have nuclei, the circulating mature red cells do not; **the nucleus has been extruded** (Fig. 14.2), usually whilst still in the bone marrow, which is where red cells develop in postnatal life.[1] The cytoplasm is normally saturated with haemoglobin. The cytoplasmic membrane is attached to a specialized cytoskeleton. Imagine a skin stretched over flexible but strong basket-work; this gives the cell its unique shape, a disc with deep concavities on both sides, resulting in a high surface-to-volume ratio which allows very efficient gaseous exchange (Fig. 14.3). It also enables the red cell to be flexible, to pass easily through the smallest blood vessels, the capillaries, which may be of a similar diameter to the red cells themselves (7–8 μm). In order to do this, the disc becomes a cone shape, travelling nose first (Fig. 14.3).

1 In the fetus, haemopoiesis occurs mainly in the liver.

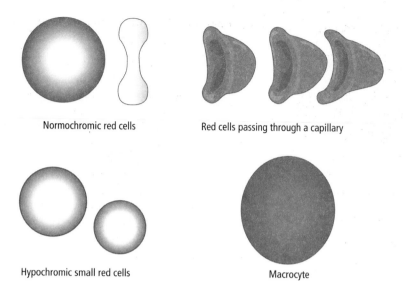

Normochromic red cells

Red cells passing through a capillary

Hypochromic small red cells

Macrocyte

Figure 14.3 Mature red cells.

Red cells normally survive and circulate for about 4 months

Oxygen carriage, and therefore health, depend upon constant production of billions of these cells which have a life-span, on the average, of 120 days. The loss of the nucleus has advantages both for individual cells, in that they can exhibit maximum flexibility, and for the cardiovascular system, since the additional mass of billions of cell nuclei need not be pumped around the body. Old red cells become less flexible and are phagocytosed by sessile macrophages, mainly in the liver, spleen and bone marrow.

Anaemia is due either to defective production or excessive loss of red cells

The disease processes which affect the production of red cells and their subsequent survival represent a microcosm of all the disease processes that can affect the whole body. Thus, anaemia can result from the effects of genetic abnormalities, environmental deficiencies and hazards from every kind of harmful agent, both animate and inanimate, or from the harmful effects of immune reactions. These various causes lead to defective or abnormal production of red cells or excessive loss; sometimes both occur together.

Red cell production defects are various (Fig. 14.4)

A wide range of disease processes can adversely affect red cell production; these include deficiencies of the cytoskeleton and abnormalities of the haemoglobin, or of the 25 or so enzymes necessary for red cell maintenance. In addition, production may be impaired by diseases specific to the bone marrow itself or more generalized disorders which secondarily affect the marrow.

REQUIREMENTS FOR NORMAL PRODUCTION OF RED BLOOD CELLS

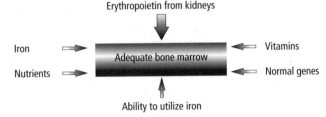

FACTORS LEADING TO ABNORMAL RED CELL PRODUCTION

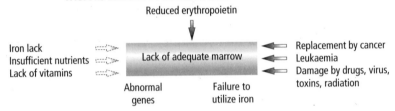

Figure 14.4 Causes of inadequate red cell production.

Interestingly, these abnormally produced red cells are often more quickly destroyed.

Red cell production requires adequate marrow stem cells

The normal precursor stem cells in the marrow may be displaced by **cancer**, either arising in the marrow itself, as leukaemias, or when a cancer has spread to the marrow from other parts of the body.

In addition, **chemicals, irradiation and viruses** are all known to damage marrow cells and can bring about depletion of variable severity and persistence. All pathways of blood cell development may be affected, or only particular ones. Human parvovirus, for example, targets the red cell precursors.

Red cell production depends upon the presence of adequate growth factors

Erythropoietin is the most important specific growth factor required for red cell development. It is made in the **kidneys**, which have a mechanism for sensing an inadequate supply of oxygen and secrete erythropoietin into the blood if the oxygen supply is low. This is how the normal red blood cell count is maintained.

When haemoglobin is inadequately oxygenated, for example at high altitudes or because of lung disease, this results in increased erythropoietin production and therefore an increase in the number of circulating red cells. This condition is known as **polycythaemia** (literally, 'many cells in the blood').

Some forms of chronic kidney disease can lead to anaemia, mainly because erythropoietin production is deficient.

Impaired synthesis of haemoglobin leads to anaemia

Impaired haemoglobin synthesis may occur because of **lack of some vital ingredient** required to synthesize normal haemoglobin or because of **genetic abnormalities** preventing accurate coding for this complex molecule, resulting in the formation of **abnormal haemoglobins**.

Inability to produce sufficient normal haemoglobin results not only in **fewer red blood cells** being produced but their **average size is smaller** and, not surprisingly, when stained and viewed under the microscope, they appear pale. When normal red cells are examined, they have a pale central area which marks the thin portion of the bi-concave disc, but when the haemoglobin content is reduced, the pale area may appear to extend to the edges of the cell (see Fig. 14.3).

Hypochromic is the word used for this decreased staining, while the term **microcytic** indicates that there is a reduction in the average diameter of the red cells, compared with those in normal (normochromic) blood (Fig. 14.5).

A deficiency of available iron is the commonest cause of hypochromic anaemia

Iron is essential for the synthesis of the haem part of the haemoglobin molecules and **this precious element is carefully recycled** within the body. However, inevitably, a small constant loss occurs in all cells shed from the body and more is lost whenever any bleeding occurs, so it may be lacking if there is insufficient iron in the diet to make up for these losses. There is also physiological menstrual loss by females during their reproductive life and, in addition, growing children have greater needs than adults. This helps to explain the

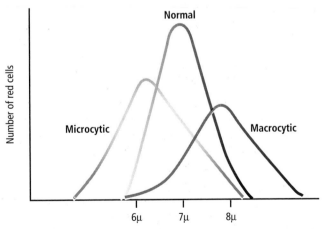

Figure 14.5 Price-Jones curves. These show the size distribution of red cells in different conditions, including the normal bell-shaped curve and the average size. Note that in the anaemias the range of sizes is wider than normal (anisocytosis).

range of levels that are regarded as acceptable in the 'normal' ranges (see Table 14.1).

An important cause of hypochromic anaemia is **chronic blood loss**, because this is a major cause of loss of iron from the body which cannot be compensated for, even by a normal dietary intake of iron. Such chronic blood loss may have a variety of causes, including excessive uterine bleeding in females or slight bleeding into the gastrointestinal tract, which perhaps goes unnoticed. For example, there may be bleeding from an unsuspected tumour of the intestine or from an infestation by hookworms, common in many parts of the world, which causes constant bleeding as the parasites injure the intestinal mucosa.

Inherited defects of haemoglobin synthesis also lead to hypochromic anaemia

Disorders which interfere with the synthesis of haemoglobin may affect only the haem part of the molecule, as does iron deficiency but, in other cases, **globin** production is genetically impaired. A large number of different abnormalities of globin synthesis have been recognized, but one important group of inherited disorders leading to hypochromic anaemia is the **thalassaemias**, in which there is reduced synthesis of either the α or β globin chains. Major and minor forms of the disease are recognized, depending upon whether the patient is homozygous or heterozygous, respectively, for the defective gene. Since α chains contribute to fetal haemoglobin, major abnormalities are fatal to the fetus, and therefore patients with the disease usually have reduction in β chain synthesis. Most of the developing cells lacking sufficient haemoglobin die within the marrow and only small, pale cells are released into the blood.

The name of the disease is derived from *thalassa*, which means sea, because it is prevalent around the Mediterranean.

Deficiencies of DNA synthesis usually present first by causing anaemia

The rapid turnover of the marrow stem cells makes them early casualties of shortage of factors essential for DNA synthesis, although other tissues are of course affected. Two of these factors are **cobalamin** (vitamin B_{12}) and **folate**. The liver stores of cobalamin are considerable and may be enough to last for 2–3 years if the normal dietary supply is curtailed, but lack of folate has effects within months because the stores are less adequate. Impairment of DNA synthesis causes both a prolonged cell cycle and a reduction in the number of cell divisions which occur in erythropoiesis, so the result is **fewer** but **larger**, misshapen red cells. The latter, which tend to be oval rather than round, are called **macrocytes** and the condition is often referred to as **macrocytic anaemia** (Fig. 14.5). It is also known as **megaloblastic** anaemia, because all the progenitor cells of the bone marrow are larger than normal.

Folate deficiency may come about because of an inadequate diet, the daily requirement being between 50 and 100μg, but it is not uncommon for the condition to develop during pregnancy, because of the additional needs of the fetus. Although some is stored in the liver, it may be inadequate to supply the increased demands of a pregnancy.[2] Another circumstance that may exhaust the store is the extra requirement that ensues when the red cells have a shortened life-span as in the haemolytic anaemias (see below). Folate absorption takes place in the upper end of the small intestine. Cobalamin (vitamin B_{12}) is absorbed from the terminal ileum, but only after it has combined with a special factor (**intrinsic factor**) which is secreted by the **parietal cells of the gastric mucosa**. There is no ileal receptor for cobalamin alone but there is one for the intrinsic factor with which it combines. Hence, anything which diminishes intrinsic factor secretion by the gastric mucosa (e.g. chronic inflammation of the stomach, or surgery) can lead to vitamin B_{12} deficiency.

One important cause of deficient absorption of vitamin B_{12} is an **autoimmune disease**, in which **antibodies develop against intrinsic factor and/or the cells that make it**, and cause injury to the stomach and its lining (**atrophic gastritis**). This results in thinning of the gastric wall and reduction in gastric acidity, because the same cells which make intrinsic factor also secrete hydrochloric acid. Because of the stores of vitamin B_{12}, the resulting anaemia develops slowly and insidiously, giving rise to the name **pernicious anaemia**.

Reduced survival of circulating red blood cells is known as haemolysis. The anaemias which result are called haemolytic anaemias

Red blood cells which are abnormal in any way do not persist as long in the circulation as normal red cells. Therefore, any defect in their production leads to a reduced life-span and many of these defects are the result of inherited disorders, like the thalassaemias already mentioned.

One group of inherited diseases affects the structure of the erythrocyte cytoskeleton or the attachment of the cell membrane to it. Very often this results in red cells which are **abnormal in shape** and often **lacking the flexibility** which is so important to their function. One example is known as **hereditary spherocytosis**, which has several variants, most showing an autosomal dominant pattern of inheritance. The defect may be of the major network protein **spectrin**, or affect its attachments to other skeletal elements such as **actin** or **ankyrin**. The much less flexible cells which result are likely to be trapped in the spleen and destroyed.

Another way that the shape of red cells can be altered, and their life-span reduced, is when they contain an abnormal haemoglobin. An example is haemoglobin S, whose deoxygenated molecules form elongated needle-like crystals which distort the entire cell. Such distorted cells have been likened in shape to a sickle and the anaemia which results is called **sickle-cell anaemia**. The rigid, elongated cells can become impacted in the microcirculation, blocking it. The abnormal haemoglobin differs from normal only by a single amino acid substitution, valine for glutamic acid in the β chain of globin, but this is enough to affect its properties profoundly. The gene responsible is found widely distributed amongst populations living in or derived from those regions where malaria is endemic. The persistence of such an apparently harmful gene is attributed to the fact that heterozygotes for it have a degree of **protection against malaria** due to *P. falciparum*, during the early years of life. The unfortu-

2 Sufficient folate and cobalamin are required for normal development of the fetal nervous system, so it is potentially dangerous for a pregnant woman to develop folate deficiency.

nate homozygotes suffer chronic haemolytic anaemia and episodic occlusion of small blood vessels.

Inherited deficiencies of key red cell enzymes affect function and survival

Since red cells lack nuclei, they are totally dependent upon the enzymes they contain when they leave the bone marrow. In cases where one or more of the enzymes is deficient, the red cells may be unable to resist the stress of oxidation or produce enough energy to maintain their membrane ionic pumps. Aggregates of oxidized haemoglobin may form or the red cell shape and flexibility may be altered—all characteristics which impede their passage through the spleen, leading to haemolysis.

Red cells are sometimes a target of autoantibodies

Antibodies can, in some cases, be shown to be directed against the combination of some drug or viral product with a large molecule in the red cell membrane but, in other cases, the cause is unknown.

Depending on the class and concentration of antibody involved, the effects are various. Their presence may lead to removal of all or part of the red cell by macrophages, or rounding up of the cells to form spheres, or cause them to stick to one another (agglutinate); other changes may also occur but all lead to reduced red cell survival.

Anaemia may be caused by microorganisms

Chronic infections may interfere with the marrow's ability to make red cells. In addition, haemolysis may be brought about by the exotoxins of various bacteria. In some infections, red cells are directly destroyed and the most conspicuous example of this is **malaria**. The parasites invade red blood cells, multiply within them and finally bring about their destruction. Unfortunately, many other red cells are also destroyed by the action of antibodies formed against antigens on the parasitized red cells.

Passage through the spleen is important for red cells

The spleen acts as a filter for the blood; as the blood passes through it, it comes first into close contact with the lymphoid tissue (white pulp), after which it is delivered into what is called the **red pulp**. This spongy splenic tissue has a framework of fine fibres, or **cords**, containing many sessile macrophages. The cords are surrounded by blood sinuses which drain back into the venous system. Although about 90% of the red cells take a fairly direct route from arteries into the sinuses, thus escaping rapidly into the venous blood, the remainder leak into the cords, **amongst the macrophages**. Their only escape route from the cords into the sinuses is through orifices in the walls, the size of which is smaller than their own diameter.

At this stage, abnormalities of shape, content and flexibility of the red cells are crucial in negotiating these orifices, because if they remain trapped in the cords for longer than the normal period, they compete with each other for the available glucose which may be insufficient for their metabolic processes. Reduced metabolic activity results in surface changes which macrophages are able to detect and this leads to their phagocytosis and destruction. In a similar way, red cells containing parasites, or with antibodies attached to their membranes, are also brought into intimate contact with macrophages during their passage through the spleen and can be recognized and removed from the circulation.

Thus, although the majority of normal red cells which become senescent are removed during their passage through the sinusoids of the liver, where the blood trickles slowly along channels lined by Kupffer cells, the spleen provides a mechanism for removing **abnormal** cells from the circulation, before their life-span is complete. Presumably, this is important because otherwise they might impede circulation in one of the important capillary beds of the body and cause significant injury.

Direct trauma can damage red cells

Premature red cell destruction may be brought about, surprisingly, by trauma. For instance, prolonged marching may cause so many red cells to break down inside the capillaries in the feet that haemoglobin is spilled into the plasma and may appear in the urine. This is only a transient phenomenon; of more importance clinically is the constant trauma that results from the presence of an artificial heart valve.

The effects of anaemia are in part direct and in part compensatory

There are direct effects upon the circulating red cells which vary with the cause of the anaemia and, most importantly, upon all the body tissues as a result of the **inadequate supply of oxygen**. This is by far the most important effect of anaemia.

Compensatory changes are quite efficient, so that slowly developing anaemia can sometimes become very severe before the patient complains of it. Probably the best example of toleration of severe anaemia is the form of vitamin B_{12} deficiency seen in **pernicious anaemia**, when the haemoglobin can fall to levels of 3–4g/dl before the condition is noticed. Such low levels can be attributed to the extremely slow evolution of the condition which allows compensatory mechanisms to operate.

Peripheral blood in anaemia

Anaemia as discussed in this account has referred to the **chronic** state, which is that usually understood by the term.

Acute blood loss, once shock has been overcome and circulating fluid volume restored, does of course lead to anaemia but the individual cells are normal, merely reduced in number, leading to lowered total levels of haemoglobin. Under normal circumstances, this would be a temporary condition.

In chronic states, some of the changes already described may be apparent when blood smears are examined; for instance, a predominance of small or large or pale-staining red cells—even red cells with abnormal shapes.

In addition, it may be possible to recognize evidence that the bone marrow has been trying to respond to the anaemia by 'hurrying the production time' and releasing less mature cells (reticulocytes) into the circulation. In fact, when the anaemia is really severe, even red cells that still retain their nuclei may appear in peripheral blood smears. This is especially likely in the haemolytic anaemias and is good evidence of the attempted compensation by the marrow.

Anaemia affects the well-being of all tissues

The most important effect of anaemia is the decreased oxygen supply to all the tissues of the body. Some effects can be recognized in mucous membranes, the skin and the nails or, if tissues are examined histologically, fatty change may be evident. To some extent, the reduced oxygen carriage can be compensated for (see below), but any tissue whose vascular supply is already reduced for other reasons, such as **arterial narrowing**, may suffer selective and sometimes fatal damage, when anaemia is superimposed.

The changes which can result may be impairment of function, the development of fatty change in severely injured cells, or even infarction.

Anaemia causes compensatory hyperplasia of the bone marrow

In all anaemias, the marrow is affected by the increased output of erythropoietin from the kidneys, as they respond to relative oxygen deficiency in their blood supply.

There is evidence of **heightened proliferative activity**, most easily recognized by the reduction in the amount of adipose tissue which is normally present in the marrow and its replacement by haemopoietic stem cells and their progeny. Not only is activity increased within those areas of marrow usually utilized for blood production but the actual **volume of productive marrow is increased**. In the normal adult, only part of the available marrow space is used for making blood cells; it is that which is found within the more central part of the skeleton (vertebrae, thoracic cage and pelvis), perhaps including a small area at the upper end of humerus and femur and a little in the skull. However, in response to prolonged stimulation, the proliferative process is extended and spreads down the humerus and femur, into marrow space normally occupied almost exclusively by adipose tissue.

Anaemia causes compensatory effects in the cardiovascular and respiratory systems

The effects vary with the degree of anaemia. Reduced oxygen carriage can be compensated for by increasing the rate at which the blood circulates. Hence, there is an **increase in cardiac output**. Blood flow is also redistributed, so that it is maintained to essential internal organs but reduced to the skin, thus contributing to the skin pallor which is characteristic of anaemia. The patient may also experience palpitations of the heart, faintness and breathlessness on exertion. Fatigue is a common early symptom.

Increased respiratory rate, maximizing the oxygenation of haemoglobin, also results from anaemia. The patient perceives this as **breathlessness**.

Summary

Anaemia can result from inadequate red cell production or excessive loss, or both. It always causes compensatory effects, in the bone marrow, cardiovascular and respiratory systems. However, its most important result is inadequate oxygenation of all the tissues.

Haemostasis and thrombosis

Haemostasis is simply **blood clotting**, normally occurring within a minute or two of a small cut or bruise. Haemostasis is obviously an important reaction to trauma, and protects against serious bleeding, whether external (**haemorrhage**) or internal (**haematoma**). The mechanisms of haemostasis are threefold: first, the **injured blood vessel contracts** (goes into spasm); second, the **blood platelets stick together** at the site of injury, tending to block the gap; and third, the plasma fibrinogen is converted to a **fibrin mesh**, which together with the aggregated platelets forms a **haemostatic plug** (Fig. 14.6).

Muscular contraction at the site of an injury is a very primitive, conserved reaction. It occurs even in the body wall of invertebrates such as hydra. Then with the evolution of a vascular system, there appeared cells called **thrombocytes** that clumped together (like platelets) at the site of injury, for example in starfish and lower arthropods. In higher arthropods came the development of protein strands analogous to fibrin, augmenting the coagulation process. The mammalian system is just a more sophisticated version of these three basic mechanisms.

Fibrin formation is an important component of haemostasis

Blood freshly drawn into a test-tube clots after a few minutes, obviously due to a mechanism **intrinsic** to the blood itself. However, if extracts of tissue are present as well, the clotting occurs in seconds—the **extrinsic** pathway. The active agent in tissue extracts is called **thromboplastin**. The **clot** that forms in a test-tube is a dark red jelly-like mass which slowly contracts and separates from a clear fluid composed of plasma constituents left over after the clotting process. This clear fluid is of course **serum**.

Fibrin formation is due to an enzyme cascade mechanism

This is like the complement system in that it consists of a cascade of compo-

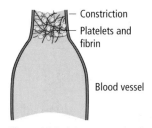
— Constriction
— Platelets and fibrin

Blood vessel

Figure 14.6 A haemostatic plug.

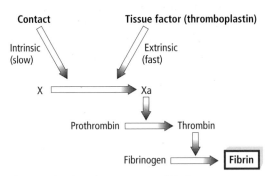

Figure 14.7 Fibrin formation simplified.

nents. Also, like complement, it can be activated in more than one way; in this case two pathways (**intrinsic and extrinsic**) converge to produce the final step, which is the conversion of the plasma protein, **fibrinogen** to **fibrin**. The various plasma proenzymes that participate in the cascade are given Roman numerals —the central point where the two pathways converge is the activation of **factor X**.

You will have noticed that essentially the extrinsic pathway is the same as that responsible for fibrin formation in an **inflammatory exudate** (see Chapter 2). Activation of factor X fills the same vital hinge role in this cascade that C3 performs in complement (Fig. 14.7).

Congenital or acquired defects in this clotting mechanism cause bleeding tendencies—excessive bleeding after trauma. One well-known clotting defect is **haemophilia**. This is a sex-linked recessive genetic defect in production of factor VIII, another protein in the cascade. Haemophiliacs bleed profusely after even trivial trauma. In the days before treatment with factor VIII injections, the disease was often fatal in childhood.[3]

Quantitative defects in clotting may also be acquired. For instance, the liver produces many of the clotting factors, so the immature liver of the newborn, or severe liver disease in later life, may cause excessive bleeding after injury. Others include shortage of vitamin K or of platelets (**thrombocytopenia**).[4]

Like any other reaction to injury, the clotting mechanism needs controls to stop it progressing too far. These are the naturally occurring **anticoagulants**, for example heparin and antithrombins, and enzymes (**fibrinolysins**) that break down fibrin, such as **plasmin**. The relative availability of these different factors therefore affects the efficiency of the process.

The blood clot that forms on a typical skin wound, if undisturbed, dries to form a **scab**. This acts as a protective layer during the healing of the underlying wound, which occurs as described in Chapter 2.

Thrombosis is haemostasis in the wrong place

Thrombosis is the formation of a mass (**a thrombus**), composed of blood constituents, which forms in flowing blood on the inside wall of a blood vessel.[5]

3 The British Queen Victoria was a carrier of haemophilia; because her numerous offspring married into other European royal houses, this disturbed the succession of more than one dynasty.

4 Vitamin K is required in the synthesis of several clotting factors by the liver.

5 A non-occlusive thrombus on the wall of a vessel is called a **mural thrombus**.

246

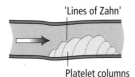

'Lines of Zahn'

Platelet columns

Figure 14.8 A mural thrombus.

A recently formed thrombus has a **structure**, which distinguishes it from clots that form post-mortem or in a test-tube.

The structure shown in Fig. 14.8 is due to columns of platelets (not truly simple as drawn here but branched, like coral) coated and linked together by fibrin strands enmeshing red and white blood cells. This structure was described in the 19th century, as were the predisposing causes of thrombosis, known as **Virchow's triad**:

1 injury to the endothelial lining;
2 slowing, or eddying of the blood stream;
3 changes in the constituents of the blood.

These still explain all the known clinical associations of thrombosis, but how these predisposing factors act was only discovered relatively recently.

Injury to the endothelial lining causes platelet activation

Hereditary and acquired abnormalities of fibrin production explain a number of haemorrhagic conditions; and anticoagulant drugs[6] that inhibit fibrin formation are partly helpful in inhibiting venous thrombosis. However, it is only since the advent of techniques to study platelet activity that we have come to understand how haemostasis and thrombosis actually begin. These techniques include electron microscopy and improved fractionation and chemistry of platelet constituents, but also, importantly, the invention of the **aggregometer**. In this apparatus, platelet suspensions, isolated from blood by centrifugation of plasma, are placed in a beam of light. The addition of various agents causes platelets to **aggregate** together in clumps. This results in a decrease in the opacity of the suspension, so the increased light transmission can be monitored as a measure of the potency of the aggregating agent (Fig. 14.9).

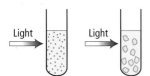

Light   Light

Figure 14.9 Aggregometry. Aggregated platelets allow more light through than normal platelets.

Aggregometry has shown that a number of biological stimuli cause platelet aggregation (Table 14.2). Low doses of these agents cause only temporary aggregation; higher doses cause a **second phase** of **irreversible aggregation**. The reason for this is that the higher doses cause not only aggregation but also the release from the affected platelets of constituents that are themselves potent aggregating agents, such as **adenosine diphosphate** (ADP) and certain **prostaglandins** (especially **thromboxanes**). Because **aspirin** and similar drugs inhibit prostaglandin synthesis, they inhibit platelet aggregation.

Platelets (Fig. 14.10) are biconcave, disc-like (about $2.5 \times 1\,\mu m$) cytoplasmic buds, with no nucleus, deriving from the cytoplasm of large cells called

6 Such as heparin or warfarin.

Table 14.2 Some platelet-aggregating agents.

Immune complexes
Endotoxin
Adenosine diphosphate
Thrombin
Adrenaline and noradrenaline
5-Hydroxytryptamine
Collagen

All these tend to be additive in their action.

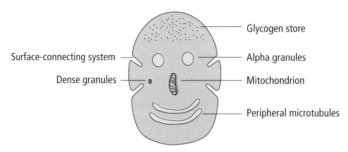

Figure 14.10 Platelet ultrastructure (schematic). The α granules are lysosomes, with stores of enzymes and of fibrinogen. The surface-connecting system is simply due to infolding of the plasma membrane. The peripheral microtubules control the shape. The dense granules store calcium, adenosine triphosphate, adenosine diphosphate and 5-hydroxytryptamine.

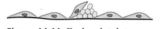

Figure 14.11 Early platelet thrombus.

megakaryocytes in the marrow. The cytoplasm of each megakaryocyte splits to give rise to 3000–4000 platelets. They then circulate in the plasma[7] for about 8–10 days until they are eventually phagocytosed and destroyed by sessile macrophages in the spleen and elsewhere. During their lifetime, they instantly adhere to any site where endothelial cells are missing. This is because they are intensely adhesive to underlying collagen which is exposed when the vessel is severed, or even when endothelial cells are lost from an otherwise intact vessel (Fig. 14.11). The latter event explains how endothelial injury can lead to thrombosis, the first of Virchow's triad. If the collagen exposed is sufficient, the adhesion leads to release of platelet constituents. This in turn leads to aggregation of more platelets at the site; and the release of platelet factor 3, which leads to fibrin formation at the site.

Thus we can explain the sequence of events in the onset of haemostasis, and the reason why thrombosis occurs after significant endothelial injury *in vivo*, for example, in severe inflammation, or due to arterial disease.

Slowing or eddying of the blood stream enhances the risk of thrombosis

In general, thrombi are commoner in veins than arteries, especially if the flow is slowed, as in venous compression, or in recumbent patients. This is perhaps because early thrombi are more easily dislodged by the rapid blood flow in arteries, which also presumably disperses procoagulant factors. Eddying, such as occurs in areas of branching, or sometimes in the heart with abnormal rhythm, presumably causes endothelial damage.

The most common site of thrombosis in humans is in leg veins, mainly in bed-ridden patients. This is due partly to the sluggish flow and partly to the calf veins being squashed by pressure of the weight of the leg on the bed.

Altered blood constituents can lead to thrombosis

The list of agents increasing aggregation (Table 14.2) shows how such factors as stress or cigarette-smoking (increasing adrenaline) or infection (endotoxin)

7 About one platelet for every 10–20 red blood cells.

may enhance thrombosis. Decreased anticoagulant factors may also sometimes play a part.

The risk of thrombosis is governed by numerous quantitative factors

It is clear from the above that the chance of a thrombus forming depends on the interplay of many factors, many of which can be influenced by the environment. This may explain why thrombosis is predominantly a disease of urban societies, with the alterations of diet and lifestyle that this entails.

Results of thrombosis

Small thrombi may lyse

Flowing blood or fibrinolysins may lead to the disintegration of small mural thrombi without significant residual effects.

Thrombi may propagate

Especially if the thrombus occludes a vessel, blood flow tends to stagnate nearby and therefore may clot, increasing the length of the occlusion. This is called **propagation** of a thrombus.

Thrombus frequently narrows or occludes the vessel

This is the major hazard of thrombosis, leading as it inevitably does, especially in arteries, to insufficiency or even total loss of blood supply to the affected tissue—known as **ischaemia**. If veins are blocked, the back-pressure on the capillaries causes **oedema** (e.g. of the ankles, in leg vein thrombosis).

Residual thrombus eventually becomes organized

Just as an area of necrosis becomes replaced by granulation tissue and scar, so does the thrombus, if it persists. The differences are that here the capillary blood vessels grow in from the endothelium that rapidly grows to cover the thrombus; and the cells providing the collagen and ground substance are not fibroblasts but smooth-muscle cells migrating from the vessel wall.

Thrombi may become infected

If a thrombus occurs in an area of infection, the microorganisms may colonize the thrombus. This can have untoward effects.

Extensive haemostasis or thrombosis may use up clotting factors

This rather unusual event may occasionally actually deplete the clotting components so severely as to lead to a haemorrhagic tendency–**consumption coagulopathy**.

Embolism

Embolism is **the passage of any mass from one part of the cardiovascular system to another**. Usually the mass (the **embolus**) is a piece of thrombus (thrombo-embolus), but not always.

Veins are the most common source of emboli

Thrombi form most frequently in veins, especially leg veins. If a piece of thrombus falls away from its site of origin it is swept away in the blood until it reaches a vessel that is too small to permit it to pass, and so lodges there. Anatomy ensures that **emboli of venous origin lodge in pulmonary arteries** (Fig. 14.12). The size of the pulmonary artery branch blocked depends on the size of the thrombo-embolus. Usually they are small and lodge in small pulmonary arteries; but sometimes an extensive thrombus from the deep veins of the leg ends up as a coiled mass blocking the main pulmonary artery. This **massive pulmonary embolism** is not an uncommon cause of death, especially in bedridden patients.

More rarely, pulmonary emboli can result from thrombi in the right atrium of the heart, especially when the heart rhythm is abnormal.

Emboli from the left side of the heart or large arteries lodge in systemic arteries

Systemic embolism or **arterial embolism** may result from thrombi in the pulmonary veins (very rare), left atrium, mural thrombosis in the left ventricle (usually the result of a myocardial infarct, and therefore common) or thrombus on atherosclerotic plaques in the aorta or its major branches (again, common). Anatomy determines that this form of thrombo-embolism will block systemic arteries (Fig. 14.13), but the artery affected is in many cases a matter of chance. Embolism to arteries supplying the brain, kidney, gut or legs is particularly serious.

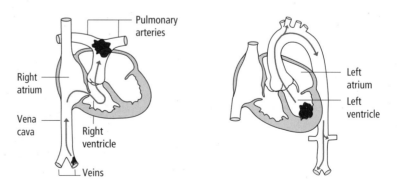

Figure 14.12 Pulmonary embolism (left).

Figure 14.13 Systemic arterial embolism (right).

Emboli from veins of the gut or spleen lodge in the liver

Blood from the gut and spleen does not pass to the lungs, as other venous blood does, but to the branches of the portal vein in the liver. Emboli are however uncommon in this part of the circulation.

Emboli are not always thrombi

Fragments of bone marrow or, more commonly, fat droplets may be sucked into ruptured veins when a bone is fractured. The resultant **fat embolism** or **bone marrow embolism** usually only blocks tiny lung vessels. Occasionally, however, showers of fat emboli may squeeze through lung capillaries to reach the arterial circulation and can even cause death by blocking numerous capillaries in the brain. Less commonly, embolism may be due to accidental introduction of air bubbles or even foreign bodies into the circulation.

The results of embolism are similar to those of occlusive thrombosis

The ischaemia resulting from embolism tends to be worse than that due to thrombosis, because the blockage is so sudden.

If tiny thrombo-emboli are infected, the result may be numerous abscesses scattered around the body. This condition, **pyaemia**, is usually rapidly fatal if antibiotic treatment is unavailable.

Summary

The processes of haemostasis and thrombosis are identical in their mechanism, and are distinguished only by the fact that the circumstances and site of the process determine whether it is helpful or harmful.

Atherosclerosis

This is a predominantly human disease, occurring in the aorta and its main branches, and consists of the gradual accumulation of focal raised patches (**plaques**) on the arterial lining. It develops slowly, over many years. Eventually its complications are **the main cause of death in urbanized societies**, because the vital arteries of the heart and brain are particularly prone to this disease.

Although it is also common in large birds, other animals are relatively spared from the disease.

Atherosclerosis is a focal disease of the intima of arteries

The artery wall has three layers (Fig. 14.14). The outermost, the **adventitia**, is simply the connective tissue surrounding the vessel. The thickest part of the normal wall is the **media**, composed of layers of **smooth-muscle cells**.

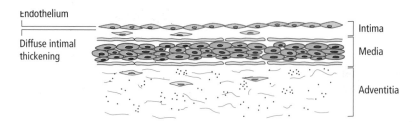

Figure 14.14 Artery wall.

These cells are of course contractile. They are also responsible, during development, for secreting ground substance, collagen and elastin fibres.[8] Layers of **elastin** are a predominant feature of the media of the aorta and its biggest branches, but much less so in medium-sized (muscular) arteries, which usually have only an internal and external elastic lamella at the borders of the media.

In the newborn the **intima** consists only of a single lining layer of flat **endothelial cells** on the internal elastic lamella. However, with advancing age, the endothelium becomes gradually separated from the internal elastic lamella by a thin uniform layer of connective tissue, referred to as **diffuse intimal thickening**.

Diffuse intimal thickening is due to migration of occasional medial smooth-muscle cells through holes in the internal elastic lamella; once in the intima they appear to revert to their former role of secretion. The resultant thickening therefore includes ground substance, collagen and elastin.

The underlying reason for this age-related change is unknown, although it is certainly accelerated by many forms of injury to the artery, such as high blood pressure, low blood flow and others. Diffuse intimal thickening of advancing age has no adverse effects that we know of, but it is upon this thickened intimal layer that the focal plaques of atherosclerosis develop.

The smallest lesions of atherosclerosis are collections of fat-filled macrophages

Young adults and even sometimes children have cream-coloured spots, called fatty streaks, visible on the aortic lining. Histology shows that these are due to groups of **foam cells**, so called because their cytoplasm is literally bulging with lipid droplets, giving the cells an appearance like a collection of soap bubbles (Fig. 14.15).

Foam cells have been shown[9] to be **macrophages**, derived from **blood monocytes** that have emigrated between endothelial cells into the intima. Occasional solitary macrophages can be found even in diffuse intimal thickening, so perhaps there may be a continuous, very slow emigration of monocytes from the blood. It is not known how the larger collections, seen as fatty streaks, arise but they do occur especially at areas where there is haemodynamic disturbance, such as at branching points.

8 Artery walls do not contain fibroblasts. Smooth-muscle cells, however, are essentially identical to fibroblasts in their ability to secrete these materials.

9 Using labelled monoclonal antibodies that distinguish different cell types by immunocytochemistry.

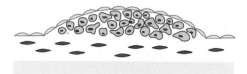

Figure 14.15 Fatty streak. (Typically 0.2–0.3 cm diameter.)

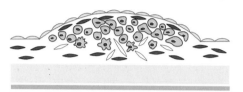

Figure 14.16 Intermediate lesion. (Bigger than fatty streak.)

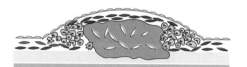

Figure 14.17 Advanced lesion. (Biggest lesion. Usually more than 0.5 cm diameter.)

Medium-sized lesions show various additional features

In the smallest lesions, the collection of macrophages is immediately sub-endothelial, on top of the smooth-muscle cells of diffuse intimal thickening. In some larger ones, however, there is a distinct **fibrous cap** containing smooth-muscle cells between the macrophages and the endothelium. How this happens is a mystery. Additional features often seen include some scattering of the macrophage foam cells among underlying smooth-muscle cells; **death** of some macrophages; and the appearance of lipid droplets in the cytoplasm of nearby smooth-muscle cells (Fig. 14.16).

Large lesions contain a lipid core

These plaques, often called **advanced lesions**, consist of a basal core, which is a pool of acellular debris, containing much lipid, including cholesterol crystals, the whole covered by a fibrous cap. Macrophage foam cells are found scattered round the necrotic mass and often in considerable numbers at the periphery, or shoulders, of the plaque (Fig. 14.17). The deeper macrophages in this area are often recognizably disintegrating at the edge of the basal lipid pool.

It is this advanced lesion that led to the name of the disease: **sclerosis** is hardening, referring to the fibrous cap; **atheros** is gruel or porridge, referring to the soft yellow material in the base.

Large lesions may show additional complications

All large lesions show the features mentioned above. Additional features often seen include areas of calcification in the necrotic area and some new capillaries. Surprisingly, however, the necrotic base does not appear to elicit an inflammatory response and is never replaced by granulation tissue. Often the media beneath the lesion shows fragmentation of elastin, and can become very thin or even completely broken. When this happens there is often chronic inflammation in the adventitia.

Advanced atherosclerosis can have dangerous effects

The small lesions are clinically completely silent, but advanced lesions have several effects, some of which can cause death.

Ischaemia

In medium-sized arteries, such as the coronary or cerebral arteries, the lumen often becomes sufficiently narrowed to make the blood supply inadequate. This may result in the potentially fatal events of **myocardial or cerebral infarction**,[10] which are the commonest cause of death in urbanized populations.[11] Ischaemia of the legs is also a serious problem in many elderly patients.

Thrombosis

The surface of an advanced plaque is particularly prone to haemodynamic damage and may even rupture completely, especially at the soft shoulders. This commonly leads to thrombosis. Because this rapidly narrows the artery even further, it often precipitates infarction.

Aneurysms

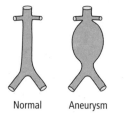

Normal   Aneurysm

Figure 14.18 Atherosclerotic aneurysm.

Atherosclerosis in the aorta is often severe, especially in the abdominal part, but the vessel is so wide that it does not lead to ischaemia even if, as often happens, there is superimposed thrombosis. What can happen, however, is that the medial thinning, beneath numerous crowded plaques, leads to such weakness of the aortic wall that it bulges outwards. This localized dilatation is called an **atherosclerotic aneurysm**—10% of elderly people have one, usually in the abdominal aorta (Fig. 14.18). Ten per cent of these aneurysms eventually burst, with fatal haemorrhage into the surrounding tissues.

Atheromatous embolism

10 You will remember that **ischaemia** means inadequate blood supply; **infarction** is necrosis due to ischaemia.

11 Nearly 50% in some surveys.

Rupture of the surface of a lesion may result in fragments of the necrotic base being swept away to lodge in small peripheral arteries. These atheromatous emboli are frequently found in the kidney and lower legs and must cause some ischaemia in these sites, mainly in the elderly.

Haemorrhage into the plaque

This may occasionally cause a sudden increase in the degree of occlusion of the artery.

Chronic inflammation

Lymphocytic and plasma cell infiltration is common in the adventitia, especially when there is much medial thinning. It probably represents an autoimmune reaction to altered large molecules in the necrotic base of the plaque. Occasionally it is accompanied by fibrosis so severe that it may block nearby hollow organs such as the ureters.

Atherosclerosis is a response of the arterial wall to injury

The anatomical sites of atherosclerotic plaques are somewhat predictable and strongly suggest that their localization depends on **haemodynamic factors**. They occur at branching points and bends in vessels exposed to high pressure, pulmonary arteries being relatively spared, veins completely so. Hypertension accelerates atherosclerosis. Normal vessels surgically transposed to a high-pressure situation often then become atherosclerotic.[12] These plaque-prone zones can be shown to have a higher than normal endothelial cell turnover rate, and increased endothelial permeability to plasma constituents.

Haemodynamic injury is therefore undoubtedly a primary factor in the disease, but it might be that some additional injurious agent has to be present as well; various suggestions include immune complexes, or viruses, but there is no proof of this and it could be that the cause of all the lesions is purely mechanical. The one and only concept that has been undisputed for over a century is that atherosclerosis represents a response to focal intimal injury.

Risk factors provide only clues to the mechanism of atherosclerosis

The epidemiology of atherosclerosis is full of pitfalls, because the severity of the disease itself is difficult to assess. However, there are many postulated associations with severity of the disease. These include the following.

1 Age: most people only begin to suffer the complications of atherosclerosis in middle or old age.

2 Gender: females tend to be spared until after the menopause, when the disease appears to accelerate.

3 Hypertension.

4 High levels of plasma cholesterol: these sometimes result from too much animal fat in the diet, but there is also a genetic disease leading to very high levels and premature atherosclerosis. This is **familial hypercholesterolaemia**, the most important example of a whole class of genetic hyperlipidaemias.

5 Diabetes.

6 Cigarette smoking.

All of these appear to be additive in their effects. Stress, lack of exercise and many others are less well-substantiated risk factors.

12 This was first done experimentally, but is now seen in humans when veins are used to bypass atherosclerotic coronary arteries.

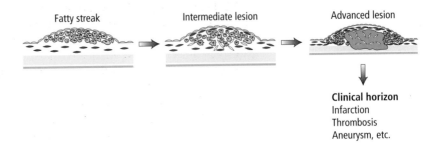

Figure 14.19 Probable stages of atherosclerosis.

The main reason for the uncertainties about such associations is that the development of **atherosclerosis in humans is silent and unmeasurable until some clinical event occurs** (Fig. 14.19).

Therefore, although one can make intelligent guesses about how a particular risk factor might affect one or more of the stages of development of the disease, it is difficult to be sure, and some might affect the onset of complications such as thrombosis, rather than atherosclerosis itself.

Theories of atherogenesis have changed over the years

In the 19th century, Carl von Rokitansky (Vienna; 1804–1878) suggested that the lesions resulted from deposition of 'formed elements' of the blood; this was revived briefly in the mid 20th century as the **thrombogenic theory**. The idea was that mural thrombi became organized and thus started the plaque; this is no longer considered likely.

Virchow, also in the 19th century, enunciated the idea that the plaque was a response to haemodynamic injury, involving increased uptake of lipid from the blood and implying also some form of inflammatory response. As we shall see, this was probably not far from the truth.

The lipids in the human lesion are rich in **cholesterol**. Therefore, early in the 20th century, attempts were made to reproduce the disease in experimental animals[13] by feeding a cholesterol-rich diet. The animals did indeed develop foam cell-rich lesions, but to this day no animal model mimics the human disease perfectly. These dietary experiments however certainly upheld the idea that the lipid in the lesion was plasma-derived and could be influenced by diet. This was also apparently supported by the fact that individuals from populations with a low mortality from atherosclerosis became susceptible when they migrated to places with a high mortality; clearly, however, it is not only the diet that changes in these circumstances.

One controversy was the origin of the foam cells, which are the principal feature of the early lesion. They are so full of lipid droplets that they are difficult to identify. The advent of electron microscopy showed, in the early 1960s, that there were certainly smooth-muscle cells in the lesions, and it became widely accepted that the foam cells must be lipid-laden smooth-muscle cells.

13 Many species have been used, but rabbits have been studied most. A pioneer in this field was Nikolai Anitschkow, the Russian physician, in the early years of this century.

This led on to a phase in which cell cultures were used increasingly in an attempt to understand atherosclerosis, and a hypothesis that was highly influential for about 10 years. It had been shown by 1970 that platelets adhere to damaged intima and that the many substances released by platelets include **platelet-derived growth factor** (PDGF). Since PDGF was known to increase smooth-muscle cell division *in vitro* and, later, was shown to be chemotactic for smooth-muscle cells, this provided an acceptable scenario. Endothelial injury → platelet adhesion and PDGF release → smooth-muscle cell division and migration into intima → smooth-muscle cell lipid uptake. In the 1980s, however, an alternative view emerged that assigned a different role to the smooth-muscle cells.

The foam cells of atherosclerosis are monocyte-derived macrophages

Starting with Anitschkow, a number of observers over the years had held the opinion that foam cells were macrophages, but this had always been a minority view. Three events coincided to confirm this, beyond reasonable doubt.

The first was the demonstration of low-density lipoprotein (LDL) receptors by Goldstein and Brown. As we saw earlier (Chapter 2), most cells take up normal or **native** LDL by receptors that are down-regulated when the cells contain sufficient cholesterol. Macrophages, on the other hand, take up **modified**, or damaged, LDL by **scavenger receptors** that are not so regulated (Fig. 14.20). Only macrophages, therefore, can become completely full of lipid droplets when surrounded by high concentrations of LDL. **Familial hypercholesterolaemia** is caused by genetically-induced inadequate expression of native LDL receptors on cells. Thus, enormous amounts of LDL accumulate in the plasma, and as it appears to become modified, it is taken up by macrophages in various sites, including the artery wall. Hence atherosclerosis is enormously accelerated in this condition. In heterozygotes, atherosclerotic complications begin in the 30s and 40s. In homozygotes, they occur even in childhood.

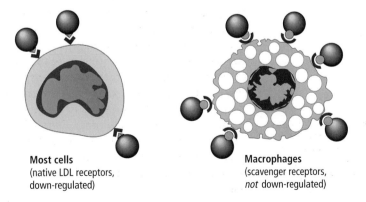

Figure 14.20 Low-density lipoprotein uptake.

Most cells
(native LDL receptors, down-regulated)

Macrophages
(scavenger receptors, *not* down-regulated)

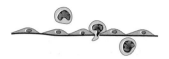

Figure 14.21 Monocyte emigration.

The second factor was the gradual realization that, in both humans and experimental animals, scanning electron microscopy of aortic lining showed that atherosclerotic plaques were **not preceded by denuding endothelial injury**, thus refuting platelet involvement in plaque initiation.

The third was the demonstration, by several groups using electron microscopy, of **monocyte emigration into experimental lesions** (Fig. 14.21). This was followed in 1985 by conclusive proof from immunohistochemistry, using monoclonal antibodies that distinguished the cell types, that **human foam cells are macrophages**.

These revelations have demanded a complete reappraisal of the development of atherosclerosis. It is possible now to regard the lesions as **a chronic inflammatory response to haemodynamic injury, in which macrophages are doing harm; the role of smooth-muscle cells may be simply a form of repair, analogous to fibroblasts in a healing wound**. Whether this is the whole truth remains to be seen.

The earliest changes caused by haemodynamic injury affect endothelial cells

It can be simply demonstrated, by counting mitoses, that endothelial cell turnover is much greater at lesion-prone sites. It seems however that a damaged endothelial cell does not fall off into the blood until its neighbours have migrated beneath it, thus avoiding exposure of collagen.

At these same sites, two additional features are seen. The endothelial permeability to large molecules, including lipoproteins, is enhanced and there is an increased tendency for monocytes to adhere to and emigrate between endothelial cells. What causes the monocyte adhesion and emigration is unknown, although there are numerous adhesion molecules and chemotactic agents that might be involved.

Macrophages take up large amounts of lipid

The main mechanism for this is thought to be the uncontrolled **uptake of modified LDL by scavenger receptors**, although the nature and site of the LDL modification are unknown. One possibility is raised by the observation that LDL is probably oxidized in the intima, perhaps by cell-derived free radicals.

Not all fatty streaks progress

Young adults develop fatty streaks in both the thoracic and abdominal aorta. In some populations, they do not usually progress beyond this stage. In those societies where lesions do progress, it is predominantly in the abdominal aorta that they do. Therefore not all fatty streaks progress and some, to judge from animal experiments, may actually become smaller.

However, advanced lesions must derive from fatty streaks because no other type of small lesion is found.

Macrophages die in advancing lesions

The lipid core of advanced lesions is a graveyard of dead macrophages, but what kills them is uncertain. One view is that it is due to the toxicity of lipids that have been oxidized by the macrophages.

Those advanced lesions with foam cells at the shoulders are probably gradually enlarging, by continuous recruitment and then death of the deeper macrophages.

Macrophages are doing harm in the lesion

This statement is at present based only on the potential activities of macrophages shown in cell cultures. They can produce substances chemotactic for monocytes, enzymes capable of damaging intimal structure, macrophage-derived growth factor stimulating smooth-muscle cell division and migration, substances that cause smooth-muscle cells to change from a contractile to a secretory function, and toxic oxygen radicals and oxidized lipids. How much of this activity is actually going on in the lesion is unknown.

What is the weakest link in the chain?

Huge efforts are being made, in research laboratories around the world, to identify one step in the complicated sequence of atherogenesis which would be vulnerable to intervention. At present, measures to decrease levels of plasma cholesterol and drugs to treat hypertension are the only weapons, coupled with advice to avoid risk factors. We must however live in hope.

Summary

Atherosclerosis is a focal disease of the arterial intima, localized by haemodynamic forces. The lesions are essentially foci of chronic inflammation in which the macrophages appear to be doing harm. The complications lead to millions of deaths every year, usually by causing ischaemia of vital organs. The way the lesions develop is incompletely understood; this is therefore one of the most urgent problems facing science today.

Heart failure

Heart failure (cardiac failure) can be defined as the **failure of the heart to maintain an output of blood** that is **adequate**. It is the **adequacy** of output that is important. In most cases, there is failure to maintain the normal cardiac output; this is called **low-output heart failure**. However there are some conditions in which the output of the heart is increased, but even so it is insufficient to match an increased demand. These include **anaemia**, in which the insufficient haemoglobin concentration leads to demand for increased flow; and **hyperthyroidism** in which all the tissues are hyperactive and require increased blood supply. If the heart can provide some increase in output, but not enough to satisfy the increased requirements, this is **high-output heart failure**.

Heart failure may be caused by: (i) **disease of heart muscle** (myocardium); (ii) **disease of the valves** of the heart; or (iii) **extracardiac causes**.

Heart failure may be acute or chronic

If the cause of failure is sudden and severe, such as a myocardial infarct, the danger to life is immediate—**acute heart failure**.

Quite frequently, however, the heart may be put under strain only gradually, for example, by progressive narrowing of a valve over a period of months or years. When this happens, compensatory mechanisms come into play which tend to relieve the difficulty and permit survival. For instance, the inadequate output would be detected by the baroreceptors[14] leading to sympathetic nervous activity; this increases the heart rate and force of contraction, and diverts blood flow from the skin and gut to the more vital organs. In this way inadequate output, even if progressive, may be tolerated over a very long period of time and, especially if treated, be compatible with long survival. This is **chronic heart failure**.

Overwork makes heart muscle hypertrophy

The thickness or bulk of the muscle in a chamber of the heart is dictated by the amount of work it has to do. Hence the atria normally have thinner myocardium than the ventricles, and the left ventricle is thickest of all. The whole myocardium of a healthy athlete becomes thicker (hypertrophied), due to increase in size of all the individual muscle fibres, and may even come to weigh twice as much as the heart of a sedentary individual. Similarly, gradually increasing work caused by a disease state will also result in gradual hypertrophy; over a period of months, the left ventricle of a patient with, for example, severe anaemia or systemic hypertension will become hypertrophied. The effect of gradual stenosis (narrowing) of the mitral valve will be hypertrophy of the left atrium; and similar rules apply according to which chamber is affected.

Therefore, **hypertrophy of a cardiac chamber shows it has had excessive work to do**.

Heart failure first affects only one chamber

Each of the four chambers of the heart relaxes and fills with blood (diastole), then expels that blood by myocardial contraction (systole). All the chambers have a valve allowing the exit of blood but not its return. The ventricles, therefore, also have a valve at their entrance (Fig. 14.22).

Essentially, therefore, a chamber of the heart fills with blood during diastole, while the exit valve is closed, and expels it by myocardial contraction during systole, when the exit valve is forced open. Normally the volume of blood received by the chamber is equal to the volume expelled. If the chamber begins

14 Baroreceptors in the aorta are collections of cells that detect changes in blood pressure.

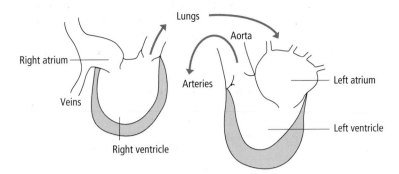

Figure 14.22 The heart as two separate halves.

to fail, it cannot expel all the blood that it receives, and retains a **residual volume** of blood. Therefore, at the next diastole it becomes slightly more distended than usual—thus **a failing chamber is a dilated chamber**.

Stretching myocardial muscle fibres causes them to contract more strongly (Starling's law of the heart), which at least temporarily can help to compensate. A failing chamber is also therefore by definition overworked, so if time allows —and that is the key proviso—the chamber will become hypertrophied. Eventually this hypertrophy may compensate for the excessive demand and, if that happens, the dilatation disappears.[15]

In summary, **hypertrophy indicates long-standing overwork. Dilatation indicates failure**.

Failure of the left side of the heart has 'backward' effects on the lung

If a chamber is failing, blood volume and pressure build up behind the failing chamber. So if the left ventricle is failing, the pressure in the left atrium will increase. This may cause failure of the left atrium in turn, unless the process is so slow that hypertrophy can compensate.

If the left atrium fails, however, the back-pressure then affects the pulmonary veins and therefore the pulmonary capillaries. This can be very serious.

The blood pressure in the pulmonary veins and capillaries is normally very low[16] and any increase in pressure causes dilatation of pulmonary veins and capillaries (**pulmonary congestion**). More important, the high pressure within the capillaries causes outflow of fluid (**transudate**) from the capillaries into the air-spaces (alveoli) of the lung. This is referred to as **pulmonary oedema**. If the left side of the heart fails rapidly (**acute left-sided heart failure**) it is this pulmonary oedema that is life-threatening; the patient may literally drown in the oedema fluid accumulating in the lungs.

Pulmonary congestion may result in scattered haemorrhages from the distended capillaries. Thus a patient with acute left-sided heart failure will be breathless[17] because of the oedema and often coughs up frothy watery fluid, which may be slightly blood-stained.

15 Unfortunately, hypertrophy increases the requirements of the myocardium for blood supply and can lead to myocardial ischaemia.

16 Less than 5 mmHg.

17 Breathlessness is sometimes called **dyspnoea**.

At the very low pressures normally encountered in lung capillaries, the difference in capillary blood pressure between upper and lower parts of the lungs may be quite significant in the erect human. The oedema tends to be worse, therefore, in the lower lobes where the capillary pressure is higher.

Failure of the right side of the heart has 'backward' effects on other organs

Just as the back-pressure due to left heart failure affects the lungs, that due to right-sided failure affects other organs of the body. Thus typically there is congestion of the liver, spleen, kidneys and other internal organs; oedema develops in the subcutaneous tissues of the lower parts of the body[18] and results in accumulations of oedema fluid (**effusions**) in the natural body cavities such as the pleural or peritoneal cavities. This combination of congestion and peripheral oedema is sometimes referred to as **congestive cardiac failure**.

The congestion of most organs is a uniform change, leading to increased size, firmness and redness of the tissue. Congestion of the liver, however, causes preferential dilatation of the sinusoids in the centre of each lobule, producing a characteristic pattern on the cut surfaces of the liver at necropsy which reminded the old pathologists of the cut surface of a nutmeg—hence the term 'nutmeg liver' (Fig. 14.23).

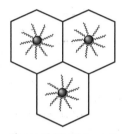

Figure 14.23 Nutmeg liver due to right-sided heart failure.

Heart failure, of whatever cause, has important 'forward' effects

The single most important effect of heart failure is inadequate perfusion of all the tissues of the body. All the organs are starved of blood (ischaemic) and therefore all of them, in varying degrees, perform inadequately. The effects are therefore far-reaching and various. Tissues with the highest demand, or those already compromised by other diseases will suffer first. In particular, most patients who develop heart failure are past middle age and their arteries are narrowed by **atherosclerosis**. Those organs supplied by the narrowest arteries are most vulnerable and may even suffer **infarction**. Indeed, sometimes the first signs of heart failure in a patient may be these distant ischaemic events.[19]

One particular forward effect has already been referred to—the sympathetic over-activity caused by decreased stimulation of the baroreceptors. Another very important one results from inadequate perfusion of the kidneys which leads to the retention of more sodium and water than normal.[20] The effect of this is to increase total blood volume, which only worsens the congestion and oedema of heart failure. Nowadays, this can be relieved by drugs increasing urine output (diuretics), but in days gone by was treated (with some success) by blood-letting, or even the application of leeches!

Causes of left-sided heart failure

1 Disease of the myocardium. The commonest is left ventricular myocardial infarction, due to coronary artery atherosclerosis. Others include myocarditis, often due to viruses.

18 Lower legs in the erect, sacral area in the recumbent patient.

19 Examples include stroke, due to cerebral infarction.

20 This is mediated by increased renin release due to poor perfusion. In turn this leads to increased angiotensin levels, which increase aldosterone release.

2 Disease of the mitral or aortic valves. Stenosis (narrowing) or incompetence (inadequate closure) of either valve may be due either to congenital deformity or acquired disease such as rheumatic fever.

3 Extracardiac conditions include those requiring high output such as anaemia or hyperthyroidism, and also systemic hypertension. Systemic hypertension is the condition in which there is sustained abnormally high blood pressure in the aorta and its main arterial branches. It is caused by generally increased arteriolar muscle tone. This arteriolar narrowing is occasionally due directly to identifiable conditions such as increased renin output in kidney disease, or catecholamine secretion by a tumour of the adrenal medulla. Usually, however, the cause is unknown—primary, or **essential hypertension**.

These extracardiac conditions usually develop gradually, and the left ventricle can usually compensate by hypertrophy long before it fails.

Causes of right-sided heart failure

Again, disease of the myocardium or valves can occur, but both affect the right side of the heart much less commonly than the left. By far the most common causes of right-sided failure are **extracardiac**. **Massive pulmonary embolism** blocking the main pulmonary arteries causes **acute right-sided failure** which is almost uniformly fatal. Less commonly, multiple small pulmonary emboli can have the same effect, but about two-thirds of the arterial tree has to be blocked for this to happen. The most common cause of right-sided failure, however, is **pulmonary hypertension** due to contraction of the pulmonary artery branches.

Pulmonary hypertension is the main cause of chronic right-sided heart failure

Like systemic hypertension, pulmonary hypertension is due to increased arteriolar muscle tone. Unlike systemic hypertension, however, it is only rarely of unknown cause (primary pulmonary hypertension). Usually it is due to one of three causes: (i) hypoxia; (ii) increased flow; or (iii) left-sided heart failure.

Decreased oxygen supply (hypoxia) causes increased contraction of small pulmonary arteries because of a direct effect on the arterial smooth muscle. When this occurs in a localized area, such as in an area of pneumonia, with exudate filling the alveoli, preventing oxygen entry, the effect is on balance beneficial. Blood flow becomes redirected to the well-aerated parts of the lungs, thus maximizing oxygenation of the blood.

There are, however, conditions in which the **oxygen supply to the whole of both lungs is insufficient**. These include living at high altitude, or diseases such as emphysema[21] and the pneumoconioses.[22] In these circumstances, oxygen supply is uniformly poor, so the whole pulmonary arterial tree is abnormally constricted and pulmonary hypertension results. If the condition persists or worsens, the right side of the heart may initially compensate by hypertrophy or it may fail. Right-sided heart strain or failure due to lung disease is called **cor pulmonale**.

Increased pulmonary blood flow can also cause arterial spasm and pulmonary hypertension. This occurs in some forms of congenital heart disease.

21 Emphysema is a chronic progressive disease in which alveolar walls break down, giving inefficient larger air spaces. It commonly results from chronic bronchitis.

22 These are diseases of industrialization. This is an example of how a mechanism that is helpful in archaic diseases like pneumonia proves harmful in the industrial environment.

Left-sided heart failure leads, as we have seen, to increased pressure in the pulmonary veins and capillaries. The pulmonary oedema that results is life-threatening, but two protective mechanisms appear to exist. The oedema impairs oxygen supply and therefore leads to arterial constriction. In addition, the increased pressure in the pulmonary veins is probably detected by baroreceptors in the veins which trigger a vagus-mediated reflex causing pulmonary artery spasm. This tends to relieve the pulmonary oedema because the arterial constriction decreases capillary pressure, but this is at the expense of increasing the pulmonary arterial pressure and putting extra work on the right side of the heart. Thus in many chronic conditions that cause failure of the left side of the heart, both sides of the heart eventually become hypertrophied. Exacerbations of such conditions, such as systemic hypertension or anaemia, therefore commonly lead to right-sided or congestive cardiac failure rather than to pulmonary oedema.

Summary

Heart failure way be acute or chronic, left-sided or right-sided. It leads to problems due to increased venous pressure behind the failing chamber but, even more importantly, to an inadequate blood supply to all tissues. Heart failure is often, but not always, due to quantitative changes in variables such as increased arteriolar tone, inadequate myocardial blood supply or anaemia.

Ischaemia

Blood supply to tissues may be inadequate in quality for a variety of reasons, such as lack of oxygen (hypoxia), lack of oxygen-carrying capacity (anaemia) or insufficient nutrients, such as decreased glucose content (hypoglycaemia). Commonly, however, it is due to insufficient quantity or volume of flow, and this is called **ischaemia**.

Ischaemia is due either to narrowing of blood vessels or to shock

The most important cause of ischaemia is **atherosclerosis** with or without **thrombosis**, causing narrowing or even occlusion of arteries. Arteries can also be narrowed by inflammation of the wall (arteritis) or rarely by external pressure from such things as tumours or tourniquets. Arteriolar spasm can result from vasoconstriction due to hormones, nerve reflexes, drugs or from extreme cold (frostbite). Veins may also be narrowed by extrinsic pressure or by thrombosis. Capillaries sometimes are blocked, for example by fat or air embolism or by extrinsic pressure.[23]

Of all of these, insufficient arterial flow is by far the most important. However, apart from arterial narrowing or occlusion, the insufficient arterial blood supply may be due to **shock**.

23 Localized pressure on skin capillaries often occurs in immobile bed-ridden patients—the resultant skin ischaemia is the cause of **bedsores**, which are skin ulcers due to ischaemia.

Shock is circulatory collapse with low arterial blood pressure

Shock may be caused by: (i) insufficient total blood volume (**hypovolaemia**) due to haemorrhage or burns;[24] (ii) **heart failure** (central or cardiogenic shock); or (iii) **endotoxin shock**. Less commonly, shock may be the result of anaphylaxis or neurogenic mechanisms.

In hypovolaemic and cardiogenic shock, increased sympathetic activity occurs. This improves blood supply to vital organs, by decreasing the supply to both the skin (which is therefore cold) and the gut. Endotoxin shock differs because it is essentially due to generalized vasodilatation, and in this condition the skin is warm. In all cases of shock however there is low blood pressure (hypotension). Whatever the cause, therefore, all tissues may be ischaemic and any organ may fail as a result. Common manifestations of shock therefore include decreased level of consciousness or renal failure.

The most important effect of ischaemia is hypoxia

Insufficient blood flow deprives tissues of essential nutrients such as glucose and allows build-up of waste products, but the limiting factor in virtually all cases is insufficient oxygen supply. This may lead to disturbance of cell function, reversible cell damage (such as fatty change) or necrosis. Ischaemia may occasionally cause necrosis of scattered cells in a tissue, such as particularly vulnerable neurons, but more commonly a localized part of an organ is completely necrotic. This zone of necrosis due to ischaemia is called an **infarct**.

The outcome of localized ischaemia is influenced by a variety of factors

1 **The anatomy of the arterial tree** is important because blockage of an end-artery (for example the retinal artery) will almost always cause infarction; blockage of an artery with many collaterals (for example a branch of the superior mesenteric artery) will not, as a rule (Fig. 14.24).

2 **The size of the block** affects the outcome because the larger the artery blocked the less likely it is that the collateral supply will compensate (for example in the superior mesenteric artery, Fig. 14.24).

3 **The degree of the blockage** is obviously crucial. Occlusion (complete blockage) is more likely to cause infarction than partial blockage, but in fact the latter is much more common.

4 **The speed of blockage** affects the outcome. Gradual narrowing of an artery by, for example atherosclerosis or mural thrombosis, is less likely to lead to infarction than sudden occlusion by an embolus. This is because in the former case collateral arteries may gradually dilate and compensate.

5 **Disease of collaterals**. The extent to which collateral arteries can compensate is limited if they too are narrowed. For instance, thrombosis of an internal carotid artery is more likely to lead to cerebral infarction if the other internal carotid artery is narrowed by atherosclerosis.

24 In severe burns, the rate of evaporation of exudate may be sufficient to cause hypovolaemia.

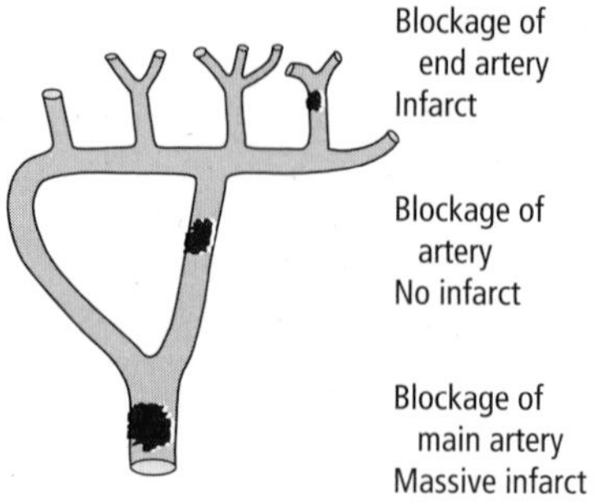

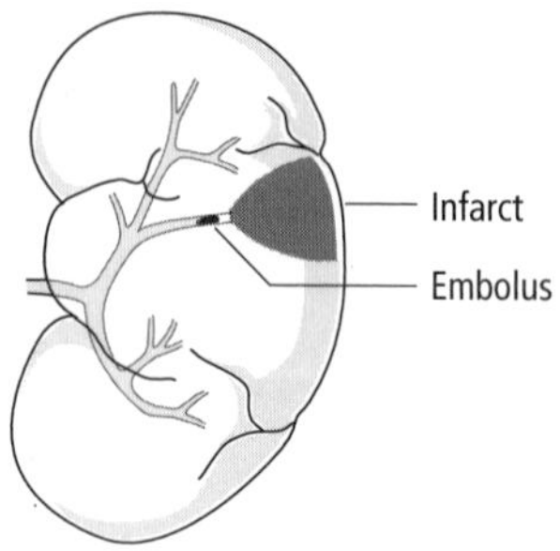

Figure 14.24 Arterial blockage (left).

Figure 14.25 Infarct of kidney (right).

6 The vulnerability of tissues influences the result of ischaemia. As mentioned before, neurons survive only about 4 minutes with inadequate blood supply; many other cell-types survive much longer.

7 The general adequacy of circulation is crucial to the outcome of arterial narrowing. This is a most important factor which is constantly underestimated or ignored, with serious results. It therefore requires emphasis. The result of narrowing of an artery (for example by atherosclerosis) is dependent upon **a law of supply and demand**. If the demand of a tissue increases, a narrowed artery may be incapable of providing the increased flow required. This explains why so often sudden exertion, such as an elderly person running for a bus, or some emotional crisis, can precipitate myocardial infarction. Conversely, and probably much more commonly, sudden decrease in general blood supply (**shock**, see above) can precipitate infarction in any tissue whose arterial supply is already compromised by atherosclerosis.

A good example of the effects of shock is **cerebral infarction**. This is the most common cause of **stroke** (sudden onset of inadequate cerebral function), mainly in the elderly. Almost all elderly people have considerable cerebral artery atherosclerosis. Cerebral infarction may therefore be caused by thrombosis due to the atherosclerosis or, less frequently, by embolism. But the **most common cause of cerebral infarction is shock**, precipitated by such extracranial events as myocardial infarction, pulmonary embolism or bleeding. The infarction is due not to the narrowing of the cerebral arteries by atherosclerosis alone, but also to the inadequate general state of the circulation, **hypotension**.

Summary

Ischaemia may have many causes but is frequently due to arterial narrowing (usually by atherosclerosis) or occlusion (usually by thrombosis or embolism). Importantly, it also results from shock. If the ischaemia is severe it may cause infarction.

Infarction

An **infarct** is a zone of necrosis due to ischaemia (Fig. 14.25). The frequency, likely causes, appearances and results of infarction vary in different organs.

In some organs, such as the kidney or myocardium, the recent infarct is very pale in colour; in others, such as the gut or lung, blood seeps into the softened dead tissue and the recent infarct is firm and dark red, because it is stuffed with blood.[25]

Infarcts, like other areas of necrosis, elicit an inflammatory reaction and eventually are replaced by a scar. An exception is the brain, where old infarcts appear as cysts surrounded by gliosis.

In the spleen and kidney, infarcts are usually small, most commonly due to thromboembolism, and not often of clinical importance.

Myocardial infarction is the most important disease of industrialized communities, and the most common cause of death. It is almost always due to **coronary atherosclerosis**, with or without thrombosis. It may be precipitated by hypotensive episodes or increased myocardial demand. Very rarely it is caused by coronary embolism. Almost all myocardial infarcts are in the left ventricle (lateral wall or septum), presumably because the thicker the myocardium, the more blood supply it needs. Myocardial infarcts may lead to heart failure, abnormal heart rhythms or sudden death. The infarcts also cause acute inflammation and may lead to thrombosis on the wall of the ventricle (mural thombosis) or to pericarditis, especially if the full thickness of the muscle is infarcted. Small infarcts tend to be subendocardial in position because of the anatomy of the blood supply (Fig. 14.26). Recent full-thickness infarcts are soft and may rupture, releasing blood at high pressure into the pericardial cavity, causing sudden death.

If a patient survives an acute infarction, the infarcts heal by scarring and the surviving myocardium develops compensatory hypertrophy. Full-thickness scars may stretch outwards because of the pressure within, forming a cardiac aneurysm (Fig. 14.27); these old infarcts frequently contain some mural thrombus but scarcely ever rupture, even though they are comparatively thin, because they are composed of tough collagen.

25 *Infarcere* (Latin), to stuff.

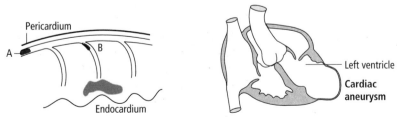

Figure 14.26 Myocardial infarction. Blockage at B—subendocardial small infarct. Blockage at A—larger, perhaps full-thickness infarct (left).

Figure 14.27 Full-thickness infarct (healed) giving rise to cardiac aneurysm (right).

Infarcts of the bowel are only seen when a major artery such as the superior mesenteric is totally blocked, or almost so, by atherosclerosis, thrombosis or thromboembolism. However, lesser degrees of bowel ischaemia can occur.

Two organs, the liver and the lung, are of particular interest because they have a double blood supply. The liver, supplied with oxygen largely through the portal vein,[26] but also through the hepatic artery, very rarely contains infarcts, and these are usually due to inadequate portal venous supply in patients with shock.

Lung infarcts are more difficult to explain. Pulmonary infarcts are not infrequent and are virtually always precipitated by pulmonary embolism. But the lung tissue gets its oxygen from the inspired air, not the pulmonary artery, which contains deoxygenated blood. This puzzle is answered by some by the observation that pulmonary infarcts only follow pulmonary embolism if the patient is in left-sided heart failure, thus compromising the bronchial artery supply. This may be true, but it is also noteworthy that in lung infarcts the alveoli are full of blood. Perhaps shutting off the pulmonary artery supply causes haemorrhage in patients with left-sided heart failure, and it is the haemorrhage itself that deprives the alveolar walls of oxygen. No one has satisfactorily explained this mystery.

Many other tissues may become infarcted in various circumstances, but the most common are described above.

Summary

The common causes, appearance and results of infarcts vary from organ to organ, but all are due to ischaemia of some sort.

Resumé of principles of cardiovascular disease

Cardiovascular diseases are caused by quantitative changes in physiological variables

We have seen that these diseases can be caused or influenced by such things as inadequate dietary iron, excess cholesterol, increased arteriolar tone, or decreased oxygen supply; the list is long. The principle is true of all other organ systems as well, but is nowhere better exemplified than here.

Many forms of injury may produce the same disease

Good examples of this include thrombosis and heart failure.

Innate reactions to injury may themselves do harm

We have seen this holds true in many other circumstances, such as the pneumoconioses, gout and hypersensitivity. We can now add thrombosis and atherosclerosis to the list.

26 The portal venous blood is a good source of oxygen for the liver because its very high flow, necessary for uptake of nutrients for the gut, is well in excess of the gut's oxygen requirements.

The different cardiovascular diseases frequently influence one another

One cardiovascular disease not uncommonly increases the likelihood of another, as shown by the arrows in Fig. 14.28. This is of course true in other organ systems, but to a much lesser extent.

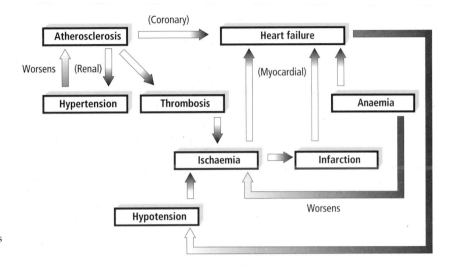

Figure 14.28 Some interactions of cardiovascular diseases.

15 Cell reactions

In previous chapters we have seen a number of examples of cellular responses to injury. If we now attempt to review the range of cells' abilities to react, it seems that they respond to external stimuli only in certain limited ways. The mechanisms involved are complicated and incompletely understood, but essentially cells can only react by changes in their **synthesis, movement, adhesion** or **division**. Some of these changes involve alterations in genetic expression but the majority do not.

Synthesis

Cells can be stimulated to alter the rate of synthesis of materials for export

All cells synthesize molecules which then leave the cell: for some of them, such as exocrine or endocrine cells, it is their main function. Such secretion is controlled, sometimes by a hormone for which the cell has receptors. Through chemical systems within the cell (messengers) the stimulus results in increased or decreased synthesis and export. In this way, for instance, adrenal cortical cells are influenced, in their rate of production of corticosteroids, by adrenocorticotrophic hormone (ACTH) from the pituitary gland, and there are many other examples.

A wide variety of diseases result from abnormalities in such systems. For instance, ischaemic damage to the pituitary, decreasing ACTH production, causes decreased secretion of corticosteroids. All such diseases in endocrine and exocrine organs follow all the rules of common sense, and will not be pursued further here. An analogy, however, is the production of immunoglobulins by B cells and lymphokines by T cells, in response to stimulation not by hormones, but by antigens.

To extend the analogy further, a rapidly increasing army of molecules (**cytokines**) is being discovered which, being secreted by one cell type, affect the behaviour of others. Some of these, such as interleukin-1 (IL-1), are stable and can act at a distance, but most are labile and therefore only affect cells close by. Examples we have seen include the macrophage-derived factors that stimulate the division and secretory activity of nearby fibroblasts and smooth-muscle cells. However, there are many more that we have not mentioned; and new ones are being discovered all the time.

Cells can be stimulated to alter the rate of synthesis of cell constituents

The cell fabric is in no sense permanent; its membranes, DNA and other constituents are constantly being degraded and replaced at variable, usually slow, rates. Sometimes we are reminded of this fact when for some reason the rate changes.

There is usually no visible evidence of this turnover, but some very long-lived cells, especially neurons and cardiac muscle fibres, are an exception. All cell constituents are at constant risk of damage by oxygen, especially oxygen radicals. Some remnants of oxidative degradation of membrane lipids are insoluble, and are deposited in a membrane-bound **autosome** in the cytoplasm. This insoluble material is a yellow-brown pigment called **lipofuscin**, and accumulates gradually in long-lived cells with advancing age—hence the old terms 'age pigment' or 'wear and tear pigment'.[1]

After various stimuli, cells may increase their rate of synthesis of cell components and become larger—**hypertrophy**. Examples include skeletal and cardiac muscle fibres when over-worked, and macrophages exposed to various chemical or particulate stimuli. Underwork, decreased nutrition, or lack of nervous or chemical stimuli can have the opposite effect—**atrophy**, in which the cell becomes smaller. Skeletal muscle deprived of its nerve supply in poliomyelitis, adipose tissue in starvation and postmenopausal ovaries are all examples. Occasionally, and understandably, lipofuscin is more abundant in atrophied cells; the small heart of an elderly wasted patient is said to show 'brown atrophy' when this is detectable to the naked eye.

Up to now we have been considering the turnover of the molecules of the cell's structure, but variations in synthesis of other molecules can also occur. **Enzyme induction** is often caused by stimuli from outside the cell. Examples include production by macrophages of enzymes suitable to degrade particular bacteria when exposed to those bacteria; and increased production of alcohol dehydrogenase by liver cells in people who drink alcohol regularly. The induction of **endonucleases**, leading to apoptosis, can be caused not only by exogenous chemicals and the activity of lymphocytes, but also in 'programmed cell death'. **Receptor expression** also depends partly on receptor synthesis, but one example we have already met, the low-density lipoprotein (LDL) receptor, reminds us that expression of the receptors on the cell membrane is influenced not only by the amounts of receptor synthesized but also on the location of the receptor molecules in the cell. This is controlled by the amount of cholesterol the cell contains and is arguably really an example of the next cell response to be considered—movement.

Movement

Cells may move in relation to other cells

We have seen that some cell types can move about in the tissues. All seem to use the same 'caterpillar tractor' mechanism described in Chapter 2 (Fig. 2.11). The leading edge of the cell finds new points of attachment; and some of the

1 These old terms are not ideal, because similar pigment can accumulate rapidly, e.g. in macrophages containing cell debris or excess lipoprotein.

rearmost attachments detach. The latter is a somewhat traumatic process; fragments of cell membrane and cell contents are left behind, much as a snail leaves a track on paving. This spillage during crawling may sometimes facilitate the cell's penetration of tissues. For instance, enzymes leaking from crawling neutrophils may help these cells to penetrate through basement membranes.

The movement of the cell also involves active assembly of new cell membrane at the leading edge and internalization of membrane at the rear. Thus you can show in culture that **the cell membrane is actually moving posteriorly over the cell, as the cell moves anteriorly**. The ways in which these complex functions are coordinated to lead to cell movement are not completely understood.

Cell types that can crawl about in tissues include fibroblasts, smooth-muscle cells, endothelial cells and all types of leukocyte. In culture, such cell types often show **random movement**, but also in general **a tendency to move to more thinly populated areas**.

The random movement of cells is influenced by various chemicals. Some, such as corticosteroids, diminish the rate of movement. Others, such as 12-HETE[2], may increase it; this is called **chemokinesis**. As we have previously discussed, directional movement, **chemotaxis**, depends upon a gradient, on the substratum, of molecules for which the cell has receptors.

Cells may show internal movements and shape-changes

The most obvious example is contraction and relaxation of muscle fibres, but really **all cells are muscle—but some are more muscular than others**. **Actin and myosin filaments** permit many cell types to contract. Examples we have seen include endothelial cells in inflammation, and fibroblasts during wound-healing. Shape change in activated platelets is a related phenomenon.

Other sorts of movements in cells include the physiological movements of cilia and sperm tails[3] and movements of membrane constituents, including **capping** of membrane structures and receptor expression.

Endocytosis and exocytosis also obviously involve cell movements. Perhaps the most remarkable cell in this regard is the macrophage, which is constantly actively sampling its environment non-specifically—**fluid-phase pinocytosis**, to be distinguished from **receptor-mediated endocytosis**. Similarly, **phagocytosis** can be non-specific (for example carbon particles) or mediated by membrane receptors for particles, or opsonins, as described previously.

Exocytosis has been mentioned as an activity of mast cells, macrophages, eosinophils, neutrophils and platelets. It obviously also occurs in various physiological processes such as exocrine secretion of various sorts and can also do harm.

Adhesion

Adhesion to extracellular materials may show variations

Epithelial cells often lose their attachment to their basement membrane when injured, and certainly if they become necrotic or undergo apoptosis, which can

2 12-Hydroxyeicosatetraenoic acid, an intermediate in leukotriene synthesis.

3 There are reasons to think that these useful appendages evolved from symbiotic spirochaetes!

make the underlying tissue more vulnerable to injury, especially if the basement membrane is damaged. Epithelium regenerating to cover such an ulcer often secretes **fibronectin** as a temporary substratum, producing proper basement membrane only later. Denuding injury to vascular endothelium is followed by perhaps the most striking example of avid cell adhesion to fibres, namely platelet adhesion to collagen.

We have also seen how adhesion of various leukocytes to particles or larger bodies leads to phagocytosis or to exocytosis of lysosomal contents.

Changes in cell–cell adhesion can take place in disease

The tendency of differentiated cells such as epithelia to adhere one to another is an important property, mediated by various structures such as desmosomes, gap junctions, tight junctions and various forms of 'intercellular cement'. This cohesion is occasionally disrupted, for instance in various virus infections of the epidermis. Another example is that immunoglobulin G (IgG) antibodies to adhesion molecules appear to be implicated in the falling apart of epidermal cells in the disease **pemphigus**.

However the most interesting instances of variations in cell–cell adhesion are seen in those cell types which normally are solitary but may be stimulated to adhere to others. **Platelets** and **leukocytes** are the most important. We have seen how platelets can be stimulated to aggregate by a variety of agents such as catecholamines, adenosine diphosphate, etc. Neutrophils are said to aggregate too, sometimes, after intravascular complement activation. When stimulated, for example by lymphokines, macrophages often clump together, as in granulomas. Here the adhesion is accompanied by membrane perturbance occasionally sufficient to cause **cell fusion**.

Mechanisms of such cohesion between blood-derived cells of a particular type may include lectin–sugar interactions, loss of net negative surface charge, or sticky molecules like fibronectin.

Adhesion of leukocytes to endothelial cells is a function vital to inflammation, the immune response, lymphocyte recirculation and 'homing', and atherosclerosis. Here too it seems that a variety of mechanisms may participate, including lectin–sugar combination, fibronectin, chemotactic factors such as C5a or leukotriene B_4 diffusing on to the luminal surface of endothelial cells; and **adhesion molecules**. This name has been coined for a whole family of molecules that are expressed on leukocytes and on the endothelial surface, particularly when the endothelial cells are stimulated, for example by IL-1.

Without going into detail, it is fair to say that the variety of adhesion molecules that have been identified is considerable. More are being discovered all the time; the variety of mechanisms that appear to be available is probably witness to the importance of the function. Much more research will be needed before we can understand the relative significance of each of the possible molecular mechanisms in various circumstances.

Summary

Although variations in cell synthesis, movement and adhesion seem to represent a rather limited range of reactions to stimuli, the variations between the reactions of different cell types, and the complexity of available mechanisms mean that an astonishingly wide range of possible reactions exist. Nevertheless, study of these reactions often throws up analogies as well as differences. There are many similarities between fibroblasts and smooth-muscle cells, between neutrophils and macrophages, and even between neutrophils and platelets. Such analogies should remind us that the complexities evolved from simple beginnings. It may even be possible one day, by studying more intensively cell reactions in lower animals, to identify those that are conserved in humans and perhaps provide some perspective among the complexities. The conserved mechanisms will probably prove to be more important; the more recently evolved may be only the icing on the cake.

Division

Cell division also includes synthesis and intracellular movement, but has to be regarded as a separate category of response from the others.

Cells are not isolated units

Each cell in a tissue is part of a complex and tightly regulated society in which there are hierarchies of development and function. The division of individual cells, differentiation and apoptosis are consequences of both environmental and genetic factors—nature and nurture operating at the cellular level. The environment of an individual cell in tissue may contain signals from both immediate and distant neighbours and these interact with the cell to activate or down-regulate cellular gene expression. Alterations in cellular division and differentiation can therefore be the consequence of environmental change altering cellular gene expression or the result of changes in the cell itself which alter its response to the environment, or both. If these changes are inappropriate and prolonged then disease can result.

Quantitative abnormalities in cell division result in too much or too little growth of tissue. Too little growth may occur *in utero* resulting in congenital or developmental abnormalities and there may be total (**agenesis,** or **aplasia**) or partial (**dysgenesis, hypoplasia**) failure of organ development. **Atrophy** describes not only a decrease in the size of cells, but also shrinkage of a tissue due to decreased cell division or increased cell loss, often by apoptosis. Changes in cellular division are not always pathological but may be quite normal physiological responses, such as in the atrophy of the ovaries in the postmenopausal woman.

The converse of atrophy due to decreased cell division is **hyperplasia**, which is **an increase in the size of a tissue due to an increase in the number of its constituent cells**. This is usually accompanied by increase in the size of individual cells and possibly their function also. The extraordinary proliferation of the ductal epithelium of the breast in pregnancy and lactation is a good example of regulated hyperplasia. The removal of the hormonal stimulus results in the breast returning to normal size and cellular numbers. A different example is hyperplasia of lymphoid tissue after antigenic stimulation. Simplest of all, perhaps, is the epidermal hyperplasia that causes the horny hand of the labourer.

Pathological hyperplasia can be the result of inappropriate hormonal stimulation, trauma or infection. For instance, viral infection may result in excessive cellular proliferation. The papillomaviruses which cause warts are an excellent example of this. Infection with these viruses causes hyperplasia of the basal layers of the infected epithelium, although the differentiation programme of the epithelium as a whole is not grossly disrupted.

Hyperplasia always occurs in response to a definite stimulus and the removal of the stimulus results in the cessation of the response.

Abnormalities in the tissue differentiation programme are seen in metaplasia—the change of one type of differentiated tissue to another type of differentiated tissue, for example when simple columnar epithelium changes to a stratified squamous epithelium—**squamous metaplasia**. This is illustrated well in the uterine cervix, at the interface between the ecto- (squamous) and endo- (glandular) cervix where squamous change occurs in the glandular component at the junction. Squamous metaplasia is seen in many sites and represents almost certainly a protective response to chronic irritation. In the bronchus of smokers, for example, it is common, with stratified squamous epithelium replacing the ciliated columnar lining. In all these sites the new squamous epithelium grows up from the basal layer, indicating that the changes in gene expression leading to the change in differentiation programme occur in the uncommitted basal cells. There is one condition in which squamous metaplasia is common but in which persistent trauma plays no part; this is hypovitaminosis A, characterized by widespread squamous metaplasia of bronchi, nose and urinary tract and hyperkeratinization of squamous epithelia.

Dysplasia is a term used to describe changes in which there is **irregular maturation of squamous epithelium** with mitosis in cell layers other than the basal layer, a loss of polarity of cells and sometimes nuclear pleomorphism (variation in size and shape).

All these growth responses involve the regulation of cell division and the commitment to differentiation. An understanding of the mechanisms involved requires a knowledge of the **control of cell proliferation**. In all mammalian cells the cell cycle of replicating cells consists of four phases (Fig. 15.1). G1 is a crucial phase in which the cell has four options:

1 to 'recycle' and embark on another round of DNA synthesis and mitosis;
2 to 'decycle' and enter a resting phase usually referred to as G0, from which the cell can re-enter the cycle if conditions demand;
3 to 'decycle' and commit itself to terminal differentiation;
4 to abort the cycle and become apoptotic.

You will remember that there are three classes of cells with respect to proliferative activity: (i) permanent; (ii) stable quiescent; and (iii) self-renewing.

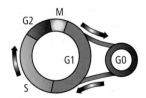

Figure 15.1 The cell cycle.

Permanent cells

These are non-replicating cells, sometimes called terminally differentiated cells. The cells lose replicative activity at the birth of the animal or in early infancy. The best examples of these are **neurons** and **cardiac muscle cells**. Because these cells are fully committed to differentiated function, their loss means a loss of function, since replacement by proliferation is not possible. These cells can only respond to increased demand by increasing the function and size of the individual cell (**hypertrophy**).

Stable quiescent cells

These cell populations can be described as **conditional renewal populations** and are exemplified by hepatocytes and fibroblasts. In these populations cells divide only rarely and are held in G0. The G0 cells however are capable of expressing differentiated function. In the face of demand because of the loss of hepatocytes caused by injury, the G0 cells enter G1 and divide to replace the lost tissue mass. When the defined tissue mass is reached the cells enter G0 again and continue as functional differentiated cells.

Self-renewing populations (labile tissues)

In these populations there is a functional differentiated fraction with a defined life-span, terminated by programmed cell death (apoptosis). There is therefore a requirement for the continuous replacement of these cells by division of the cells in a **self-renewing compartment**. Self-renewing populations always consist of at least three compartments:

1 proliferating–self-renewing;
2 maturation and commitment;
3 functional, non-proliferative, differentiated.

The tissues which consist of such populations include all epithelia and bone marrow. Self-renewal in these populations depends upon the existence of **stem cells**–cells which maintain their own numbers throughout the lifetime of the animal despite the removal of some of them in the process of differentiation. When a stem cell divides, one daughter retains the parental phenotype and the other may embark on a programme which will result in maturation and differentiation into functional end cells. Almost all that is known about stem cells and their properties comes from studies on the bone marrow using a functional stem cell assay known as the **spleen colony-forming unit assay**. In this assay a mouse is irradiated with a dose which kills bone marrow cells. It is then injected with bone marrow from a healthy donor. Within the donor marrow are healthy stem cells which will colonize the sites of haemopoiesis within the mouse, one of which is the spleen. When the spleen is examined 2 weeks after the procedure there are many nodules, each of which represents a colony consisting of proliferating haemopoietic cells. These nodules can be counted and a measure of the stem cell number obtained.

Using this assay, combined with *in vitro* culture, some of the characteristics of haemopoietic stem cells and their growth regulation are known. These cells are very few in number, they have a long cell cycle time and at any one time only a few marrow stem cells are in cycle; the remainder are held in G0. Stem cell self-renewal is dependent upon a **stem cell niche** provided by a different cell type, the marrow stromal cell. The niche consists of the local environment produced by the stem cells and the extracellular matrix which they secrete. The role of the niche is not clear. It may protect cells from cytokines which induce differentiation whilst exposing them to growth factors which promote proliferation. The niche environment may be one which biases to the G0 state and a prolonged cell cycle which may be crucial for these cells to carry out genetic housekeeping such as the sorting and repair of damage in old DNA strands.

In the small intestine, at least in the mouse, there is a single slow cycling cell at the base of each crypt. This maintains the epithelium of each crypt through a population of transit cycling cells which finally become committed to maturation and function. In the epidermis the existence of distinct functional units, **epidermal proliferative units (EPU)**, has been demonstrated kinetically. In each EPU the proliferating cells are in the basal layer firmly attached to the basal lamina. Included in this proliferating population are rare slow cycling cells—the putative stem cells. Movement and detachment from the basal lamina is the signal for commitment and maturation and the cells move up steadily through the epidermal layers to mature, and eventually fall off.

Each of these examples reveals an exquisitely regulated programme of birth, commitment, the expression of differentiated function and death. The systems can respond to increased demand, for example in infection when granulocyte numbers increase, or in wound repair when re-epithelialization and fibroblast proliferation can occur, but there is always a retention of the spatial and functional architecture and a return to normal when the emergency is over.

Summary

As in cell synthesis, movement and adhesion, cell division is normally carefully controlled. Cell populations behave in a highly disciplined manner, although we do not yet know all the rules they obey. In general, the more one looks at cell behaviour, the more one can find similarities between cell types rather than differences. The controls on cell behaviour include large numbers of molecular messengers that have recently been discovered. Only a few of these have been mentioned, for the sake of simplicity. Many more await discovery, and this is an exciting challenge.

Unfortunately, this exquisite discipline can break down, and then cell division becomes uncontrolled. The result is cancer.

16 Cancer

Cancer is a familiar and rather sinister term

It is commonly taken to mean abnormal growths of tissue that are always potentially fatal. In fact it is not really a scientific term. It refers to the nastier end of a spectrum of diseases that have in common the development of abnormal swellings or **tumours**.[1] The swellings begin for no apparent reason, but the vast majority of them soon cease to grow and do not threaten life. We therefore need a term that covers all these unexpected new growths of tissue. The correct term is **neoplasia**, literally 'new growth', and the abnormal swelling is called a **neoplasm**.

Not all neoplasms are alike

Neoplasms were described in antiquity. It was soon noted that in some cases the growing mass destroyed tissues around it and seemed to spread through the patient, appearing in distant sites of the body. This dreadful disease led to death and these growths can be described as **malignant neoplasms**, malignant tumours, or cancer.

However, not all tumours pursued this aggressive course and, although they could interfere to some extent with the patient's well-being, they grew slowly or ceased to grow altogether and did not spread away from the place in which they had first appeared. Tumours having these characteristics were unlikely to bring about death and were therefore called **benign neoplasms**, or benign tumours.

Benign and malignant are terms indicating the natural history of neoplasms

These are old terms but they have been retained. Their use suggests that all neoplasms are either 'good' or 'bad' but the reality is that neoplasms are found across a whole **spectrum of different behaviour**, with 'good' at one end and 'bad' at the other. It is also true that some neoplasms can move along that spectrum, with a change from 'good' towards 'bad'. This does not mean that the terms benign and malignant are therefore useless. If not treated as absolutes, they can be useful concepts to describe the nature and predict the behaviour of neoplasms.

Thus, with experience, we can draw up a set of guidelines by which to judge, from the macroscopic and microscopic features of any particular tumour, whether its behaviour will be benign or malignant.

1 You will remember that the Latin word *tumor* means a swelling of any kind, not necessarily a neoplasm.

279

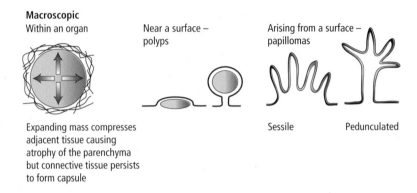

Macroscopic

Within an organ

Expanding mass compresses
adjacent tissue causing
atrophy of the parenchyma
but connective tissue persists
to form capsule

Near a surface –
polyps

Arising from a surface –
papillomas

Sessile   Pedunculated

Figure 16.1 Macroscopic
features of benign neoplasms.

Benign tumours may often be recognized by their macroscopic features

The abnormality in a benign neoplasm is usually that its constituent cells are dividing more than the other cells which make up the parent tissue. In certain cases, the cells may not divide much more frequently but they may undergo less programmed cell death, by the process of **apoptosis**, than the normal population. In either case, there is a local increase in the number of cells.

If the tumour begins within a solid tissue, the new cell mass gradually expands and as it does so may bring about pressure atrophy of adjacent normal cells. The fibres of the supporting connective tissue do not atrophy; they become stretched around the expanding tumours. In this way, a **capsule** may be formed (Fig. 16.1). Usually the benign neoplasm is roughly spherical and obviously different in some way from the normal tissues surrounding it; it may be different in colour, or texture, or both.

If the expanding mass is close to a surface, either internal (e.g. mucosa of gastrointestinal tract) or external (skin), it may project and lift the skin or mucosa over it. This may result in a dome-shaped projection but sometimes it protrudes on a stalk of normal tissue. Such a projecting mass is called a **polyp.**[2] When it has a broad base, it is a **sessile** (sitting) polyp but if a stalk, or peduncle is present, it is a **pedunculated** polyp (Fig. 16.1).

What macroscopic features will be seen when a benign neoplasm develops from epithelium covering a surface? At the site of origin, there is no longer enough room for the increased number of cells so the new epithelium grows outwards, either into an internal lumen or away from the skin.

Again, two major growth patterns can be distinguished. The site of origin may be broad, giving rise to another type of **sessile polyp**, although its surface will not appear smooth, but irregularly heaped-up like a range of mountains. In other cases, the mass is supported by a narrow stalk. Again however, such a pedunculated polyp does not have a smooth convex surface because it is made up of the excess neoplastic epithelium, thrown into complex folds, a feature which can often be seen easily with the naked eye. Tumours with these finger-like projections are described as **papillomas** (Fig. 16.1).

2 Like 'tumour', the term 'polyp' is non-specific. Some polyps are not neoplastic, such as inflammatory polyps in the nasal spaces.

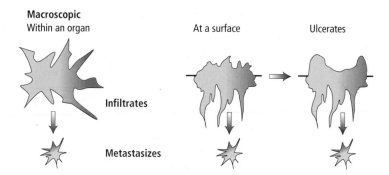

Figure 16.2 Macroscopic features of malignant neoplasms.

Some malignant neoplasms have characteristic macroscopic features

At the junction of the neoplastic and normal tissue, the relationship is different when benign and malignant growth patterns are compared. The malignant neoplasm does not merely compress; it destroys and infiltrates into the normal tissue in an irregular manner.

The result of this is not a round mass, but one which has irregular processes extending out into the nearby tissue (Fig. 16.2). It was this appearance which gave rise to the name **cancer** (Latin for crab). The tissue of the neoplasm may have a variegated appearance due to varying amounts of grey fibrosis, yellow necrosis or red haemorrhage, all possible complications of a malignant tumour.

Where a malignant tumour abuts on to a surface, it projects as an irregular mass, which often undergoes secondary ulceration, infection or bleeding. There may be loss of tissue as a result of necrosis and often this can result in a profile resembling a broad volcano, with a rim of viable malignant tissue raised above the surrounding normal surface and a central crater with an ulcerated base (Fig. 16.2).

Malignant neoplasms metastasize

Another sinister feature may be seen macroscopically. Masses of neoplasm may be present, growing at a distance, and quite separate from the original mass. They are often found in lymph nodes nearby, which become enlarged, firm and on the cut surface contain pale or variegated tissue, different from that of normally reactive lymph nodes. These are referred to as **secondary** neoplasms as opposed to the **primary** tumour at the site of origin. They are also called **metastases**[3] or metastatic spread. Other common sites for metastases to occur are liver, lungs and bone marrow.

The property of metastasis is probably the most important characteristic of malignant neoplasms. It depends upon malignant cells gaining access to lymphatics and blood vessels, with **embolism** to distant sites. Metastases may be early, distant and unpredictable, making it very difficult to treat them

3 *Meta-stasis*: standing at a distance.

successfully. Surgical removal of the primary neoplasm is of little use if the distant metastases are already established.

Summary

The gross or macroscopic appearance of tumours, especially if they have been present for some time and the features described have had a chance to develop, often betrays their nature. Precise recognition however depends upon the **microscopic appearance**.

Microscopically, benign neoplasms closely resemble the parent tissue

The concept of a benign neoplasm is that there is an abnormality present in the cells which results in the production of too many of them. However, each individual neoplastic cell still closely resembles the differentiated tissue cell from which the clone originated, although often they are larger (Fig. 16.3).

The other important feature is that the new population of cells is not just jumbled up together to form a haphazard mass, for just as there is **cytological differentiation**, there is also **tissue differentiation**.

Thus, the cells take up an orderly relationship to one another which resembles that in the normal tissue. For example, if the neoplasm arises from mucus-secreting, columnar cells of the large intestine, then the new cells form tubular structures resembling normal glands and secrete a supportive basement membrane.

Both the cytological features and the degree to which the arrangement of the cells resembles normal tissue are taken into account when commenting upon **differentiation** of a neoplasm. Part of the definition of a benign neoplasm is that it is **well differentiated** because it so closely resembles the tissue of origin.

Depending upon the tissue, there may be evidence of products specific to the particular cell type. In the benign tumour arising from the large intestinal mucosa, mucin is synthesized and secreted. Neoplastic cells originating from the β-cells of an islet of the pancreas may synthesize and secrete insulin.

Microscopic
Close resemblance to tissue of origin but cells are larger and may be crowded

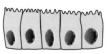

Normal columnar epithelium

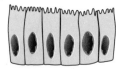

Large bowel adenoma

Figure 16.3 Microscopic features of a benign neoplasm.

The names for benign neoplasms are derived mainly from Greek with some Latin

Usually the name ends in-oma, a Greek suffix meaning a tumour. (You have already met this term in a non-neoplastic context, granul-oma.) There are some general rules about the names, so that usually the Greek or Latin name of the tissue of origin precedes -oma, but as with all rules there are exceptions.

Here are some examples of nomenclature which do obey the rules:
1 adenoma—a benign neoplasm derived from glandular epithelium;
2 chondroma—a benign neoplasm derived from cartilage;
3 lipoma—a benign neoplasm derived from adipose tissue.

The microscopic appearance of malignant neoplasms is much more variable than that of benign ones

Differences in the microscopic appearances of various benign neoplasms are only because of their **different tissues of origin**, but that is not always true for their malignant counterparts. The molecular abnormalities that underlie their development lead not only to **an increase in the number** of cells present but also have an effect upon **the degree to which those cells differentiate**.

As a result malignant neoplastic cells, although capable of rapid cell division, may not progress beyond certain phases of the normal differentiation pathway. They may even be diverted along abnormal pathways and express genes whose products are not normally present in the tissue from which they arise.

Therefore, even **malignant neoplasms arising from identical tissues can have very different microscopic appearances**. Some may vary only a little from what has already been described for benign tumours, whilst others show greater degrees of deviation from the parental phenotype. This affects the appearance of individual cells; their size, shape, nuclear/cytoplasmic ratio, mitotic activity and characteristics of their cytoplasm; it also affects the ability of these cells to form themselves into the layers, glands or other special structures that were present in the tissue of origin (Fig. 16.4).

Indeed, in some cases, the neoplastic cells appear to lose completely the ability to reproduce the parental pattern and this loss goes hand in hand with a failure to differentiate at the cytological level. The result, of course, is a whole range of histological appearances. In order to express this range in a useful form, it is usually simplified and we describe **well-**, **moderately** and **poorly differentiated** malignant neoplasms.

A **well-differentiated** malignant neoplasm is made up of cells of easily recognizable type, arranged in configurations that resemble quite closely the structure of the tissue of origin. This represents a degree of **orderliness** within the tumour and may be accompanied by evidence of normal cellular products, such as **keratin** in a **squamous cell** tumour (Fig. 16.5) and **mucin** in a **glandular** tumour (Fig. 16.4). These good features, however, are outweighed by the fact that they infiltrate and metastasize.

Mucin within cytoplasm

Mucin in pools outside cells

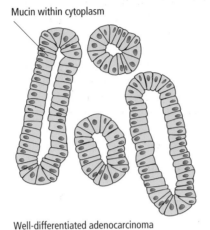

Figure 16.4 Differences in differentiation in adenocarcinoma.

Well-differentiated adenocarcinoma

Poorly differentiated adenocarcinoma

Forming keratin

No keratin formed

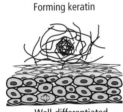

Figure 16.5 Differences in differentiation in squamous cell carcinoma.

Well-differentiated squamous carcinoma

Poorly differentiated squamous carcinoma

A **poorly differentiated** malignant neoplasm is characterized by great variation in the size and shape of both cells and their constituent nuclei (**pleomorphism**), or in some cases by a monotonous population where the cells show little variation and no resemblance to any normal tissue cell. Accompanying either of these cytological appearances is **disorderliness**—poor organization into any structure or pattern. This may be the result of failure of the neoplastic cells to express surface molecules, which allow them to bind to one another and to the extracellular matrix.

Intermediate between these two extremes are neoplasms whose histological appearances show reasonable mimicry of the parental tissue, and in these cases, '**moderately differentiated**' is the most appropriate term.

Malignant neoplasms are named according to whether they are of epithelial or non-epithelial origin

As with the naming of benign neoplasms, words derived from the Greek predominate. For those arising from epithelium, the terminal suffix **carcinoma**[4] is used. When **glandular** epithelium is the source, the term is an **adenocarcinoma**.

4 *Carcinos* (Greek)—crab.

In both cases, the suffix is preceded by the name of the tissue of origin or perhaps an adjective derived from that name, but there are no strict rules and other terms can be used.

Thus:

1 gastric adenocarcinoma, or adenocarcinoma of the stomach;

2 bronchogenic carcinoma, or carcinoma of the bronchus;

3 squamous cell carcinoma, or squamous carcinoma;

4 mammary carcinoma, or carcinoma of the breast.

Non-epithelial malignant tumours usually have the suffix of -sarcoma

Usually the Greek name for the tissue precedes the suffix, but variations are used in some cases.

Thus:

1 osteosarcoma, or osteogenic sarcoma or sarcoma of bone;

2 chondrosarcoma, or sarcoma of cartilage;

3 leiomyosarcoma, or smooth-muscle sarcoma;

4 liposarcoma, or sarcoma of adipose tissue.

The natural history of benign neoplasms is to grow slowly, causing disease but rarely death

Benign neoplasms may cause significant disease, by several different mechanisms.

1 By occupying space: this effect is most damaging where space is limited, such as inside the skull. Most of the available space is already occupied by the brain. A **meningioma** is a benign neoplasm arising from the meninges. Usually it has a firm texture and indents the brain, causing pressure atrophy. The precise effect depends upon the location, but is may be quite serious.

2 By causing obstruction: this may involve a blood vessel or a hollow organ or duct. The tumour may press from the outside, project into the lumen as a polyp, or develop within the wall itself.

3 By ulceration or bleeding: these complications are more likely at a surface, when there may be trauma, for example, in the bowel or the skin.

4 By secretion of synthesized products: the differentiated neoplastic cells may be capable of making and releasing the same substances as the original tissue. If that product is active and normally under homeostatic control, such excess secretion can have serious effects. Often the activity of neoplastic cells escapes normal control mechanisms. Therefore, a benign tumour arising from the β-cells of the islets of Langerhans can release insulin into the blood stream. Because this release is uncontrolled, the patient may suffer severe hypoglycaemia.

5 By being a precursor to a malignant tumour: at some sites, especially the colon, a malignant neoplasm can arise from a benign one.

The natural history of malignant neoplasms is to grow and spread, tending to bring about death as well as causing disease

This is a broad generalization, because there is enormous variability in their behaviour and effects upon the host. Rates of growth of tumours and their propensity to metastasize are very different and the rate of progress is often linked to the degree of differentiation, the better differentiated ones tending to be slower-growing.

Malignant neoplasms can cause disease by the same mechanisms as benign tumours but also in other ways

1 By occupying space and destroying tissue: it is important that malignant tumours do not merely compress adjacent tissue, but infiltrate into it.

Normal cells are destroyed, due partly to pressure and disruption of their blood supply.

The loss of normal tissue may be serious. Not only is the patient deprived of its function but, for instance, complete destruction of the wall of the gastrointestinal tract may lead to perforation and peritonitis.

2 By becoming ulcerated, and hence infected or bleeding: this is much more likely to occur with malignant than benign neoplasms. Infection may spread; or chronic blood loss (e.g. into the bowel) may lead to iron-deficiency anaemia.

3 By obstruction: again, this is much more likely with malignant as opposed to benign neoplasms. It is a not uncommon event for a carcinoma of the bronchus to prevent drainage and cause a persistent infection as a result.

Adenocarcinoma of the colon can also cause obstruction. This may result from a tumour projecting into the lumen, but some types provoke a dense fibrous reaction, causing stenosis (narrowing).

There may also be pressure from outside a hollow organ. Lymph nodes enlarged near the liver, or an adenocarcinoma in the head of the pancreas, can both constrict the common bile duct. Since this prevents the normal excretion of bile, the patient becomes jaundiced[5] (Fig. 16.6).

4 By destroying tissues distant from the primary tumour: it has already been mentioned that the bone marrow is a common site for secondary neoplasms. It often seems to provide a particularly favourable environment; the normal haemopoietic tissue is displaced and, as a result, the patient may suffer from a deficiency in red cells, platelets and white blood cells.

Destruction of bony tissue as a result of metastasis can lead to fractures, occasionally of long bones, but more commonly collapse of vertebral bodies.

5 By causing pain: numerous mechanisms are responsible for pain. These include release of inflammatory mediators, bony destruction, pressure and direct infiltration around nerves.

6 By the secretion of synthesized products: as with benign neoplasms, occasionally differentiation of a neoplasm allows a product to be formed and released from the cells, independently of normal control mechanisms.

Particularly interesting, in malignant neoplasms, is that the differentiation

5 Jaundice is yellow pigmentation of the tissues, including skin and sclerae, because of the excess bilirubin present.

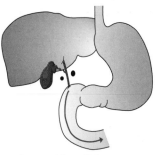

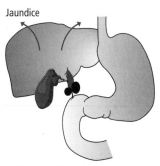

Jaundice

Figure 16.6 Obstruction to biliary outflow causes jaundice.

Unobstructed flow of bile into the duodenum

Enlarged nodes at the porta hepatis obstruct biliary outflow

pathway may have been altered with resultant synthesis of a product not usually associated with the parent tissue. Most of such documented examples of unorthodox secretion concern carcinomas of the bronchus. Two of the best known examples are secretion of adrenocorticotrophic hormone or antidiuretic hormone by bronchial carcinomas.

Other products released by malignant neoplasms are those associated with a less differentiated state and may even represent products normally typical of early stages in fetal development. Examples are carcinoembryonic antigen, produced by many tumours of the bowel and pancreas, and α-fetoprotein secreted by carcinomas of the liver and germ cell tumours.

These products have no biological effects, but are useful in diagnosis as they can be detected in the serum.

7 By causing thrombosis: especially as malignant neoplasms become far advanced, clumps of cells and fragments of necrotic tissue can gain access to the circulation and activate the thrombotic cascade.

In some cases this leads to venous thrombosis, which may be further complicated by embolism.

8 By an ill-defined state, cachexia: this term means no more than wasting of muscles and a generally poor state of health and as such is not exclusive to malignant disease since it also complicates some chronic inflammatory diseases. It involves weight loss and weakness, perhaps mental as well as physical.

No doubt cachexia is multifactorial, contributed to by loss of appetite, anaemia, infection, pain, release of neoplastic cells and necrotic fragments into the blood and sometimes psychological factors.

9 By many other mechanisms: each particular malignant neoplasm can exert many other effects, depending partly upon the site. For instance, fluid can accumulate within body cavities when these are invaded. Other so-called paraneoplastic syndromes are described, the pathogenesis of which is ill-understood. They tend to affect skin, nerve and muscle and whether they are mediated by toxins or immunological mechanisms is speculation.

A neoplasm contains components other than the neoplastic cells themselves

Our description so far has referred only to the neoplastic cells, their varying appearance and behaviour in so far as they arrange themselves and do or do not move from the site of origin. A moment's reflection is enough to make one ask how such complex collections of cells are maintained and enabled to survive.

Neoplastic cells have supporting connective tissue (stroma) and a blood supply

Like the neoplastic cells, both these elements are **new**. The study of how neoplastic cells are able to induce the host to provide these elements, which are so necessary for their survival, is of great practical as well as theoretical interest, since if therapies could be tailored which would interfere with the development of stroma and blood vessels, then that might be just as effective as destroying neoplastic cells directly.

Understanding the two processes may come from a study of the normal responses of body tissues to injury. In granulation tissue (Chapter 2), growth factors are synthesized which bring about the ingrowth of endothelial cells to establish a blood supply, followed by fibroblasts which secrete supporting connective tissue. The newly formed connective tissue later loses its vascularity and its cellular content to a large extent, leaving mainly collagen fibres which form a scar.

It seems likely therefore that growth factors having similar activities are responsible for the formation of connective tissue stroma and blood vessels in tumours. These need not be synthesized directly by the neoplastic cells but could be produced locally by other cells, in response to the presence of the neoplasm. In this way tumours could hijack normal mechanisms in order to survive. It is not known what governs the widely differing vascularity and stroma formation which occurs in different tumours. The arrangement of stroma may have particular patterns in particular neoplasms, so that a tumour may be composed of mainly its own neoplastic cells with negligible connective tissue present or, in other cases, extremely dense collagenous tissue may be interspersed with only sparse neoplastic cells.

Neoplasms do not develop a new lymphatic drainage

This may be important in relation to the tendency for malignant neoplasms to develop areas of necrosis. Perhaps this is due in part to compression of their haphazard, thin-walled vasculature by their own growth but, in addition, the blood vessels leak fluid into the tumour from which it has no means of escape, so it accumulates and hence increases the pressure still further. Obviously, pressure will also be increased if there is haemorrhage within a tumour.

A crucial characteristic of malignant neoplasms is invasion, leading to spread

Invasion means that malignant cells spread amongst normal tissue cells. Initially this may be within the same tissue type but then it extends into those which are different, including connective tissue, other kinds of parenchyma or epithelia and the walls of veins and lymphatics. **Arterial walls are rarely invaded**.

This haphazard intermingling of cell types which occurs in invasion is in marked contrast to both normal embryonic development and the aggregation of cells in culture, when it is found that like tends to stay together with like. We know almost nothing about the molecular mechanisms which are involved in invasion; it has been suggested that neoplastic cells move more than their normal counterparts, so that **they behave more like wandering cells**, such as phagocytes. They lose their normal contacts with each other and the surrounding stroma and are no longer subject to normal inhibitory signals from their surroundings. Perhaps they also express surface molecules of the type that allow phagocytes to adhere to and 'crawl' through a variety of tissues.

Another hypothesis is that the secretion of enzymes, mainly proteases (again like phagocytes), aids the process of invasion, but up to now searches for such enzymes have been inconclusive. Certainly some tissues, **particularly collagen and cartilage**, are resistant to invasion and it has been suggested that this is because malignant cells lack suitable collagen- or cartilage-dissolving enzymes.

In general terms, the pattern of invasion is along **the line of least resistance**. Thus a pre-existing channel or space is exploited, especially if the normal contents move. Examples would be spread via lymphatics and veins; it is found that **carcinomas tend to enter the lymph early** and thus reach the draining lymph nodes, only later using the blood as a mode of spread, but **sarcomas tend to invade veins early** and therefore become widespread in the body more quickly. The resistance of arteries to invasion may be due to their thicker walls, but the effect of pulsatile pressure within them is probably more important.

Body cavities are sometimes a ready means of spread, especially if the neoplastic cells are capable of implantation within them. Other viscera may then be invaded in turn. A well-known example is spread from an adenocarcinoma of the stomach, via the peritoneal cavity to reach the ovaries, where the latter seem to provide a welcoming environment and large secondary tumours can develop.

Neoplasms elicit inflammatory and immune responses

Many neoplasms, particularly malignant ones, are infiltrated by inflammatory cells. Neutrophils in malignant neoplasms are usually elicited by necrosis or infection, but there is some evidence that the lymphocytic and plasma cell infiltration which is common in malignant tumours may represent an immune response to the tumour itself. In breast carcinomas, the presence of a florid lymphocytic infiltrate correlates with a better outlook (prognosis) for the patient.

It is often claimed that there are antibodies to malignant tumours. There is even a school of thought that many early neoplasms are eliminated as a result of an immune response, and therefore are never detected. This theoretical concept is often referred to as **immune surveillance**. It implies that any tumour that becomes big enough to be recognized must have somehow escaped any immune response. One type of skin tumour, the **keratoacanthoma**, is histologically identical to a squamous carcinoma but, after reaching the size of about 1 cm or more, becomes heavily infiltrated by lymphocytes, shrinks and disappears completely.

Unfortunately, however, the concept of immunity to cancer is disputed and no way has yet been found to augment immune responses to eliminate neoplasms.

Carcinomas developing within an epithelium may be confined by the basement membrane

In a sense, some epithelia can be viewed as being 'outside' the other tissues of the body. This is because their **basement membrane separates them from the underlying tissues**, vasculature and lymphatic drainage and their metabolic processes rely entirely upon the process of diffusion. This does not mean that certain specialized cells cannot enter and leave the epithelium, penetrating the basement membrane to do so, but the epithelial cells themselves do not normally enter the tissues and are usually shed from the surface at the end of their life-span.

Examples include squamous epithelium at its many sites, including the skin and lining some hollow internal organs. If a malignant neoplasm develops within such an epithelium, it must cross this tough basement membrane before it can invade. In most cases, destruction or breaching of the membrane probably occurs soon after the appearance of the neoplasm. It is suggested that the process requires close adherence to the basement membrane, followed by the secretion of collagenase to allow passage of the neoplastic cells. However, at certain sites in the human body, epithelial neoplasms are recognized which, for a time at least, do not penetrate the basement membrane.

Carcinoma confined to its site of origin is known as carcinoma-*in-situ*

Probably the most thoroughly studied example is squamous carcinoma-*in-situ* affecting the cervix uteri, which will be discussed in more detail below, but similar conditions occur at other sites, including the breast and the skin.

Dysplasia is a term which has been used very loosely

Also sometimes used to describe developmental disorders, the word dysplasia means **disturbed growth or form**. Since these are features which also characterize neoplasia, the term is often used by histopathologists for cellular abnormalities suggesting that, although neoplasia is not present as yet, it may be expected to develop in the future.

Sequential, apparently preneoplastic changes are seen in squamous epithelium

In both the bronchus and the endocervix, a series of epithelial changes **in response to injury** is well-documented. The normal lining epithelium, respiratory in the bronchus and columnar in the cervix, is replaced by tougher squamous epithelium, a process known as **squamous metaplasia**. Sometimes this **metaplastic** epithelium can be further altered to more rapidly growing and less orderly epithelium, which is then described as **dysplastic**.

The lack of order shows itself in the loss of the normal layer of uniform basal cells having a regular vertical arrangement, and the failure of those cells to change from a vertical to a horizontal orientation as they move towards the surface.

In normal squamous epithelium, mitoses are initiated only in cells which remain in contact with the basement membrane. Stem cells, the dividing component of each proliferating unit of squamous epithelium, require this anchorage in order that the cytoskeleton can be rearranged for cell division. But in abnormal squamous epithelia, cells no longer have this rigid requirement and mitotic figures can be seen well above the basal layer. This may be accompanied by persistent large nuclei, often more densely stained than the normal ones and abnormally shaped (Fig. 16.7).

When the whole thickness of the squamous epithelium has this disorderly appearance, then the epithelium has many of the features of a **malignant neoplasm** and the condition is called **carcinoma-*in-situ*** (Fig. 16.8).

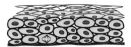

Normal squamous epithelium

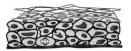

Dysplastic squamous epithelium

Figure 16.7 Normal and dysplastic squamous epithelium.

Normal squamous epithelium

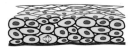

Carcinoma *in situ* – Thick
    Disorderly arrangement of cells
    Mitoses above the basal layer
    Individual cells form keratin beneath

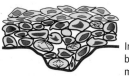

Intact
basement
membrane

    the surface
Pleomorphism
Increased nuclear/cytoplasmic ratio

Figure 16.8 Normal squamous epithelium and carcinoma-*in-situ*.

The uterine cervix is a good model of sequential changes within epithelium

The changes described above have been best studied in the endocervix because they occur in a small, well-defined area and the tissue is readily accessible to study, by scraping off cells (cervical cytology) and biopsy. Also local forms of treatment are applicable and their results can be assessed.

In the cervix, before sexual activity begins, the endocervical canal is usually tightly closed and lined by columnar, mucus-secreting epithelium which changes abruptly to squamous epithelium covering the ectocervix (Fig. 16.9). Squamous epithelium is multilayered, tough and waterproof. It lines the vagina and ectocervix and is presumably the most suitable barrier between the internal tissues and the environment of the vagina. When sexual activity begins, but even more after pregnancy, the lower end of the endocervical canal becomes everted to a variable degree. Thus the delicate mucus-secreting columnar epithelium of the endocervix is exposed to the hostile environment of the vagina with its bacterial flora and acid pH.

Its response to this injury is to undergo **squamous metaplasia**. The tall endocervical cells give way to a type of squamous epithelium, the change appearing first in the basal layers with gradual development of multilayering. The original mucus-secreting cells can be observed being displaced towards the surface where they are shed. The result is therefore both an increase in cell proliferation and a change in phenotype.

Other factors may now operate, especially if there are multiple sexual partners. Besides the venereal acquisition of bacterial and chlamydial infections, **viral** infections have become much more widespread. A number of different types of **papillomavirus** have been discovered to be transmitted in this way and they successfully enter and replicate within the metaplastic squamous epithelium of the cervix, in some cases.

The presence of such viral infections promotes further cell division and at the

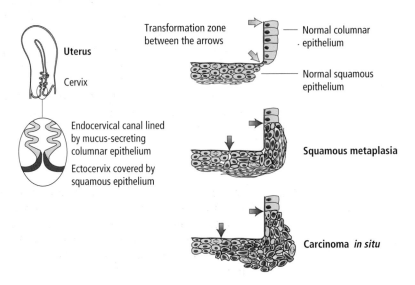

Figure 16.9 Squamous metaplasia of endocervical epithelium usually precedes development of carcinoma-in-situ.

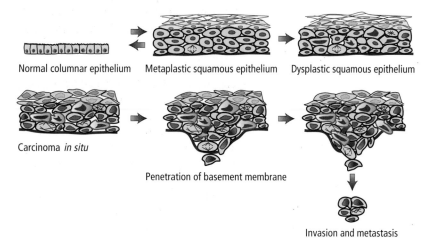

Normal columnar epithelium · Metaplastic squamous epithelium · Dysplastic squamous epithelium

Carcinoma *in situ*

Penetration of basement membrane

Invasion and metastasis

Figure 16.10 Stages in the development of invasive carcinoma in the cervix.

same time there may be characteristic effects on the cytological appearance of the cells, many of which resemble the changes we have already described as **dysplasia**. Unfortunately, it appears that a number of these papillomavirus infections, in particular types 16 and 18, do have a true potential to contribute to the development of neoplasms and indeed carcinoma-*in-situ* does develop in the endocervix (Fig. 16.9) and has a steadily increasing incidence in young women.

The *in situ* stage of carcinoma is of great clinical importance

If carcinoma-*in-situ* is detected it can be treated successfully. How long the non-invasive stage of cervical carcinoma persists is not clear, but it is probably usually several years, since invasive carcinoma (Fig. 16.10) tends to occur in women in an age group about 10 years older than those who have the *in situ* form of the disease.

Its clinical accessibility has made the cervix the best-studied example of carcinoma-*in-situ* but the bronchus can undergo a similar train of events, attributable mainly to cigarette smoking, which can also be detected by cytological examination and biopsy. However, finding it is much more difficult, since it is not restricted to a single defined site and treatment is therefore much less successful.

Carcinoma-*in-situ* is not uncommon in the breast

The breast is the most frequent site of carcinoma in women (if skin is excluded) and characteristic forms of *in situ* disease are recognized.

Unfortunately, access to the preinvasive cancer is difficult but some cases can be recognized because necrotic cancer cells in the middle of ducts may calcify, giving rise to tiny radiopaque cylinders, visible on X-ray examination (Fig. 16.11).

293

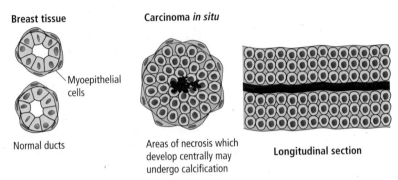

Breast tissue

Carcinoma *in situ*

Myoepithelial cells

Normal ducts

Areas of necrosis which develop centrally may undergo calcification

Longitudinal section

Figure 16.11 Carcinoma may arise from the epithelium lining the ducts of the breast.

An *in situ* phase of squamous carcinoma can also be recognized in the skin

The epidermis becomes irregularly thickened, with nuclear pleomorphism, disorderly cell maturation and mitotic figures high above the basement membrane. Often it is known under the eponym of Bowen's disease.

The large intestine is a frequent site for malignant neoplasms

Again, a sequence of changes seems to be the common underlying pattern.

At first, a benign tumour (adenoma) appears, but within it there may develop a focus where the epithelium has a different cytological appearance; the cells are larger, more mitotically active, more pleomorphic and densely packed together (dysplasia). Following a phase of further growth, the pattern of glands in the dysplastic area becomes very irregular, accompanied by a change to invasive behaviour. Thus many malignant tumours of the large intestine are thought to be preceded by adenomas (Fig. 16.12).

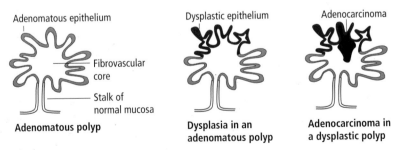

Adenomatous epithelium

Dysplastic epithelium

Adenocarcinoma

Fibrovascular core

Stalk of normal mucosa

Adenomatous polyp

Dysplasia in an adenomatous polyp

Adenocarcinoma in a dysplastic polyp

Figure 16.12 Stages in the development of carcinoma arising from an adenomatous colonic polyp.

Is there any other evidence for such a progression?

Further evidence is that often, when an adenocarcinoma of the colon is re-moved, one or more separate adenomatous polyps may be found nearby. Moreover, it has been found that when adenomas and adenocarcinomas occur simultaneously, both types of tumour contain the same set of mutations, but the malignant neoplasm has some extra ones.

Another important piece of evidence is provided by an inherited disease called **familial adenomatous polyposis** which shows an autosomal dominant pattern of inheritance. Affected individuals develop numerous adenomatous polyps of the colon by their early 20s and have a high risk of colonic adenocarcinoma by the time they are 30. Only total removal of the colon at an early age can prevent the patient's untimely death.

Neoplasia also occurs in blood cell precursors

So far in this chapter, we have referred only to neoplasms which develop from tissues which are **fixed at a particular site**. But neoplasms can also occur in the haemopoietic cells of the bone marrow. In fact, because of the enormous amount of cell proliferation which takes place there, one might perhaps have predicted that marrow would suffer the greatest frequency of genetic errors and hence neoplasms but, for some reason, this is not so.

Nevertheless, neoplasms can arise from the marrow precursors of leukocytes. Like their normal counterparts, the neoplastic cells leave the mar-row and circulate in the blood. The result, which has been called a circulating metastasis, is **leukaemia**. Much more rarely, neoplasms of the precursors of red cells or platelets also occur. The leukaemias tend to take over the marrow, so that other cell series are depleted. The result is that leukaemia patients are deprived of red cells, platelets and effective white cells. Death is usually due, therefore, to anaemia, haemorrhage or infection.

It is fortunate that leukaemias are rare, because all of them are life-threatening, although some types are more malignant than others. The degree of malignancy seems to depend on the stage of cell development at which the neoplasm originates. **Neoplasms of blast cells** (e.g. lymphoblasts or myeloblasts) give rise to circulating blast cells, never normally found in the blood. This is **acute leukaemia**, so called because it can kill within months. Neoplasms in which the cells mature to some extent cause more slowly progressive disease—**chronic myeloid or lymphocytic leukaemias**. The latter is the most benign leukaemia, and patients may survive for many years. The leukaemic cells may not only be found in the blood, but are also deposited in the tissues. Spleen and lymph node enlargement occurs in some types of leukaemia but localized tumour masses in other tissues are rare.

Most blood cells do not divide after leaving the marrow, but lymphocytes are an exception. Therefore neoplasms (**lymphomas**) can occur in peripheral lymphoid tissues such as lymph nodes or gut. These neoplasms can arise from T cells or B cells at any state of development, so once again there is a range of degree of malignancy. Lymphomas therefore come in many varieties. Multiple myeloma, the tumour of plasma cells, is one example we have talked about previously.

Although some lymphomas behave rather like other solid tumours, and give rise to metastases, the majority seem to be widespread early on, in keeping with the fact that lymphocytes normally circulate through the body.

Summary

We have now considered the natural history of neoplasms, their varied behaviour and the host–tumour relationship. We must now examine how they arise.

17

Cancer: the genes

Cancer is a disease caused by alteration of a cell's genes

Neoplasms are the result of **loss of control**: loss of control of cell division and loss of organization of cells into tissues. The processes of division and of organization into tissue are controlled by genes. Tumours arise because some of these genes get altered or rearranged, so that the cell divides too many times and loses its correct place in the tissue.

The idea that alteration in a cell's genes caused cancer has been around since early this century, but until the 1980s it was just a hypothesis that could reasonably be questioned. We can now state with confidence that the major cause of neoplasia is alteration of the genetic material in a cell.

Koch's postulates can be applied to identifying the cause of neoplasia

One way to test the evidence is to draw an analogy with infectious disease and use Koch's postulates to demonstrate that a specific cause is responsible for a specific disease.

1 Alteration of genes has been demonstrated in many types of tumour, and the alterations have been studied by sequencing the DNA. In many cases, it has also been shown that the mutation is present in the tumour cells but not the normal cells of the patient.

2 The altered DNA sequences can be isolated from tumours and large numbers of copies made by recombinant DNA techniques. This is analogous to propagating a pathogen *in vitro*, in the case of an infectious disease.

3 When the altered genes that have been isolated are introduced into cells in tissue culture they often upset the cells' control of cell division. In a few cases it has been possible to go further and introduce an altered gene into an animal tissue and show that it causes the tissue to develop tumours. For example, when an altered form of the gene *myc* was inserted into cells of the mammary epithelium of a mouse, the epithelium became hyperplastic—its growth was increased.[1] It appeared that it had taken a step towards becoming a tumour. Then, when an additional altered (mutated) gene, *ras*, was introduced into these hyperplastic cells, abnormal epithelium formed which gave rise to true neoplasms.

Thus, the agent causing the disease has been isolated, grown *in vitro* and shown to be able to cause the same disease in a new host— Koch's postulates have been satisfied. In fact, the argument can be carried beyond the fact that

1 Conventionally gene names are given in italics, e.g. *myc*, while their protein products are normally written with a capital initial letter, e.g. Myc.

Koch's postulates have been satisfied, because we have some idea of how the alterations to the genes upset the mechanism of growth control in the cell—in other words, we have some idea of the **molecular pathogenesis of tumours**.

So there is no longer much doubt that alteration of the genes of a cell is the major cause of neoplasia, although there may also be other things happening that we do not yet know about. For convenience, we will refer to damage to genes as mutation, using mutation in the most general sense, not just to mean a change of sequence but also, for example, to include deletion or even addition of new sequence.

Several gene changes are needed to give a malignant tumour

A single mutation is not enough to cause a normal cell to develop into a tumour cell.

$$\text{normal cell} \quad \underset{\text{mutations}}{\to \to \to \to \to \to \ldots} \quad \underset{\text{tumour}}{\text{benign}} \quad \underset{\text{mutations}}{\to \to \ldots} \quad \text{malignant tumour}$$

(each arrow represents the alteration of a gene)

At the time of writing, analysis of the DNA in different types of tumour is progressing rapidly. The current estimate is that cells in a typical colon carcinoma, which is probably representative of tumours in general, **have at least five critical genes altered**, and this estimate seems more likely to increase than decrease as more research is done. This is consistent with several lines of older evidence that many mutations or steps are required: for example, the chromosomes of cells from solid tumours are grossly abnormal, usually with many additions, deletions and translocations, showing that many genetic alterations have occurred. Many tumours progress through recognizable precursor stages; for example, in the cervix we see a spectrum of abnormalities ranging from squamous metaplasia through dysplasia and carcinoma-*in-situ* to fully invasive carcinoma. In the large bowel, adenomas of varying degrees of abnormality often precede carcinomas, and these adenomas have many of the mutations found in the carcinomas. It now seems certain that these different abnormalities are stages on a pathway to a malignant tumour.

Because a number of mutations are needed for a tumour to develop, they usually take a long time to accumulate, and most cancers occur more frequently with age: breast cancers, for example, are very rare in the under-30s, and when they do develop at this early age, it is likely that the women are genetically predisposed.

Tumours are clones of cells that evolve in stages as their genes are altered

A model of how a tumour might develop from a normal cell is shown in Fig. 17.1. The effect of each successive mutation is to give first a single cell, and then

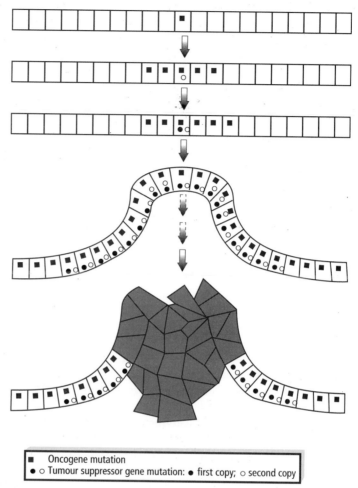

Figure 17.1 Imaginary history of a tumour. Schematic representation of the possible sequence of events in the development of a tumour, showing how successive mutations that give a clone of cells a selective advantage over their neighbours lead to successive stages of overgrowth of clones. The time scale may be many years. Two types of mutation are shown; ■ represents an oncogene being mutated, [●] and [○] represent, respectively, the first and second copy of a tumour suppressor gene being mutated. The shaded cells in the final drawing represent a malignant tumour with perhaps five or more genes mutated. Note that inactivating one copy of a tumour suppressor gene has no effect on growth.

its progeny, a growth advantage so that it forms a clone of cells that grows more than its neighbours. The process is then repeated: one cell of that clone undergoes a further mutation to give a more vigorously overgrowing clone;

and so on. Beyond a certain stage the tissue is distorted by the overgrowing clone and we may recognize the growth as some form of tumour.

Only a few particular mutations contribute to tumour development

Damage to the DNA in our cells is occurring all the time, for example from natural radiation and mistakes that happen during the replication of DNA, but most of this damage either has no effect or disables the cell and actually makes it less likely to divide. Only extremely rare mutations make cell division more likely and so contribute to the development of a tumour cell.

Tumours develop because of alterations in the normal genes that control cell division and tissue organization

The genes which are affected by the mutations that cause tumours are not special cancer genes: they are genes that function in normal cells and are involved in controlling cell division and the arrangement of cells in tissues. Mutations in growth-control genes cause the cell to divide, either by giving it false signals that tell it to divide or by blocking signals or feedback controls that should tell it not to divide.

At least part of the control of cell division is through signals that reach the cell from outside, in the form of growth factors and hormones. These are received by receptors either at the cell surface or in the nucleus. The receptors in turn pass signals to other proteins in the cell until ultimately they reach the machinery in the nucleus that organizes DNA replication and the actual process of cell division. Figure 17.2 is a simplified schematic representation of our current understanding of the steps in this process.

A wide range of the proteins involved may be altered by gene changes that occur in tumours. We will consider here just a few examples.

Tumour cells may produce their own growth factors

The simplest case is where alteration of a gene induces a cell to secrete a growth factor that stimulates that same cell to divide. For example, the peptide **platelet-derived growth factor** (PDGF) stimulates cell division in most mesenchymal cell types, as we saw in wound healing. A key discovery in the development of tumour biology was that in one model system where sarcomas (tumours of mesenchymal cells) were induced by a retrovirus, the retrovirus caused expression of the gene for PDGF in affected cells. These cells then continuously stimulated their own division.

Tumour cells may have aberrant receptors for growth factors

A similar effect occurs when a tumour cell has a mutated gene for a growth factor receptor, so that either the receptor is over-sensitive to the growth factor, or the receptor behaves as though it was permanently stimulated, even when

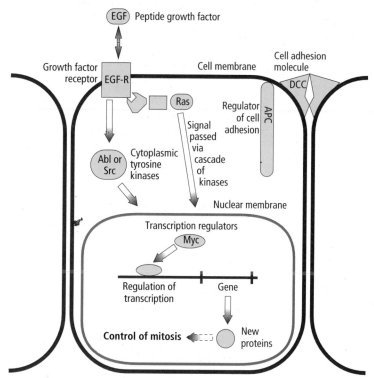

Figure 17.2 The role of some oncogenes and tumour suppressor genes in controlling cell division. Simplified diagram of how cell division is controlled, showing the role of some of the oncogene and tumour suppressor gene proteins discussed in the text. Arrows represent flow of signals between proteins. Growth factors such as epidermal growth factor (EGF) and platelet-derived growth factor (PDGF) bind to receptors at the cell membrane such as the EGF receptor. These in turn activate proteins in the cytoplasm such as Ras, Abl or Src, which are components of signal pathways that communicate between the receptors and the nucleus. Also at the cell surface are molecules that make or detect interactions with neighbouring cells or extracellular matrix, such as the tumour suppressor genes *DCC* and *APC*. How these affect cell division is not yet known. The effect of growth-controlling signals on the cell nucleus is often to alter gene expression. Myc for example is an oncogene protein that regulates expression of as yet unknown genes.

the growth factor is not there. For example, a mutation in the gene *erb-B*, that codes for the epidermal growth factor (EGF) receptor, removes a section of the protein-coding sequence. The resulting receptor protein behaves as though it was constantly being stimulated by EGF.

Components of the growth-controlling mechanisms within the cell may be altered

An example of a protein located inside the cell, that is involved in controlling cell division and found to be frequently altered in tumours, is the Myc protein.

The production of Myc seems to encourage DNA replication; it is thought to achieve this by binding to DNA and regulating gene expression. Alterations in *myc* are found in a variety of tumours, including breast carcinomas and neoplasms of B lymphocytes. As a result, the Myc protein may be produced all the time, or at a higher than normal level, causing the tumour cells to divide more often than they should, or perhaps persist when they should die.

Another gene involved in some way in controlling DNA replication is *Rb-1*, so called because it was discovered first during work on retinoblastoma, a rare childhood tumour. Rb-1 protein is produced in many or all cells and its presence seems to inhibit DNA synthesis and mitosis. To remove this inhibition, the Rb-1 protein has to be inactivated in some way, probably by phosphorylation. Loss of both copies of the *Rb-1* gene in a cell results in no Rb-1 protein being produced, and so it cannot inhibit cell division.

Other growth controls are also affected

It seems likely that there are other mechanisms controlling cell growth which we cannot yet relate to the pathways in Fig. 17.2, but which are also altered by tumour mutations. In particular, both intercellular junctions and attachments between cells and the extracellular matrix must be involved in controlling growth and differentiation. There are already examples of alteration of these structures in tumours. For example, a gene called *DCC*, that is often lost by adenomas and carcinomas of the colon, is one that codes for a cell–cell adhesion molecule. Also in some of these tumours, the cells seem to have lost the ability to bind to components of extracellular matrix such as collagen.

Gene changes responsible for malignancy and metastasis have not yet been identified

We know almost nothing about what causes some tumours to begin to invade and metastasize, partly because we know very little about how cells are normally organized into tissues. Malignant behaviour is presumably also caused by changes in genes, but what these genes might be is controversial. The conventional view is that the change from a non-invasive tumour, such as a carcinoma-*in-situ* of the cervix or an adenoma of the colon, to an invasive tumour, is different from the change from normal tissue to a benign tumour and presumed to require mutations in different kinds of gene. Popular candidates include genes for the proteases and protease inhibitors, because proteases are thought by some to be necessary for cells to escape from their normal position in tissue. Another large class of genes thought to be important are those which code for proteins involved in cell–cell or cell–extracellular matrix interactions, as cells may have to interact differently with their environment to make their escape or to survive in alien tissue. According to this view, the **most important cancer mutations, the ones that lead to malignancy, are yet to be identified**.

The alternative view, less popular but compatible with the limited evidence available, is that malignancy might be caused simply by the **accumulation** of a critical level of mutations of **exactly the same kind** that are found in benign tumours, rather than by the acquisition of new mutation(s) specific to malignancy.

Genetic changes in tumour cells may affect one or both copies of a gene

Mutations in tumours can be divided into two main categories. Cells have two copies of each gene, one originally from the mother, the other from the father (except some of the genes on the sex chromosomes). Tumour mutations can be classified according to whether they exert their effects through changes to only one or to both copies of the gene involved (Fig. 17.3).

In some cases, alteration to only one of the gene copies is enough to change the behaviour of the cell. These can be considered dominant mutations (Fig. 17.3a). An example is a mutation of the gene for a growth factor receptor so that the receptor protein constantly stimulates the cell to divide. Although the other copy of the gene still makes normal receptor, that does not prevent the effect of the mutant gene. Generally, these dominant mutations affect genes whose protein product stimulates cell division and the mutation increases the activity of the protein. These mutations are **oncogene** mutations.

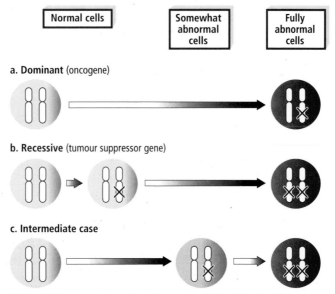

Figure 17.3 Types of mutation in tumours. Mutations leading to development of tumours may need to affect one or both copies of a gene. In (a) mutation of one copy of a gene causes abnormal behaviour of the cell. Such a mutation is dominant in the cell, and the mutant gene is an oncogene. In (b) the cell's behaviour is only altered when both copies of the gene are affected. The gene affected is called a tumour suppressor gene. In the intermediate case (c), mutation of one copy of the gene alters the cell's behaviour to some extent, but the loss of the remaining normal copy of the gene enhances the effect. Genes affected by such mutations have not yet been given a distinctive name; they are currently also called tumour suppressor genes.

The second kind of mutation (Fig. 17.3b) has to affect both copies of the gene to cause the cell to behave differently. These can be considered recessive mutations. For example, the *Rb-1* gene codes for a protein that in some way restrains DNA synthesis and cell division. If a single copy of the *Rb-1* gene is inactivated, the other copy can still make the Rb-1 protein, which is enough to restrain cell division. Only if the second copy of the *Rb-1* gene is also lost will the cell be released from its control. In contrast to the first category of mutations, the genes affected by this kind of mutation generally code for proteins that restrain cell division, and the mutations generally inactivate the gene or its product. These are **tumour suppressor gene** mutations.

The genes affected by the two types of mutation have been called oncogenes and tumour suppressor genes

The names oncogene and tumour suppressor gene were given for historical reasons, and they are misleading and inconsistent. Where changes to a single copy of a gene can alter the cell's behaviour, the gene affected is called an **oncogene**. More precisely, the term should be applied to the mutated, overactive form of the gene; the correct name for its normal precursor is **proto-oncogene**, although most people call the normal form an oncogene too. This is sensible because in human tumours the mutation that results in a gene being overactive is often simply many-fold reduplication (amplification) of the gene, so the distinction between proto-oncogene and oncogene becomes rather academic.

The term 'oncogene' is unfortunate: it was originally coined to name an imaginary, evil gene that was usually silent and hidden in the genome but popped out to cause cancer when activated. This original oncogene theory has long been abandoned. The name was then applied to cancer-causing genes in retroviruses, before it was realized that they were mutated cellular genes picked up during infection. We now realize that **proto-oncogenes are normal genes** coding for normal components of the cell's division-controlling machinery, and that the **oncogenes are nothing more than mutated forms of these genes**. Taking as our example again the gene *erb-B*, the receptor for EGF: the normal gene is the proto-oncogene, and the mutant, truncated form that behaves as though it is constantly stimulated is an oncogene.

The term **tumour suppressor gene** is used for genes that are affected by the second category of mutation, where mutation only affects the behaviour of the cell when both copies of the gene are altered. Thus *Rb-1* is a tumour suppressor gene.[2] Note that the name is applied to the normal, unmutated form of the gene, which restrains cell growth. Since the most common kind of mutation of a tumour suppressor gene is deletion, the mutant form of the gene is often nothing! Although 'tumour suppressor' conveys the growth-restraining nature of the protein product, these genes are not of course there just to suppress tumour formation. They are components of the machinery that regulates normal cell division and tissue organization.

The oncogenes were discovered before the tumour suppressor genes and much more is known about them, so most of the examples we will discuss are taken from the oncogenes. It seems likely that the products of both kinds of

2 An alternative suggestion was 'anti-oncogene', but mercifully this name seems to have been abandoned.

gene will be found throughout the systems regulating cells, the only difference being that the products of the oncogenes will generally have a stimulatory role, while those of the tumour suppressor genes will generally restrain growth. One thing is already clear: mutations of both types of gene are important in human tumours.

There is probably a category of mutation intermediate between dominant and recessive

As in most of biology, the true picture is probably more complicated; in some cases, when one copy of the gene is mutated, the cell gains some growth advantage, but when the remaining normal copy of the gene is also mutated, the cell is affected much more (see Fig. 17.3c). At the moment there is no special term for such genes. At the time of writing, the best candidate for a gene of this intermediate category, the *p53* gene, is referred to as a tumour suppressor gene, and this makes sense because such genes have much in common with true tumour suppressor genes; in particular they restrain cell division.

Oncogenes and tumour suppressor genes can be mutated in many ways

The mutations that can activate oncogenes or inactivate tumour suppressor genes are as diverse as the genes themselves. Table 17.1 lists the main categories of change in DNA sequence that have been discovered so far. These are described below.

Point mutation

A number of genes found in tumours are altered by a point mutation, a change in a single base-pair of the DNA sequence. The best known example is the *Ha-ras* oncogene, where a point mutation alters a single amino acid in the Ha-Ras protein and makes it overactive. There are three genes in the *ras* family, *Ha-ras*, *Ki-ras* and *N-ras*. All three can be mutated in this way in human tumours. Point mutations can also give recessive mutations. They can change an amino acid, disrupting the protein's function, or have a more drastic effect such as introducing a stop codon to give a shortened protein.

Gross rearrangement of protein-coding sequence

More substantial changes to a protein sequence can be made by deleting part of its coding sequence, or creating a hybrid protein by joining parts of two unrelated proteins together. We have already encountered a striking example of deletion of part of a protein-coding sequence in *erb-B*, the gene for the EGF receptor. In a mutant form of *erb-B* found in a retrovirus affecting birds, most of the extracellular portion of the protein product has been deleted to leave a truncated receptor that is permanently activated. A similar mutation has been found in some brain tumours in humans.

Table 17.1 Examples of mutation that occur in tumours.

Type of mutation	Example of gene affected	Example of human tumour in which mutation has been recorded
Oncogenes		
Point mutation	*ras*	Carcinomas of bladder and colon, acute myeloid leukaemia
Gross alteration of protein		
By truncation of protein	*erb-B*	Brain tumours
By fusion of unrelated proteins	*abl*	Translocated chromosome in chronic myeloid leukaemia
Inappropriate expression		
Inappropriate promoter inserted	*myc*	Burkitt's lymphoma
Deletion of regulatory sequences	*myc*	Burkitt's lymphoma
Amplification (multiple copies)	*myc*	Many, including squamous and breast carcinoma
Tumour suppressor genes		
Deletion	*Rb-1*	Retinoblastoma, breast carcinoma
Insertion of short sequence	*DCC*	Colon carcinoma
Point mutation		
Altering protein sequence	*p53*	Colon, breast and lung carcinoma
Altering splicing of message	*Rb-1*	Breast carcinoma
Prematurely terminating protein sequence	*APC*	Colon carcinoma

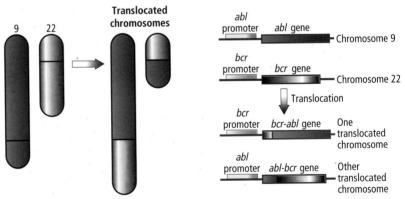

Figure 17.4 Fusion of genes in the chromosome translocation of chronic myeloid leukaemia. Most cases of chronic myeloid leukaemia have the characteristic reciprocal chromosome translocation that creates the Philadelphia chromosome. Parts of chromosomes 9 and 22 are interchanged (left). On one of the resulting chromosomes the 5' end of the *bcr* gene is joined to the 3' end of the *abl* gene to create a new hybrid gene. The expression of this hybrid is controlled by the *bcr* promoter region (right).

Fusion of unrelated proteins occurs as a result of some chromosome translocations. In chronic myeloid leukaemia a characteristic chromosome translocation occurs in which parts of chromosomes 22 and 9 are interchanged (Fig. 17.4, left). The effect of this is to join together part of the genes *abl* and *bcr* (Fig. 17.4, right), which were originally on the two separate chromosomes, to create a new gene *bcr-abl*. Normal Abl protein is a tyrosine kinase, an enzyme that adds phosphate groups to tyrosine residues in proteins, which in some way transmits signals that encourage cell division (see Fig. 17.2). When joined to Bcr, the Abl protein becomes a more active kinase. The new *bcr-abl* gene is also an example of the next type of mutation, because its expression is also affected by the translocation.

Altered expression of a gene

The expression of a gene may be altered, by changes in the sequences that control expression. Examples of this in human tumours are in chromosome translocations. Cells of Burkitt's lymphoma, a neoplasm of B cells, have a chromosome translocation that fuses the *myc* gene with part of the gene for immunoglobulin heavy chain. This can have several consequences: one is that one of the 'enhancer' sequences that direct high-level expression of immunoglobulin may be placed close to the *myc* gene and increases its expression, and another is that sequences in *myc* that control messenger RNA (mRNA) synthesis and stability may be removed. As already noted, Myc seems to be necessary for cell division and in normal cells its synthesis is very elaborately regulated. The overall effect of the chromosome translocation is that Myc protein is produced at inappropriate times or at too high a level, or both, and the B lymphocyte which is affected gains a growth advantage.

Another example is in the translocation that creates the *bcr-abl* hybrid gene. *abl* is not expressed much in normal myeloid cells, while *bcr* is expressed vigorously. The DNA sequences that control the expression of a gene are usually found upstream of the protein-coding sequence, so the *bcr-abl* fusion gene has the expression-controlling sequences of *bcr* and is expressed well in the leukaemic cells. The overall effect is that the Abl tyrosine kinase is expressed in an overactive form, in a cell that normally has little or no Abl.[3]

Amplification

Perhaps the simplest way an oncogene can be activated, and possibly one of the most frequent in human tumours, is for the whole gene to be reduplicated a number of times to give gene amplification, which apparently causes overproduction of the protein. This is well-documented for a number of (proto-) oncogenes; for example, *myc* and *erb-B2* (a gene related to *erb-B*) are each amplified in about 20% of breast carcinomas.

Inactivation of tumour suppressor genes

Tumour suppressor genes may be inactivated by similar or quite different mechanisms. The simplest of these is deletion of part or all of the gene. A more

3 *bcr* is probably a tumour suppressor gene, so the translocation may enhance cell proliferation even further by disabling the *bcr* gene.

subtle change with a similar effect has already been discussed — the case where a single base change alters a sequence that directs the splicing of mRNA so that an entire section of protein-coding sequence is lost from the mRNA produced. Another mechanism is the insertion of a sequence into the tumour suppressor gene. This has been described for the *DCC* gene, which is inactivated in colon carcinomas, where some examples have a short sequence inserted into a particular region of the gene. The nature of the inserted sequence is not yet known, but it could be a transposable element, one of a class of DNA sequences that can move around in the genome.

From every viewpoint the genetic damage that causes tumours is diverse

The genes that are altered in tumours code for all kinds of components of the pathways which control cell growth (see Fig. 17.2); the ways in which the alteration of the gene causes the gene to be overactive or inactive are very varied; and the alterations of the DNA sequence can also vary widely (Table 17.1). A cell can produce its own growth factor by changing the control of expression of the gene; two protein sequences can be joined to make a new protein with enhanced kinase activity; a sequence regulating the stability of mRNA can be lost from a gene that itself regulates gene expression; a DNA sequence may be inserted into a gene (*DCC*) encoding a cell–cell recognition protein, and so on. But we should not be surprised by this diversity — any mutation that can give a cell a growth advantage could be a tumour mutation, and that is the only thing we should expect to be a common factor.

Genetic instability is important in cancer development

Cells which have defects in their machinery for protecting and repairing DNA are particularly prone to mutation and so are more likely to become fully malignant tumour cells. It seems likely that **most tumour cells are genetically unstable** because only cells that are unstable could accumulate the number of mutations needed to give a fully malignant cell. It follows that some key mutations in the development of tumours may be genetic instability mutations rather than mutations that increase cell division. Mechanisms for repairing DNA can reverse some types of damage as long as they are able to act before replication occurs. In order to protect DNA, there are systems that stop its replication when it is damaged, allowing repair to proceed first. **Cells can therefore be cancer-prone if they have mutations in either their DNA-repair or DNA-protection genes.** Recently some of the causes of genetic instability in tumour cells have been identified. In particular, p53 seems to protect DNA by arresting cell division following damage to DNA, preventing replication until the damage has been repaired. Mutations in p53 will allow replication of damaged DNA, and have been shown to lead to an increased rate of DNA alteration. p53 is mutated in many, probably more than half of all human tumours, so is probably a key source of instability.

In hereditary cancer, individuals inherit mutations that predispose to tumours

Some individuals have a hereditary predisposition to cancer, which becomes obvious when several members of a family develop tumours, often of the same tissue. Those affected inherit from one of their parents a mutation that either causes genetic instability, as we have just discussed, or is one of the mutations contributing to tumour development, such as a mutated oncogene or tumour suppressor gene. As a result, all their body cells have that mutation.

A number of such hereditary predispositions or **hereditary cancer syndromes** are known or suspected. The first kind includes **hereditary non-polyposis colon carcinoma**, where a defective gene for one kind of DNA repair is inherited; and **Li-Fraumeni** syndrome where a mutation in p53 is inherited. Amongst the latter cases, examples include **retinoblastoma** and **adenomatous polyposis coli**. Hereditary retinoblastoma is important because, although it is a rare condition, it gave crucial insights into the nature of tumour suppressor genes. Retinoblastoma is a tumour of the eye which occurs in childhood, and 40% of cases are in individuals with the inherited predisposition. Nearly all who inherit the gene develop retinoblastoma—in fact they usually get multiple tumours. For a tumour to develop, a retinoblast has to have lost the influence of both copies of the gene *Rb-1*. This may result from either mutation or actual loss of the gene. In hereditary cases, the individual inherits one mutant copy of the gene and it only requires a single retinoblast to lose the remaining normal copy for a tumour to arise. In non-hereditary cases, both genes must be affected after conception. In familial adenomatous polyposis coli (APC), affected individuals develop large numbers of adenomas of the colon in early adult life as a result of inheriting a mutant *APC* tumour suppressor gene. Of more practical importance, in breast and ovarian cancer, statistical models suggest that perhaps 10% of cases occur in patients who have an inherited predisposition. Most of these women have inherited a mutant gene, either one called *BRCA1* on chromosome 17 or one on chromosome 13 called *BRCA2*, which give a probability of developing breast cancer of over 50%. Overall, these predispositions are not just rare curiosities; they may well account for over 10% of all cancer.

DNA tumour viruses mimic tumour mutations

So far we have made the slight oversimplification that tumours are caused by damage to DNA, and have ignored the possible contribution made by DNA tumour viruses to such tumours as Burkitt's lymphoma and carcinoma of the cervix (see Chapter 18). DNA tumour viruses such as Epstein–Barr virus and certain human papillomaviruses have specialized genes that affect cells in much the same way as tumour mutations, so that the virus takes the infected cell one or more steps along the pathway to neoplasia. The virus genes add to the complement of genes controlling the cell's behaviour, so our concept that cancer is a disease of altered genetic information embraces this effect of DNA tumour viruses.

In fact, the effects of some DNA tumour viruses may mimic tumour mutations very closely. Some of the papillomaviruses, for example, have transforming proteins that interact with the protein products of the tumour suppressor genes *Rb-1* and *p53*. Presumably the transforming proteins inactivate the Rb-1 and p53 proteins, and their effects on the cell will be similar to inactivation of both copies of these genes.

Summary

Cancer is caused by damage to a cell's genes. The evidence for this is now very strong: neoplasms have characteristic changes to their genes that are found only in the neoplasms and not in neighbouring normal cells; and when the altered forms of these genes are introduced into normal cells they confer neoplastic properties. **Several, probably five or more genes have to be altered to give a fully malignant cell.** The mutations occur in genes that normally regulate cell division and tissue architecture. For example, a receptor for a growth-stimulating signal may be mutated so that it permanently stimulates cell division, or a protein that halts cell division may be lost because its gene is deleted. The genetic changes found in neoplasms may be classified according to whether they are dominant or recessive mutations in the cell, and they are called respectively **oncogene** and **tumour suppressor gene mutations**. Both are important in human cancer. Neoplastic cells often have damaged systems for repairing or protecting DNA so they are unusually susceptible to mutations. This makes it possible for the cell to acquire sufficient mutations to become malignant. Some individuals are predisposed to developing cancer because they inherit either an oncogene or tumour suppressor gene mutation, or a defect in DNA repair.

18

Cancer: the causes

Perhaps the most important topic in the study of cancer is its causation, because to identify and control its causes would be far more valuable than struggling to treat the disease. Unfortunately, the overall message of this section is that we have made very little progress on this front and are still largely ignorant of the important causes of human cancer, with the exception of smoking tobacco. **Tobacco smoke is estimated to cause at least 30% of cancer** in the UK, and allowing for the effects of smoke on non-smokers, the figure could be higher. One consequence of our ignorance overall is that there are many popular myths about carcinogens. A recurring theme of this chapter is the unreliability of both the myths and our scientific information about carcinogens.

Cancer incidence is largely determined by environment

The incidence of different neoplasms varies between human populations. This could be due to genetic differences or to environment and behaviour. To distinguish between these, epidemiologists have studied the **diseases of migrant populations** such as Japanese immigrants to the west coast of the USA, who changed from having the Japanese pattern—a high incidence of stomach cancer but a low incidence of breast cancer—to the American pattern, which is the reverse. Also, some neoplasms common in the developed world, e.g. those of the large bowel and breast, are generally relatively uncommon in under-developed countries, whereas the opposite is true for others such as primary liver carcinoma. From such comparisons it is argued that perhaps 90% of carcinomas of the colon and 80% of breast carcinomas in the USA are caused by avoidable factors in the environment, or possibly behaviour.

One important misconception is that much of our present cancer incidence in the western world is caused by contemporary environmental problems, such as pollution and food additives. The incidence of the most important cancers has in fact changed very little since the beginning of this century—certainly not by as large a factor as separates different cultures. The main exception to this is lung cancer, attributable to smoking.

Mutagens are the major but not the only causes of cancer

Cancer results from alteration of DNA sequences, so many of its causes are probably **agents that damage DNA directly**, such as chemicals that react with DNA and alter its structure, and nuclear radiation, which breaks strands of DNA. However it is important to remember that there may be other factors that do not directly damage DNA, but make that damage more likely, or encourage the growth of cells that have been mutated. In addition, some human tumours are caused in part by viruses which, as well as altering the genetic programme of a cell, may make mutation more likely because of increased cell turnover.

These are the causes of cancer.

1 Agents that directly damage DNA–radiation, ultraviolet light and mutagenic chemicals.

2 Agents that do not directly damage DNA: non-mutagenic chemicals or promoters.

3 Other causes: chronic irritation, damage to tissue or abnormally high cell turnover; aberrations of DNA replication and cell division.

4 Tumour viruses.

There is some overlap between these categories. For example, non-mutagenic chemicals and tumour viruses may both act by causing chronic irritation, damage to cells or increasing cell turnover.

Agents that directly damage DNA

Radiation

Radiation, or more correctly **ionizing radiation**, occurs in various forms and comes from various sources. They include X-rays, which can come from medical sources and electrical equipment; and the products of radioactive decay and cosmic rays, which include γ-rays, neutrons, β particles (free electrons) and α particles (charged helium nuclei).

Radiation damages DNA by producing free radicals and ions as it passes through tissue, which then react with DNA and alter the structure of bases or cause strand breaks.

Exposure to radiation is measured as the amount of energy absorbed per unit of tissue: the unit in current use is the **gray** (Gy)[1] which is joules absorbed per kilogram tissue. Different types of radiation give more or less damage for a given amount of energy absorbed, as illustrated in Fig. 18.1. **α Particles** leave dense tracks of ions and radicals, so that if they pass by a DNA helix they are likely to cause double-strand breaks or multiple chemical changes. γ-**Rays** on the other hand leave scattered ions and radicals and so will usually only damage one residue on one strand of a DNA molecule. As we shall see, **damage to DNA can often be repaired**, but single hits or strand breaks are much more readily repaired than double or multiple ones. As a result, α particles are much more likely to cause permanent damage to DNA than γ-rays, for a given dose measured in grays. To make some allowance for this, the measure of exposure to radiation in grays is often multiplied by a **quality factor** for the particular type of radiation, to give an approximate measure of biological damage or **dose equivalent**, which is measured in **sieverts** (Sv). Quality factor is 1 for X-rays and γ-rays and ranges up to 20 for α particles.[2]

In the UK, annual exposure of the general population to radiation is estimated to average 2.5 mSv. Half of this comes from the radioactive gas **radon**, which is formed by natural radioactive decay of minerals in the earth and seeps out of the ground into the air in houses. About one-eighth results from medical

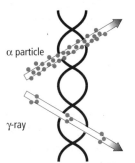

Figure 18.1 Damage done by different kinds of radiation. Schematic illustration of the ionizing events along the track of an α particle and a γ-ray photon, in comparison with the size of a DNA molecule. The α particle will almost inevitably damage the DNA and may cause double-strand breaks, while a γ-ray will leave occasional radicals and ions and the damage will usually be milder.

α particle

γ-ray

1 The gray supersedes the rad: 1 Gy = 100 rad.

2 1990 recommendation. Values for the quality factor are revised from time to time.

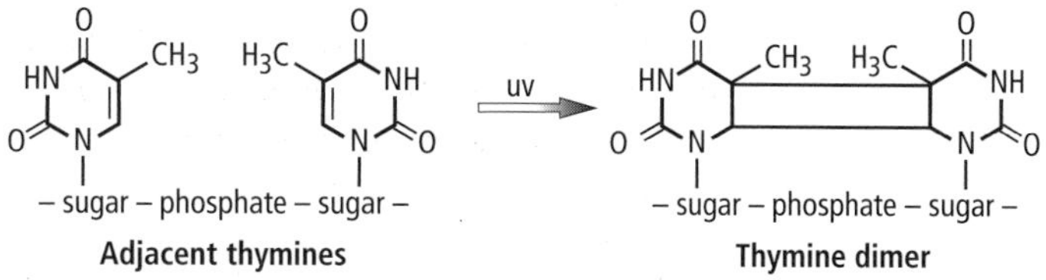

Figure 18.2 Formation of thymine dimers. Ultraviolet light can cause adjacent thymines to dimerize.

exposure and around one-hundredth from fallout, including that from the Chernobyl disaster. This average exposure of 2.5 mSv/year is probably not a very important source of cancer overall.

Ultraviolet light

Ultraviolet light, principally from sunlight, but also from synthetic sources, is another important mutagen. It is presumed to be the cause of the high incidence of skin cancers in white Australians. Its principal effect is to photoactivate pyrimidine residues in DNA so that they form dimers in which two thymines or a thymine and a cytosine occur sequentially in the DNA (Fig. 18.2), and base-pairing can be disrupted.

Mutagenic chemicals

Among the chemicals that we know are potent carcinogens, most are mutagenic, and many of these fall into the categories illustrated in Fig. 18.3.

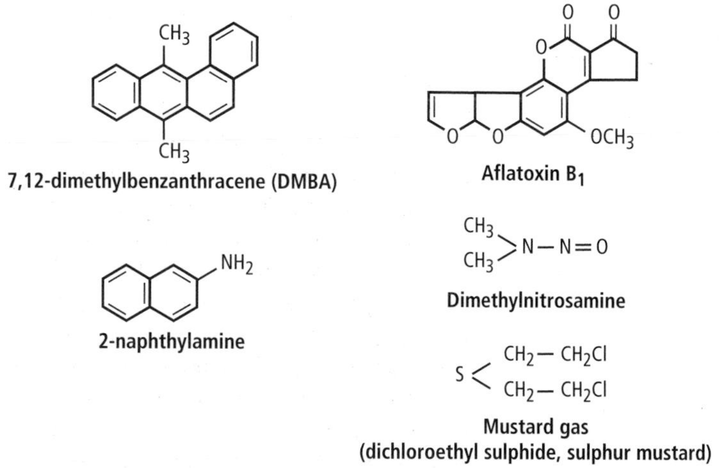

Figure 18.3 Examples of known chemical carcinogens. Many known carcinogens fall into one of the groups of substances shown here: the aromatic hydrocarbons, such as dimethylbenzanthracene (DMBA); the aromatic amines such as 2-naphthylamine; more complex aromatic compounds such as the natural product aflatoxin B_1; the nitrosamines such as dimethylnitrosamine; and the alkylating agents such as mustard gas.

The first group of carcinogens shown in Fig. 18.3 are the **aromatic hydrocarbons** such as dimethylbenzanthracene (DMBA), which occur in smoke and coal tar. Closely related are the **aromatic amines** such as **2-naphthylamine**, which are used in the dyestuffs industry. Other more complex aromatic compounds include the **aflatoxins**, naturally occurring products of fungi.

The **nitrosamines** are quite different, formed by the condensation of an amine and nitrous acid. Such reactions can occur in the acid environment of the stomach. The resulting nitrosamines are probably too unstable to occur in the environment.

Then there are a group of chemically very reactive compounds, called the **alkylating agents** because they tend to add alkyl groups to other molecules. The classic example is **mustard gas**.

There are other carcinogens that do not fall into any of these groups.

One of the compounds in Fig. 18.3 explodes another myth about carcinogens —that they are synthetic. **Aflatoxin B$_1$ is possibly the most powerful carcinogen known**, at least when assayed in rats, and it is a natural substance, produced by the fungus *Aspergillus flavus*, a contaminant of ground nuts (peanuts), which may grow on the nuts when they are stored in warm humid conditions. The toxin was discovered as a result of a widespread outbreak of liver failure in turkeys that had been fed peanuts. When the toxicity was investigated, it was found that lower doses over longer periods caused carcinoma of the liver. It is thought that aflatoxins or similar fungal products may be important as contributory causes of human cancer, particularly in Africa and China, where carcinoma of the liver is relatively common.

Mutagenic chemicals usually need to be metabolized to an active form

The most potent chemical carcinogens are more or less inert chemically, in the form to which we are exposed, and are only **metabolized to an active form by the cell**. The carcinogens formed in this way are so highly reactive that, if introduced as such into the body, they would react with something else before they reached the DNA. The one example in Fig. 18.3 that does not need to be activated by metabolism is mustard gas, and it is a much less potent carcinogen than the others.

Ironically, the cellular enzymes that activate carcinogens are generally part of systems that have evolved to render harmless or **detoxify lipid-soluble molecules** that the body needs to eliminate, by making more soluble derivatives, that can be excreted. Examples of carcinogens created by such enzymes are shown in Figs 18.4 and 18.5. A hydrogen atom attached to a carbon may be replaced by a hydroxyl group. Alternatively, a carbon-carbon double bond may be oxidized to an epoxide which can then be hydrated to give two hydroxyl groups. Hydroxyl groups may then have the sugar acid, glucuronic acid, added to them. All these steps increase the water-solubility of the compound. Unfortunately, some of the epoxides **created as intermediates are highly reactive with DNA**—aflatoxin is activated in this way (Fig. 18.4).

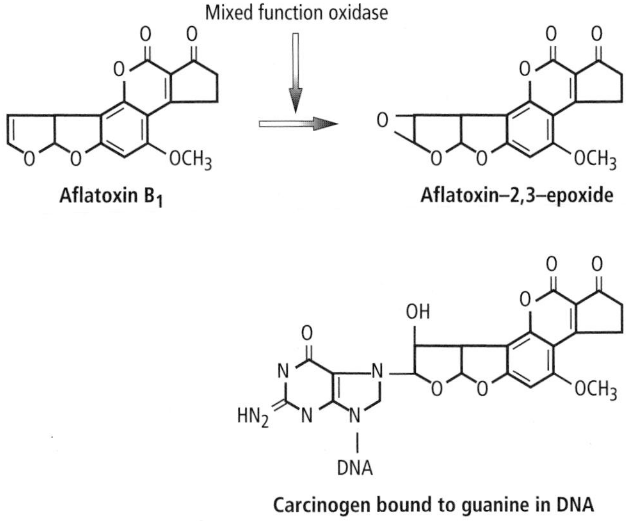

Figure 18.4 Activation of aflatoxin by metabolism. Aflatoxin is activated to a highly reactive epoxide by oxidases, enzymes that add oxygen atoms to substrates. The epoxide can react with a DNA base as shown.

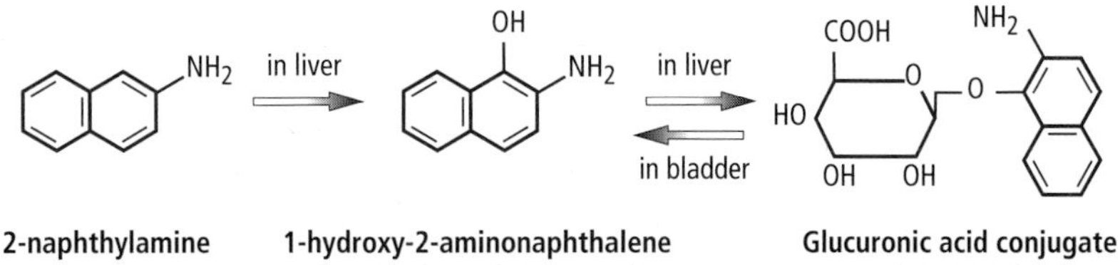

Aflatoxin B$_1$

Mixed function oxidase

Aflatoxin–2,3–epoxide

Carcinogen bound to guanine in DNA

2-naphthylamine

in liver

1-hydroxy-2-aminonaphthalene
(reactive form of carcinogen)

in liver

in bladder

Glucuronic acid conjugate
(unreactive)

Figure 18.5 Activation of 2-naphthylamine by metabolism. 2-naphthylamine is activated by addition of a hydroxyl group in the liver. It is then rapidly converted to a harmless derivative by addition of a glucuronyl group, and is then excreted in the urine. However, in certain species, the glucuronyl group is later removed in the bladder to regenerate the reactive compound.

Mutagenic chemicals tend to be tissue-specific in action

Many carcinogens have a characteristic target tissue. For example, **2-naphthylamine** can cause cancer in the bladder in humans, because the bladder activates the molecule to create a carcinogen (Fig. 18.5). Some carcinogens not only act specifically on a tissue but the stage of development of the animal can change their specificity. When **nitroso-methyl-urea** is fed to pubescent female rats it causes mainly mammary tumours but, when it is fed to pregnant rats, the principal effect is that their offspring develop tumours after birth, predominantly in cells of the nervous system. What causes this tissue-specificity is not fully understood, but one factor is tissue-specific metabolism, as in the case of 2-naphthylamine. Another major factor may be that the target tissue is in a particularly receptive state, typically because of rapid cell proliferation. For example, in pubescent female rats the mammary gland is at a peak of cell growth as the glandular epithelium develops and, in the pregnant

315

animals, it is the cells of the fetal nervous system which are proliferating rapidly.

Mutagenic chemicals often show species-specificity

The potency of carcinogens often varies between species. For example, 2-naphthylamine is a potent bladder carcinogen only in species that have bladder glucuronidase, such as dogs and humans. Another example is **benzidine**, which is a bladder carcinogen in humans but causes mainly liver tumours in rats. Again the mechanism is not fully understood, but differences in metabolism are likely to be the major factor. Different species tend to have different detoxifying enzymes. These may have evolved to deal optimally with particular substances to which that species tends to be exposed.

Not all mutagenic chemicals damage DNA by reacting directly with its bases

The reactive molecules discussed so far generally attach to the bases of DNA. For example, aflatoxin, after metabolic activation, reacts with guanine to produce a large derivative which is unable to take part in normal base-pairing (Fig. 18.4). But not all mutagens have to react chemically with the DNA, though they may interact with it: one important class of mutagens inserts or **intercalates between the bases of the helix**; in other words, they bind non-covalently between successive bases. If this occurs during replication or repair of the DNA, the intercalated molecule may be taken to be a base and another base may be inserted or deleted to compensate for it. As a result, if the altered DNA encodes a protein sequence, the reading of the genetic code gets out of phase and a **frame-shift mutation** occurs. An example of a molecule that intercalates and causes frame-shift mutations is **diaminoacridine**.

DNA may be damaged spontaneously

Finally, it is worth remembering that occasional damage to DNA occurs without any direct intervention by outside agents—as in errors of replication, recombination during mitosis, and even spontaneous hydrolysis by water. It has long been observed that aberrant mitoses occur in tumours, so the later mutations in the development and progression of tumours may well arise because the dividing neoplastic cell has become prone to such spontaneous genetic accidents.

Damage to DNA can often be repaired

Cells have a variety of enzyme systems that can repair different kinds of damage. For example, pyrimidine dimers formed by ultraviolet light (see Fig. 18.2) can be recognized by an enzyme, removed, and replaced by new thymine residues synthesized using the complementary strand as template. The sequences of reactions that achieve this are shown in Fig. 18.6.

The importance of DNA repair is shown when hereditary deficiencies of particular repair systems occur. In **xeroderma pigmentosum**, patients inherit

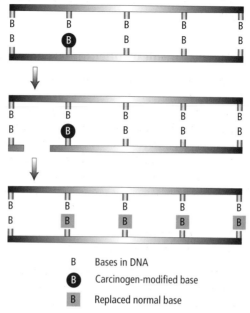

B	Bases in DNA
B	Carcinogen-modified base
B	Replaced normal base

Figure 18.6 An example of a DNA repair pathway. One pathway by which damaged DNA can be repaired; it is used for example to remove thymine dimers. The initial event is cutting of the altered strand adjacent to the aberrant base. A few residues are then removed by an exonuclease, the missing nucleotides are resynthesized by a DNA polymerase, and the strand is rejoined by the enzyme ligase.

an inability to repair pyrimidine dimers (Figs 18.2 and 18.6), so they are very sensitive to mutation by ultraviolet light, and develop skin cancers unless protected. Another hereditary DNA repair defect produces the complex syndrome **ataxia telangiectasia**, which probably includes predisposition to breast cancer.[3]

The success of DNA repair depends on the type of damage. To take a simple example, a large modified base can be identified and removed accurately but, if a double-strand break occurs, repair mechanisms can probably only rejoin the DNA without knowing which strand should join to which and, in many cases, opposite strands will be joined. If one base is replaced by another so it cannot pair properly, the DNA repair mechanism will alter one of the mismatched bases, but whether it alters the faulty one or the correct one may be a matter of chance.

DNA repair can only occur when the helix is recognizable as imperfect

It is a common misconception that DNA repair mechanisms can correct an altered DNA sequence. This is wishful thinking. Repair mechanisms work only by recognizing that there is something structurally wrong with the DNA helix —a strand is broken, a pair of bases on opposite strands is not properly matched, or a base has an alien structure. The repair enzymes cannot recognize an altered sequence of bases if base-pairing is correct. So repair to damaged

3 These repair defects are recessive mutations and so sufferers are rare. However, carriers are more common, and they may be predisposed to cancer.

317

DNA can only occur while the DNA structure is incorrect. Once the helix structure has been corrected, even though occasionally the sequence of bases may have been changed, DNA repair mechanisms are unable to take any further action.

Promoters increase the effect of mutagens

Apart from mutagenic chemicals there are other chemicals that **promote** the development of tumours without damaging DNA. They were originally discovered by studying carcinogenesis in mouse skin. Test substances were painted on the skin of mice, and those giving rise to squamous papillomas were called carcinogens. It emerged that two kinds of carcinogenic substances could be distinguished, which were called **initiators** and **promoters**. A high yield of papillomas could be obtained by using a combination of initiator and promoter. Their properties are compared in Table 18.1. **The initiators are chemical mutagens** like DMBA and are **effective when applied in a single dose**. In modest doses on their own they produce a negligible number of papillomas. The tumour promoters, of which the best known example is tetradecanoyl phorbol acetate (TPA), **only have an effect if applied after an initiator and have to be painted on repeatedly** over a period of time to be effective. The **effect of an initiator is permanent**, and months can elapse before application of promoter. There is no threshold dose nor plateau above which increasing dose of initiator produces no further papillomas. **Promoters on the other hand elicit a drug-like dose–response**: there is a threshold concentration below which they have little activity and their effect plateaus above a certain dose. All these findings are consistent with the initiator being a mutagen and the promoter acting like a drug to encourage outgrowth of mutated cells. Recently it had been shown that, in the mouse skin system, the critical mutation caused by the initiator is often activation of an oncogene of the *ras* family. TPA is indeed drug-like: it is an activator of protein kinase C, an enzyme inside cells involved in transmitting mitogenic signals. It can therefore reduce the extent of communication between neighbouring cells through gap junctions; this may allow a clone of abnormal cells to escape from the restraining influence of their normal neighbours.

Table 18.1 A comparison of the properties of initiators and promoters.

	Initiator	Promoter
Example	DMBA (dimethylbenzanthracene)	TPA (tetradecanoyl phorbol acetate)
Dose schedule needed	Single dose	Repeated application
Effective alone?	No effect alone, unless very large dose	No effect alone, only works after initiation
Reversible?	Irreversible	Reversible
Dose dependence	Dose-dependent, no upper limit or threshold	Threshold and plateau
Overall character	Mutagen	Drug

Just as the most potent mutagenic carcinogen known, aflatoxin, is a natural product, so are the most potent promoters. TPA is the active principle of croton oil, which comes from the seeds of the tropical plant *Croton tiglium*.

Many kinds of agent or circumstances may be promoters

Anything that increases the number of neoplasms that develop, without directly causing mutation, can be considered to be a tumour promoter. For example, anything that increases cell division could be a promoter, because **tumours tend to develop more readily in dividing cell populations**. This may be because dividing cells are more susceptible to carcinogens, or a large cluster of mutant cells may escape from the controlling influence of surrounding cells. Among agents that are likely to act as promoters we may therefore include anything that causes cell death and regeneration, particularly over a long period, as in chronic inflammation.[4]

Some examples will show the range of agents that might be considered as promoters. One is the tendency for actors and singers to get carcinoma of the larynx. Hormones may also act as promoters. There has been concern, for example, that the contraceptive pill might act as a promoter of breast cancer. One of the best-known carcinogens is **asbestos**, which can cause **mesothelioma**, a neoplasm of the pleura. It seems rather unlikely that asbestos fibres are mutagenic, so they should probably be considered as a promoter. They may act by damaging cells and causing increased cell turnover, though more complex mechanisms have been proposed. It has also been argued that cigarette smoke might act as a promoter as well as a mutagen, on the grounds that people who give up smoking get less lung cancer than might be expected if smoke was only acting as a mutagen.

Summary

Cancer incidence varies between human populations and most of this variation seems to be environmental. Agents known to cause cancer include mutagens—mutagenic chemicals, ultraviolet light and ionizing radiation—but also a variety of non-mutagenic chemicals, certain viruses, and other agents or circumstances that cause increased cell turnover, such as in chronic inflammation. The potent mutagenic carcinogens are mostly rather inert chemically until activated by metabolism. Typically they are lipophilic molecules that are metabolized in cells to more water-soluble derivatives, via intermediates that are highly chemically reactive. Some carcinogens show tissue-specificity and often also species-specificity, partly because of variations in metabolism. Ionizing radiation creates ions and radicals that react with DNA. DNA that has been damaged by chemical mutagens or radiation can often, but not always, be repaired. Non-mutagenic chemicals that help the development of cancer are called promoters. They may for example increase cell division or allow mutant cells to escape from the restraining influence of neighbouring cells.

4 Agents that cause inflammation might also encourage tumour development by causing phagocytic cells to produce radicals which might be mutagenic.

Identifying causes of cancer and assessing their importance

There are great difficulties in trying to test substances to see if they are carcinogens of significance to human populations. The size of the problem is enormous. It is estimated that we are exposed to 60 000 different natural or synthetic chemicals. In investigating the system, **we need to know two things**: first, whether a substance is **capable** of acting as a mutagen or promoter; and second, how **potent** it is—how much exposure to it can be considered safe. We need to know how potent mutagens are because it is unrealistic to attempt to eliminate all of them from our environment. For example, among the substances that have been shown to be mutagenic are oxygen and tomatoes: exposure to oxygen is unavoidable and we would not want to give up tomatoes until we knew how much they increased our risk of cancer. Also there are sometimes dangers in eliminating a carcinogen: a fungicide that was used to stop growth of moulds on agricultural produce was judged to be a mild carcinogen on the basis of animal tests, and was therefore banned. This may have caused 50 times as many cancers as it saved, because the increased growth of fungus may have contaminated food with carcinogens like aflatoxins. A further problem is that, although we have some methods for testing for mutagenicity, we do not have assays for promoter action.

Epidemiology can sometimes suggest a cause of cancer, but has its limitations

Most of the carcinogens that are known to cause cancer in humans were discovered because particular people exposed to them developed particular kinds of tumour. For example, some workers in the dyestuffs industry exposed to 2-naphthylamine developed bladder cancer and some workers exposed to asbestos developed mesothelioma. Unfortunately, this approach has only revealed about 20 carcinogens and in general they are not substances that cause a significant amount of cancer in the general population. This is inevitable because, to identify carcinogens using this method, people exposed have to be clearly identifiable and the cancer they suffer has to be either very frequent, which is unlikely, or of an unusual type so that the extra cases are obvious. Thus it is unlikely that we could use this approach to identify a substance that causes a common cancer, because we are probably all exposed to it.

Tobacco smoke is an exception to the generalization that epidemiology has limited power to identify important carcinogens. The reason that it has been so clearly identified as a carcinogen is that it is easy to distinguish people who are heavily exposed (smokers) from those who are only lightly exposed (non-smokers), and it is the cause of most carcinomas of the bronchus, so the link was easily established. Even so, it has been impossible so far to estimate reliably the number of cancers caused by passive smoking (i.e. non-smokers inhaling tobacco smoke) because essentially everyone is exposed. One approach had been to compare cancer incidence in non-smokers who live in smoking and non-smoking households: this approach suggests that non-smokers exposed to tobacco smoke have significantly increased risk of cancer—two- to threefold according to some studies.

Animal experiments can identify carcinogens

Since we cannot test potential carcinogens on human beings, the most straight-forward alternative is to test on animals. The technique is to expose animals to as high a dose as possible for as long as possible and monitor tumour development. Large doses are used in the hope of demonstrating a significant tumour incidence, so that it is not necessary to use very large numbers of animals. In the standard test, 50 animals of each of two species, usually mice and rats, of each sex, are exposed for 2 years. Although testing on animals is the next best thing to testing on humans, we would obviously prefer to minimize the use of animals for such work, and the tests are slow and expensive.

In vitro testing is more humane, cheaper and quicker, but less satisfactory

Many attempts have been made to devise *in vitro* tests for carcinogens. In general they are simpler, more reproducible, quicker and cheaper, but they are so artificial that it is difficult to know how useful they are. In particular they have only limited ability to reveal carcinogens that require metabolic activation.

Bacterial mutagenicity testing

The simplest tests use bacteria and test directly for mutagenicity. The strategy generally adopted is to isolate a bacterium containing a small mutation that prevents it from growing on a certain medium. A large number of these bacteria are exposed to a test chemical. Mutagens that can reverse the small mutation will then convert a small number of the bacteria to wild-type cells that will multiply on the medium to form colonies, thus revealing the mutagenic activity.

The most important known limitation of this assay is the absence of metabolism of the potential carcinogen. An attempt to solve this problem is to add crude preparations of enzymes from mammalian cells to the assay. Unfortunately, since we don't know what the carcinogens are that we need to discover, we have no way of confirming that they would give positive results in such an assay.

Tests on mammalian cells in culture

Tests for mutagenicity can also be performed using mammalian cells in culture, which may mimic more accurately conditions in the human body. Mutant cells can be selected that have defects in metabolic pathways, and used to test for mutations that reverse the defect, as in bacterial assays. Alternatively, chromosome damage can be assessed.

Unfortunately, the **tests on mammalian cells in culture are far from satisfactory**. Mammalian cell culture is technically difficult and uses expensive materials and equipment; it is difficult to derive mutant cell lines for tests on reversion; and assessing chromosome damage is very laborious. Another major problem is how poorly cell culture mimics the properties of cells in an organism. Cells in culture usually lose most of the detailed differentiated characteristics of cells in living tissue. A particularly important example of this is the rapid and almost complete loss of the metabolic characteristics of liver cells in culture. The detoxifying enzymes that are central to the activation of carcinogens are almost entirely lost in conventional cell culture. In addition all interrelationships of different cell types are lost in tissue culture, so for example it could not reveal the action of 2-naphthylamine (see Fig. 18.5).

Interpreting the results of carcinogenicity testing is extremely difficult

It is difficult to interpret the results of carcinogenicity testing, even in animals, and even more difficult to decide how to use the information. A recent review found that, of 800 compounds that had been tested, 65% gave a significant increase in tumours in at least one organ. A substantial proportion of these actually lowered the incidence of tumours in another organ, so it is not clear whether overall they should be considered harmful. We would like to play safe and consider all the 65% that give an increase in tumours as hazardous. However, this is of no practical value because not only can we not afford to ban 65% of chemicals in use, but if 65% of all 60 000 chemicals in use are carcinogens, they individually, on average, only cause 1/40 000th of cancer, so individually they are not dangerous enough to matter. A further problem is that only 70% of the chemicals that give a positive result in rats give a positive result in mice, and vice versa. Since mice and rats are far more closely related to each other than either are to humans, there is doubt about extrapolating the results to humans. The precise difficulty here is that the **compounds concerned are carcinogens in certain circumstances, but the dose at which they are effective is completely unknown, so the risk they pose is unknown**.

Estimating the risk of exposure to agents that cause cancer

As already discussed, we need to know not only what agents can cause cancer but how much cancer they will cause in real situations. This is best discussed in terms of the risk of cancer to people exposed in real situations. To estimate the hazard of exposure to a carcinogenic agent we need to know how many mutations or tumours are caused by a certain dose, and how this relates to the doses received in practice. Usually the data come from the effect of a relatively large dose that causes a high incidence of cancer, because then the rate of extra cancers can be clearly measured above background. However, we are most interested in doses that cause a small increase as these are likely to be of practical importance. Extrapolating from the effects of high doses to the effect of a small dose is a very uncertain process, the most obvious question being whether the number of extra cancers is linearly related to dose of carcinogen, as we shall debate in detail for radiation exposure (Fig. 18.7).

The only cancer-causing agent for which the risk of exposure has been estimated in detail is ionizing radiation, because for chemical carcinogens we

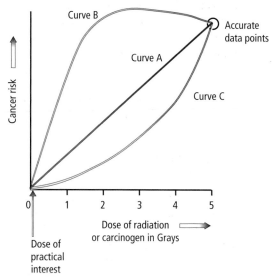

Figure 18.7 How much cancer can a cancer-causing agent cause? The problem of extrapolating from high exposure to low exposure. We need to know how much cancer risk there is from exposure to an agent that causes cancer, but usually the only data we have are from the effects of high doses of the agent, so we have to extrapolate down to low doses. Data for radiation exposure are accurate at doses of several Grays, but we want to know, for example, what the effect of exposure to radon in houses is where the dose may be 0.01 Gy. Unfortunately, we do not know how this extrapolation should be done, as different experimental models give different curves for genetic damage versus dose. Curve A is the linear relationship and is found when the number of chromosome aberrations in cultured cells is measured following exposure to neutrons. Curve B is the incidence of myeloid leukaemia in mice irradiated with X-rays. Curve C is the incidence of chromosome aberrations in cultured cells exposed to γ-rays.

generally have little information about how many tumours a given dose will give. In considering how the calculation is done for radiation, bear in mind that we would like to make the same calculation for all carcinogens.

Estimating the risk of cancer due to radiation

Data on the effects of radiation come from people exposed to relatively high doses. Up to about 3 Sv irradiation has no gross effect on humans. Individuals who receive between 3 and 8 Sv suffer serious damage to bone marrow, but they may recover if protected from infection, impaired blood clotting due to loss of platelets, etc. Above 8 Sv, diarrhoea and vomiting occur and bone marrow failure ensues. Above about 12 Sv damage to the gut is likely to be fatal. **People exposed to irradiation show an increased incidence of leukaemia,** which begins to appear about 2 years after exposure. **Later there is an increase in solid tissue tumours,** which is only evident after about 15 years.[5] For example, some patients with ankylosing spondylitis (a disease of the spine) were treated with X-rays in the period 1935–1954. On average they received about 3 Gy and they later showed about a fivefold increase in leukaemia incidence.

5 The stage of development of tissue affects its radiation sensitivity. For example, a given dose of radiation is more effective at generating breast cancer in younger women.

323

By far the largest body of information comes from detailed studies of 120 000 survivors of the atomic bombs dropped on Hiroshima and Nagasaki in 1945. Unfortunately, the interpretation of this crucial data depends on estimating the radiation that reached the ground. Simulations were therefore performed in the Nevada desert in western USA. The conclusions of this study were reported in 1965 and form the basis of much of our estimates of the carcinogenicity of radiation. It was then realized that an important correction needed to be applied to the data to account for atmospheric conditions. A new study was begun in 1980 and published in 1987. The revised estimates of radiation dose received by the survivors were lower by up to a factor of 10 — in other words this later study suggests that radiation is substantially more carcinogenic than the earlier estimates. At the time of writing, much of the data in use are still based on the earlier calibration.

But the uncertainty surrounding the data is only part of the problem in estimating the effect of the low doses of radiation that we might receive during, for example, transatlantic flights or as a result of the Chernobyl accident. These doses are of the order of 0.01 Gy. The only way to estimate the effect of such doses is to extrapolate from high to low doses. Consider Fig. 18.7: we have to draw a line from the data at high doses to a low dose — but should the line be straight, or a curve up, or a curve down? A straight line (A) would imply that the effect of a particle of radiation was independent of other particles, but often this is not the case. DNA repair may cope better with individual hits than a shower of hits occurring in a short time, and we have already seen (Fig. 18.1) that particles that leave dense tracks of ions and free radicals are more likely to create double-strand breaks which are less likely to be correctly repaired. These effects tend to give an upward curve to the dose-effect curve — curve C in Fig. 18.7. On the other hand, at high doses of radiation a significant number of cells are killed or disabled and are unable to form the beginning of a tumour. This effect causes the reverse curvature, like curve B in Fig. 18.7. Experimentally, all of these patterns can be found. Figure 18.7 shows the straight-line relationship for the incidence of chromosome damage in cultured cells, caused by radiation that leaves a dense track of events, while the upward curve C is taken from the results of the same experiment for γ-rays. Curve B shows the downward curve obtained for radiation-induced leukaemia in mice. The data for increased leukaemia in the ankylosing spondylitis patients fit this curve slightly better than the straight line. The raw data for Hiroshima and Nagasaki are too scattered to fit one curve best.

In conclusion, although much care and thought goes into estimates of radiation carcinogenicity, there remains enormous uncertainty. While we can say with some confidence that **for the vast majority of people radiation presents a negligible hazard**, we are on much shakier ground when it comes to deciding how much radon we should tolerate in our homes, or how many deaths the fallout from Chernobyl will cause.

This also shows how difficult it will be to arrive at the effect of a certain dose of a chemical carcinogen, even when we have solved the problem of estimating the number of cancers caused in humans by a high dose.

Summary

We do not have satisfactory ways of identifying carcinogens that are important to the general human population. We need two kinds of information: whether a substance is carcinogenic, and how potent it is. Epidemiology has shown that tobacco smoke is the most important known carcinogen and has identified some carcinogens of industrial importance, but in general is ineffective in the identification of carcinogens to which most of the population is exposed. Animal tests and *in vitro* tests using bacteria or cultured cells have been devised to show whether a substance can be carcinogenic, but they have severe limitations, giving too many positive results, and only a few of the substances to which we are exposed have been tested. There is no reliable method of estimating the potency of carcinogens. Quantitative estimates of the effect of exposure are more advanced for radiation than for carcinogens, but even in this case we are uncertain how to extrapolate from the measurable effects of high doses down to what we most need to know — the effect of low doses.

Viruses in human cancer

There has been much debate over the role of viruses in human cancer

Since 1911, when Rous discovered a virus that caused sarcoma in chickens, there has been debate about whether viruses cause cancer in humans. The **Rous sarcoma virus** is a retrovirus, and a variety of other retroviruses that cause tumours in mice, rats and chickens have been discovered since. Subsequently a variety of DNA viruses were discovered that cause tumours in animals, for example, the **Shope papillomavirus** which causes papillomas (warts) in rabbits; the **SV40 virus** and **adenoviruses** which cause tumours in young rodents; and **Marek's virus** which is a herpesvirus that causes tumours in turkeys.

These discoveries led some to argue that viruses must be important in human cancer, while others felt that most of these viruses were only relevant to domesticated animals, and were misleading. As a result, the importance of viruses in human cancer has remained controversial until recently.

Viruses do play an important role in certain specific human cancers

Two sorts of evidence implicate viruses in the development of some human neoplasms. The first is the **presence of viral nucleic acid sequences in tumour cells**: the second is an **epidemiological link** between infection by a particular virus and the incidence of a particular neoplasm. Thus, the consistent finding of **Epstein–Barr virus** (EBV) DNA in nasopharyngeal carcinoma cells convinces us that EBV must be involved in the cause of this tumour. By contrast, the evidence that **hepatitis B virus** (HBV) is oncogenic is that infection with HBV is associated with a high risk of primary liver cancer in all populations regardless of racial or environmental factors.

Our current view is that **viruses are involved in the development of only a few human neoplasms**, notably **liver cancer, carcinoma of the cervix** and **nasopharyngeal carcinoma**, and there is no evidence at present to link viruses with other tumours such as those of the breast, lung or colon. However, worldwide, the virus-associated tumours are among the most frequent and, as there are practical hopes for prevention of a virus-induced cancer, by immunizing or preventing transmission, they are the subject of much research.

Viruses contribute to cancer development in humans, but they cannot cause tumours on their own

Other events as well as virus infection are necessary for tumour development. For example, EBV infects most people in the world, and in the vast majority causes, at worst, the disease infectious mononucleosis (glandular fever). But in Chinese populations and in children exposed to malaria, some infected individuals develop particular cancers.

Viruses can contribute to the development of cancer in two ways

Just as chemical carcinogens can cause cancer either by acting as mutagens or promoters, so viruses can contribute to cancer development either by **changing the genes of a cell** or by **causing long-term cell turnover** so that the outgrowth of mutated cells is encouraged. Viruses can alter the genes in two ways, either by introducing new genes from the viruses or by disrupting the genes of the cell.

Causing cancer is incidental to the virus life cycle

It is of no advantage to a virus to cause tumours in some of its hosts. It is probably an incidental side-effect of virus infection, and usually only a small proportion of infected individuals develop tumours. As noted in Chapter 10, many viruses carry genes which alter the host cell so that it favours virus replication, and among these are genes that promote cell division or cell survival. So, for example, EBV causes proliferation of B lymphocytes and extends their life-span. This enhances the survival of the virus, but quite incidentally generates cells which may be more likely to become lymphoma cells.

Certain viruses are known to be major contributors to human cancer

EBV carries genes for several proteins that interfere with replication and survival of infected cells, so it is easy to understand how it can contribute to tumour development. It causes two kinds of tumour. In **Chinese populations** it causes squamous carcinomas of the nasal and pharyngeal epithelium— **nasopharyngeal carcinoma**. In **West African children** exposed to both malaria and EBV at an early age it causes **Burkitt's lymphoma**. Nasopharyngeal carcinoma in particular is a major killer, affecting hundreds of thousands of people in China and South-East Asia. Why the virus causes these specific tumours in these populations, while causing virtually no tumours in most of the rest of the world's population, is not clear, but it is thought that something else in the environment cooperates with the effects of the virus. Burkitt's lymphoma is strongly associated with exposure to malaria; it may be that ethnic Chinese are exposed to particular carcinogens. Recent evidence suggests that EBV might also contribute to Hodgkin's lymphoma.

Chronic infection with HBV is very strongly associated with the development of **primary liver cancer** (hepatocellular carcinoma), which is a major killer in China and Africa. The mechanism of action of the virus is uncertain but tumours develop after years of chronic HBV infection, and the main effect of the virus is probably to cause continual cell death and renewal over a long period. This view is given credence by the fact that other agents that cause chronic liver damage, such as alcohol, also raise the incidence of primary liver cancer.

There are a large number of **human papillomaviruses**. The most familiar cause common **warts**, which are small squamous papillomas that rarely, if ever, develop into carcinomas. A small group of the papillomaviruses are, however, associated with **carcinoma of the uterine cervix**, which is the commonest cancer of younger women worldwide. Carcinoma of the cervix has long been known to have the epidemiology of a sexually transmitted disease, and it now seems that sexual transmission of certain human papillomaviruses is responsible for most, though probably not all, of these neoplasms. Again, infection with human papillomavirus alone does not lead to cancer—it leads to the hyperplastic epithelium which may go on to become carcinoma over a number of years. Again, there is good reason to think that persistent infection is necessary. The viruses carry several genes that modify the cell division and differentiation of the host squamous epithelial cells to produce the tumour precursor cell population.

The human T lymphotropic viruses, HTLV1 and HTLV2, are currently the only retroviruses known to cause neoplasia in humans. Human immunodeficiency virus infection has been associated with development of tumours such as Kaposi's sarcoma, but this is probably because a weakened immune system makes the infected individual more susceptible to other cancer-causing viruses. HTLVs are present predominantly in Japanese and Caribbean populations. A small proportion of infected individuals develop T-cell leukaemias after many years of infection.

Evidence that these viruses contribute to human cancer comes from epidemiology and the biological properties of the viruses

With the exception of EBV, these tumour viruses have all been identified because of striking associations between infection and tumour development. In a large study of Taiwanese, hepatocellular carcinoma was found to be about 50 times more common in people chronically infected with HBV than in uninfected individuals. Certain human papillomavirus types are found in cervical carcinomas, and there is strong evidence that the disease behaves like a sexually transmitted disease. As long ago as 1842, Regioni-Stern noted that nuns did not get cervical carcinoma—except one, whom he had found had been a prostitute before taking the veil! Similarly, HTLV infection is strongly associated with a rare kind of T-cell leukaemia. The story of the discovery of EBV is ironic, because Burkitt showed that Burkitt's lymphoma had the epidemiology of an infectious disease, but the disease concerned now appears to be malaria. The epidemiology of EBV-induced cancer has not been very helpful in identifying its role.

The other kind of evidence that these viruses contribute to cancer development comes from studying the virus proteins. The human papillomaviruses and EBV have powerful transforming genes which would take the infected cell at least one step down the road to being a tumour cell.

Summary

Most human cancer probably has nothing to do with viruses. However, a few specific neoplasms are associated with particular viruses. The viruses that are currently known to contribute to human cancers are EBV, HBV, human papillomaviruses and HTLV. Virus infection alone is not enough to cause a tumour. Other changes, probably mutations, have to occur in the cells, so that many individuals infected with the viruses will not develop a tumour, and tumour development often requires several years of chronic or persistent infection.

19 Disease in the modern world

We began this book by noting that diseases in Nairobi are different from those in New York. The reasons for this are to be found in many places in these pages, but it is time to sum up.

Every disease is an interaction between injuries and the body's reaction to those injuries

The genetic and environmental causes of disease are so numerous that we have looked at only a small selection of them. The defences against disease are qualitatively the same throughout a species: the inbuilt defences, and the four major responses—inflammation, the immune response, regeneration and haemostasis.

The diseases that are easiest to understand are those in which a specific environmental hazard, such as trauma or a pathogenic microorganism, does the damage and the defences are protective. These are the archaic disease types that led to the evolution of the defence mechanisms; we might well call them **orthodox diseases**. In these diseases, survival depends upon the responses overcoming the injury.

Geographical differences may be due to relative prevalence of the injurious agents

Many tropical diseases are due to the existence there of particular parasites, or insect vectors. Where poverty exists, disadvantages such as overcrowding and poor sanitation increase the spread of pathogens. But poverty, through undernutrition, also affects the ability of the body to react efficiently to trauma or microbes. So the dice are doubly loaded for many of the poor of this world.

Needless to say, the geography of disease depends also on heredity. Genetic diseases such as the haemoglobinopathies are clear examples, but there are many more subtle genetic effects on resistance to orthodox diseases.

Social customs can affect disease

Examples include the effects of smoking, promiscuity, male homosexuality and many others.

The variables are clearly complicated, but orthodox diseases are always a battle between the severity of the injury and the ability of the host to respond.

329

Disease is affected not only by geography, but also by history

Urbanization, and especially industrialization, have changed patterns of disease incidence in many ways, in many places. The most obvious effects come from improvements in nutrition and sanitation; but prosperity brings with it also a gradual decrease in overcrowding. The benefits of immunization, organized medical care and sophisticated treatments have transformed the prospects for the richest populations, with a corresponding increase in life expectancy.

On the whole, therefore, infective disease has declined with urbanization, but industry has brought with it more trauma and many new hazards, including poisons, carcinogens, novel antigens and industrial dusts. Once these are recognized as harmful, they can sometimes be minimized by eliminating their source or by measures to decrease population exposure to them. These precautions are in fact similar to those used in avoiding infections.

The worst diseases in rich countries are unorthodox

Most morbidity and mortality of developed countries is due to diseases of obscure cause that also appear to have been increased by urbanization. Atherosclerosis and its complications, thrombosis, many forms of hypersensitive and autoimmune diseases and perhaps some forms of cancer are in this category. All of them are rare in animals and in non-urbanized human societies. All of them differ fundamentally in their nature from the orthodox diseases of poorer societies; they appear to be due not to a specific injury from the exterior nor to gene abnormalities, but to inappropriate activity of a defence mechanism. We could call them unorthodox diseases.

The clue to their cause comes from diseases, like gout, pneumoconioses and hypersensitivity, which are demonstrably due to activation of the inflammatory and immune responses caused by exposure to external stimuli which are themselves harmless. They are caused by tissue damage due to spillage of phagocyte contents, or to other activities of the inflammatory response.

Although we do not yet understand the pathogenesis of these diseases, it appears at present that atherosclerosis is an inappropriate inflammatory response, thrombosis is harmful activation of haemostasis, the connective tissue diseases, like rheumatoid arthritis, are due to immune mechanisms and some forms of cancer result from mutations occurring in the process of regeneration.

Orthodox and unorthodox diseases

Table 19.1 shows some examples of diseases categorized according to the defence mechanism primarily involved and whether they are orthodox or unorthodox.

The orthodox diseases cause disease and death in wild animals as well as in all human communities. The causes are trauma and pathogenic microbes. Apart from simple avoidance of the injury, modern countermeasures include antimicrobial therapy, vaccination and the elimination of disease reservoirs, or of communicability.

Table 19.1 Examples of orthodox and unorthodox diseases.

	Orthodox	Unorthodox
Inflammation and healing	Infections, trauma	Gout Pneumoconioses Atherosclerosis
Immune response	Infections	Hypersensitivity Autoallergy
Haemostasis	Trauma	Thrombosis
Regeneration	Most forms of injury	Cancer?

The unorthodox diseases occur mainly in the different circumstances of industrialized communities. Where the triggering cause is known, as in the pneumoconioses and some forms of cancer and hypersensitivity, the individual can be protected by simple avoidance. But many of these diseases are of unknown cause. Some, as we have seen, can be imperfectly managed by the use of anti-inflammatory or immunosuppressive agents. Against many of them, however, no suitable treatment exists.

It can be argued that these unorthodox diseases might have existed for thousands of years, but because they occur mainly in relatively old age, they would be a major problem only in modern long-lived populations. This would also explain the long historical persistence of such diseases, because evolution is unconcerned by deaths occurring after the period of child-rearing.

An alternative explanation is that some of the changes in the environment caused by civilization and industrialization are actually increasing the incidence and severity of the unorthodox diseases. This interpretation has become increasingly likely as we have learned more about the epidemiology of these diseases and about the complicated mechanisms of the reactions to injury.

How might unorthodox diseases happen?

We have seen that some unorthodox diseases can be triggered by exposure to novel environmental agents such as industrial dusts or carcinogens. This does not, however, seem to be true of all of them, by any means, and more subtle factors can be involved. One example that illustrates this well is thrombosis.

Once a method had been invented for measuring the aggregation of platelets, it became clear that the aggregation was enhanced by a variety of molecules, and that these in turn were influenced quantitatively by environmental factors. Thus aggregation is measurably increased, for instance, by high concentrations of catecholamines (and hence by stress and cigarette-smoking) and of saturated fatty acids (and hence by the diet). So here is evidence that the activity of a defence mechanism can be increased by quantitative environmental changes. Therefore not only haemostasis but also thrombosis is enhanced by these environmental influences. This suggests that the molecular mechanisms of other reactions, and the diseases that can result from them, may be influenced by quite subtle changes in the environment of the industrialized community.

Many of the unorthodox diseases, especially those affecting the cardiovascular system, share this unusual form of origin. That is, they are not caused by a novel exogenous stimulus, as measles is due to the measles virus. Rather they result from quantitative changes in physiological variables. Examples of these variables include vasomotor tone, platelet stickiness, concentrations of plasma lipids and so on. All of these are influenced by environmental changes, which might be deficiency of one factor or excess of another, and which may therefore, singly or in combination, produce unorthodox disease.

Atherosclerosis is a particularly good example. Over 200 risk factors have been described by epidemiologists, although most are probably spurious. The disease itself is more complicated than thrombosis, and difficult to study because in the patient it is subclinical for many years. It seems to be a chronic inflammatory response of the artery wall to haemodynamic injury. Most authorities readily accept the importance of some of the risk factors, such as smoking, or animal fats in the diet, and advise against them. Other factors are more contentious. For instance, recently a school of thought has arisen that because lipid oxidation appears to be an important factor in atherogenesis, this may mean that the dietary balance of different lipids may be inappropriate, or that dietary antioxidants are deficient in some urbanized societies. This is one example of a general notion that there may be specific dietary imbalances in our industrialized communities, and this is more difficult for some to accept. The difficulty stems from the widespread belief that healthy human adults eating a balanced diet cannot by definition have a dietary deficiency. Unfortunately this ignores the fact that in our society every 'healthy adult' is developing atherosclerosis, and half will die of it.

It can be argued, therefore, that many of the diseases of civilization are due to the blind reactions to injury being activated inappropriately in two circumstances: when they are elicited by novel but harmless stimuli, or when their mechanisms are themselves accentuated somehow by quantitative environmental alterations, such as changes in diet. These environmental changes have occurred during what, in evolutionary terms, is a very short time indeed.

When we send a man to the moon, we provide him with oxygen for that alien environment. If we wish to continue to create more and more alien surroundings for ourselves on earth, and yet avoid these unorthodox diseases, we may have to take some appropriate precautions rather urgently.

Index

Page numbers in *italics* refer to figures.